# GER
# NOTES



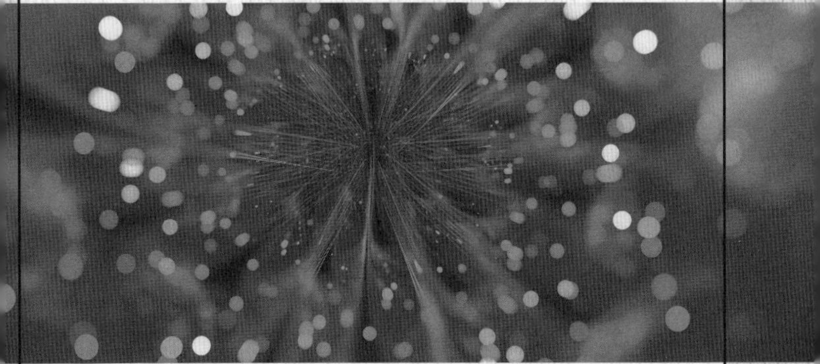

JAMIE W. SMITH, MSN, RN, FNP-C
BRADLEY J. GOAD, DO, CMD, FACP

JONES & BARTLETT
LEARNING

*World Headquarters*
Jones & Bartlett Learning
5 Wall Street
Burlington, MA 01803
978-443-5000
info@jblearning.com
www.jblearning.com

Jones & Bartlett Learning books and products are available through most bookstores and online booksellers. To contact Jones & Bartlett Learning directly, call 800-832-0034, fax 978-443-8000, or visit our website, www.jblearning.com.

Substantial discounts on bulk quantities of Jones & Bartlett Learning publications are available to corporations, professional associations, and other qualified organizations. For details and specific discount information, contact the special sales department at Jones & Bartlett Learning via the above contact information or send an email to specialsales@jblearning.com.



**Production Credits**
VP, Product Management: David D. Cella
Director of Product Management: Amanda Martin
Product Manager: Teresa Reilly
Product Assistant: Anna-Maria Forger
Production Editor: Daniel Stone
Production Manager: Carolyn Pershouse
Marketing Communications Manager: Katie Hennessy
Product Fulfillment Manager: Wendy Kilborn
Composition: S4Carlisle Publishing Services
Cover Design: Kristin E. Parker
Rights & Media Specialist: John Rusk
Media Development Editor: Troy Liston
Cover Image (Title Page, Part Opener, Chapter Opener): © (Photo) © Ideas_Studio/iStock/Getty Images; (Graphic Image) © tofutyklein/Shutterstock
Printing and Binding: McNaughton & Gunn
Cover Printing: McNaughton & Gunn

**Library of Congress Cataloging-in-Publication Data**
Names: Smith, Jamie, 1986- author. | Goad, Bradley J. (Bradley Jackson), author.
Title: Geriatric notes / Jamie Smith, Bradley J. Goad.
Description: Burlington, MA : Jones & Bartlett Learning, [2019] | Includes bibliographical references and index.
Identifiers: LCCN 2018032146 | ISBN 9781284153828 (pbk.)
Subjects: | MESH: Geriatrics--methods | Aged | Handbooks
Classification: LCC RC952.55 | NLM WT 39 | DDC 618.97--dc23
LC record available at https://lccn.loc.gov/2018032146

6048

Printed in the United States of America
22 21 20 19 18 10 9 8 7 6 5 4 3 2 1

# Dedication

This book is dedicated to my family, Kellen and Madelyn, my parents, Robin and Rodney, and all my contributors and coauthor for your support. Thank you to Jones & Bartlett Learning for making my dream of writing a book become a reality.

**Jamie W. Smith**

# Table of Contents

# Preface

This book is intended to be a practical, concise, and up-to-date guide specific to geriatric medicine. It is not exhaustive; however, it is a convenient resource on common conditions/diseases, symptoms, and topics encountered to guide practitioners in their clinical setting. Given that the medical field is always changing with new research, theories, and recommendations, this book is to be taken as a guide only. Every patient scenario is unique; therefore, it is recommended that clinicians use their judgment to direct their ultimate decision according to their practice standards.

# Contributors

**Marie Shockley English, MPAS, PA-C**
Carilion Clinic
Roanoke, VA

**Casey Henritz, DO**
Iora Health
Atlanta, GA

**Danny R. Huff, PhrmaD, MBA, BCGP**

**Arneda Faye Lyons, RN, FNP, DNP**
Dublin, VA

**Holly Roy, MPAS, PA-C**
Roanoke, VA

**Pamela Ruppel, MSN, PMHNP-BC**
Roanoke, VA

**Angela R. Stiltner, MD, HMDC**
University of Virginia Health Systems
Charlottesville, VA

**Fannie F. Utz, MSN, RN, FNP-BC**
Hospice of the Piedmont
Charlottesville, VA

# Reviewers

**Sola Aina-Popoola, PhD, RN**
Assistant Director
Tuskegee University, School of Nursing and Allied Health
Tuskegee, AL

**Diane Anderson, DNP, MSN, RN, CNE**
Assistant Dean
Chamberlain College of Nursing
Downers Grove, IL

**Kathleen Anderson, DNP-C**
Associate Professor
Binghamton University, Decker School of Nursing
Binghamton, NY

**Susan Beck, PhD-C, MSN, CNS, RN**
Assistant Professor
Bloomsburg University
Bloomsburg, PA

**David J. Carter, PhD**
Professor
University of Nebraska
Lincoln, NE

**Diane M. Champa RN, BSN**
Nursing Instructor
Greater Lowell Technical School of Practical Nursing
Tyngsborough, MA

# Reviewers

**Jacqueline F. Close, PhD, APRN**
Professor, Program Coordinator
University of San Diego
San Diego, CA

**Rachel W. Cozort, PhD, MSN, RN, CNE**
Associate Professor of Nursing
Pfeiffer University
Misenheimer, NC

**Jason T. Garbarino, DNP, RN-BC, CNL**
Clinical Assistant Professor
University of Vermont
Burlington, VT

**Tracy P. George, DNP, APRN-BC, CNE**
Assistant Professor of Nursing
Francis Marion University School of Health Sciences
Department of Nursing
Florence, SC

**Sheila C. Grossman, PhD, APRN, FNP-BC, FAAN**
Professor, Family Nurse Practitioner Coordinator; Director, Faculty Scholarship & Mentoring
Egan School of Nursing & Health Studies
Fairfield University
Fairfield, CT

**Angela Groves, PhD(c), RN-BC, CNE**
Adjunct Professor
Utica College
Utica, NY

**Kathleen Hall, PhD, APRN, GNP-BC**
Assistant Professor of Nursing, Co-coordinator of the Doctor of Nursing Practice Program
Colorado Mesa University
Grand Junction, CO

**Deborah L. Hopla, DNP, APRN-BC**
Director MSN/FNP Program
Francis Marion University
Florence, SC

**Roseann Kaminsky RN, MSN, BSN, BSEd**
Associate Professor
Lorain County Community College
Elyria, OH

**Linda J. Keilman, DNP, GNP-BC, FAANP**
Associate Professor; Gerontological Nurse Practitioner
Michigan State University, College of Nursing
East Lansing, MI

**Shirley Levenson, PhD, FNP-BC**
Professor
Texas State University
San Marcos, TX

**Dr. Susan E. Lowey, PhD, RN, CHPN**
Associate Professor & Advisement Coordinator
State University of New York College at Brockport
Brockport, NY

**Renee Mirovsky DNP, ANP-BC**
Professor
Oakland University
Rochester, MI

**Geri Budesheim Neuberger, RN, MN, EdD**
Professor Emerita
University of Kansas, School of Nursing
Kansas City, KS

**Sandra Oliver-McNeil, DNP, MSN, ACNP-BC**
Associate Clinical Professor
Wayne State University, College of Nursing
Detroit, MI

**Brenda Olmos, APRN, MSN, FNP-C**
Instructor in Clinical Nursing
The University of Texas at Austin
Austin, TX

**Patti A Parker, PhD, RN, CNS, ANP, GNP, BC**
Assistant Clinical Professor
University of Texas at Arlington College of Nursing and Health Innovation
Arlington, TX

**Tiffany A. Phillips, DNP, NP-C**
Assistant Professor of Nursing
Francis Marion University
Florence, SC

**Sue Polito, MSN, ANP-C, GNP-C**
Specialist Professor
Monmouth University
West Long Branch, NJ

**Marisue Rayno, RN, MSN, EdD**
Professor
Luzerne County Community College
Nanticoke, PA

# Reviewers

**Dr Faith Richardson, DNP, RN**
Clinician/Educator/Researcher
Kindle Health/Trinity Western University
Langley, BC, Canada

**Joy A. Shepard, PhD, RN-BC (Gerontological Nursing), CNE**
Clinical Associate Professor
East Carolina University College of Nursing
Greenville, NC

**Amy L. Silva-Smith PhD, APN**
Professor, Associate Dean for Academic Affairs and Operations
University of Colorado, Colorado Springs
Colorado Springs, CO

**Denise Vanacore, PhD, CRNP, ANP-BC, PMHNP-BC**
Director, NP and DNP Programs
Associate Professor of Nursing
Gwynedd Mercy University
Gwynedd Valley, PA

**Barbara Schwitz White, DrPH, A/GNP**
Associate Professor Emerita
School of Nursing/California State University, Long Beach
Long Beach, CA

**Virginia M. White, MN, RN, FNP-BC, CEN**
Professor
Olympic College
Bremerton, WA

**Ann Marie Zvorsky, MSN, RN, CNE**
Medical-Surgical Nursing Instructor
Joseph F. McCloskey School of Nursing
Pottsville, PA

SECTION I

# Prevention and Health Promotion

| Topic | Sex/Age | Recommendation |
|---|---|---|
| Abdominal Aortic Aneurysm | Men 65–75<br>Women 65–75 | Per US Preventive Services Task Force (USPSTF):[1]<br>• Screen with a one-time abdominal ultrasound with a smoking history.[1]<br>• Screening is not recommended in women with no history of smoking; in those who have smoked, the evidence is insufficient to support screening.[1] |
| Alcohol Use | All Adults | Per USPSTF:[1]<br>• Screen for alcohol misuse.<br>  • AUDIT, AUDIT-C, or single-question screening (e.g., "In the past year, have you had four or more drinks in 24 hours?")<br>• Counsel on the health risks associated with alcohol.<br>  • Stress risk of liver disease and malignancy of the mouth, esophagus, pharynx, liver, and breast.[1,9]<br>• Screening interval not determined.[1]<br>• Dependent drinkers should be referred to alcohol treatment programs; consider prescribing naltrexone to aid in drinking cessation.[6] |

| Topic | Sex/Age | Recommendation |
|---|---|---|
| Aspirin for Cardiovascular Disease (CVD) Prevention and Colorectal Cancer | Adults ≥ 50–69 | Per (USPSTF):[1,2]<br>• Aspirin 81 mg daily *(optimal dose unknown; lower dose is just as effective as higher doses).*<br>  • Consider the risks of bleeding (e.g., upper abdominal pain, gastrointestinal [GI] ulcer, concurrent use of anticoagulant and/or NSAID) vs. benefits.<br>• Use with a ≥ 10% 10-year CVD risk (http://tools.acc.org/ASCVD-Risk-Estimator/).<br>• Use if patient plans to take medication daily and has a life expectancy of at least 10 years.<br>• Use of aspirin in adults ≥ 70 years should be individualized (current evidence is insufficient). |
| Cancer Screening – Breast | Women 50–74 | Per USPSTF:<br>• Mammogram recommended every 2 years.[1,6]<br>• Evidence is not sufficient to continue screening beyond the age of 75.[1] |
| Cancer Screening – Cervical | Female > 65 | Per USPSTF:[1]<br>• Screening not recommended in those with:<br>  • Prior history of negative cervical cytology and human papillomavirus results<br>  • No cervix (and without a history of cervical pre-cancer or cervical cancer) |

| Topic | Sex/Age | Recommendation |
| --- | --- | --- |
| | | • Screen if prior screening results have been inadequate and if patient would be able to tolerate cervical cancer treatment (if tested positive).[6] |
| Cancer Screening – Colorectal | Adults 50–75 | Per USPSTF:[1]<br>• There are several screening strategies:[1,6]<br>  • Annual fecal immunochemical test (FIT)<br>  • Colonoscopy every 10 years<br>  • CT colonography every 5 years<br>  • Flexible sigmoidoscopy every 10 years plus annual FIT<br>Screening for those age 76–85 is individualized; not recommended if life expectancy is less than 10 years.[6] |
| Cancer Screening – Lung | Adults 55–80 | Per USPSTF:[1]<br>• Screen annually with a low-dose computed tomography in individuals at high risk for lung cancer:[1]<br>  • Heavy smoker (30 pack-year) and<br>  • Currently smokes and/or stopped in the past 15 years |
| Cancer Screening – Prostate | Men | USPSTF recommends against prostate-specific antigen (PSA)-based screening.[1,6,22]<br>American Urological Association (AUA) recommends screening in those between age 55–69 every 2 years with life expectancy of at least 10 years.[6,32] Not recommended in men over age 70, unless in excellent health.[32] |

| Topic | Sex/Age | Recommendation |
|---|---|---|
| | | American Cancer Society (ACS) recommends having discussions regarding PSA screening (i.e., risks, benefits); men above age 50 can be screened if life expectancy at least 10 years.[6,31] |
| Cognitive Impairment and Dementia Screening | Adults > 65 | Per USPSTF, evidence is insufficient to screen for cognitive impairment.[1]<br>The Medicare Annual Wellness visit (part of the Affordable Care Act) requires routine assessment to detect for cognitive impairment.[13,25] Recommended algorithm:[13]<br>• Alzheimer's Association Medicare Annual Wellness Visit Algorithm for Assessment of Cognition |
| Depression | All Adults | USPSTF recommends to screen periodically (optimal interval time unknown) in all patients regardless of risk factors.[1,12]<br>American Geriatrics Society (AGS) recommends screening with the Patient Health Questionnaire (PHQ)-2 initially; if positive, the PHQ-9 or 15-item Geriatric Depression Scale can be used.[30]<br>Once depression is identified, the patient will need treatment, which includes psychotherapy, medications, or a combination and close follow-up to ensure treatment is effective.[1] |

| Topic | Sex/Age | Recommendation |
|---|---|---|
| Diabetes Mellitus Type 2 and Abnormal Blood Glucose | Adults 40–70 | Per USPSTF:<br>• In obese or overweight individuals, screen for diabetes with a fasting plasma glucose, HbA1C, or oral glucose tolerance test every 3 years in low-risk individuals or yearly if high risk.[1,10,11] HgbA1c is more convenient.[1,20]<br>Per AGS, a target HbA1C goal in older adults is 7.5%–8.0%; may consider a goal of 7.0%–7.5% in healthier patients with few comorbidities. In frail older adults with limited life expectancy or extensive comorbidities, an A1C goal of 8.0%–9.0% is appropriate.<br>• The American Diabetes Association (ADA) guidelines are slightly more stringent.[20,37,38] |
| Fall Prevention | Adults ≥ 65 | Per USPSTF, assess for risk of falling:[1]<br>• Prior falls history<br>• Balance and/or gait issues<br>Implement strategies to prevent future falls:[1]<br>• Exercise or physical therapy evaluation/consultation to assess gait, balance, muscle weakness.[1,21]<br>• Have vision tested and treated.[1,21]<br>• Test and treat orthostatic hypotension.[1,21]<br>• Consider vitamin D[21] and/or protein supplement.[1]<br>• Determine risk factors for falls in the home setting (i.e., rugs, cluttered floor, slippery surface).[21]<br>Per AGS, screen for falls annually.[19] |

| Topic | Sex/Age | Recommendation |
|---|---|---|
| Heart Health – High blood pressure<br>NOTE: Determining appropriate blood pressure goals in older individuals is controversial. | All Adults | Per USPSTF:<br>• Yearly screening recommended in individuals ≥ 40 years and in those with high-normal pressures *(systolic 130–139; diastolic 85–89 mm Hg)*, who are overweight, or black.[1,3]<br>• Office blood pressures are performed while the patient is sitting, using a manual or automated sphygmomanometer. The mean of two measurements is taken with an appropriately sized arm cuff; allow for at least 5 minutes from entering office and blood pressure measurement.<br>• Blood pressure monitoring at home can be used; however, 24-hr ambulatory blood pressure monitoring (ABPM) is preferred for confirming hypertension.[1,3]<br>• Adults ≥ 60 years old: Target blood pressure should be 150/90 mm Hg.[1,3]<br>The Joint National Committee (JNC 8) recommends a blood pressure goal of < 140/90 mm Hg in adults > age 60 years who have diabetes and/or chronic kidney disease; in the absence of these conditions, the goal is < 150/90 mm Hg.[33]<br>The American College of Cardiology/American Heart Association (ACC/AHA) new blood pressure goal is < 130/80 mm Hg.[34,35] |

| Topic | Sex/Age | Recommendation |
|---|---|---|
| Heart Health – Lipid disorders | Adults ≥ 40–75 | Per USPSTF:[1]<br>• Low-moderate dosed statin therapy recommended in those *without* known heart disease (i.e., symptomatic coronary artery disease or ischemic stroke) with ≥ 1 CVD risk factors, including a calculated 10-year risk of a cardiovascular event of more than 7.5%, most especially if ≥ 10%.[1]<br>  • CVD risk factors: dyslipidemia, diabetes mellitus, hypertension, smoker[1]<br>• Initiating statin therapy in adults ≥ age 76 years for primary prevention should be individualized (current evidence is insufficient).<br>In individuals > 75 years old without arteriosclerotic cardiovascular disease (ASCVD), shared decision making is recommended regarding statin therapy. If you foresee the patient having a future CVD event and he or she is relatively healthy, life expectancy not poor, and have low burden of medication and co-morbidities, statin therapy is likely appropriate.[5]<br>In the presence of clinical ASCVD, moderate-intensity statins are recommended (ACC/AHA guideline).[27] |

| Topic | Sex/Age | Recommendation |
|---|---|---|
| Hepatitis B Screening | All Adults | Per USPSTF:<br>• Screen in individuals at high risk, such as:<br>  • Having sex with persons infected with hepatitis B<br>  • Injection drug use<br>  • Individuals with human immunodeficiency virus (HIV) infection or weakened immunity<br>• Screening tests: hepatitis B surface antigen (HBsAg), hepatitis B surface antibody (anti-HBs), hepatitis B core antibody (anti-HBc). |
| Hepatitis C Screening | All Adults | Per USPSTF:<br>• Order a one-time screening for hepatitis C for those born between 1945–1965, including those at high risk of the infection (i.e., injected drug use, recipient of blood transfusion prior to 1992, multiple sex partners, tattoo with unclean needle).[1]<br>• Screening tests: Anti-HCV antibody testing (high sensitivity > 90%) followed by confirmatory polymerase chain reaction. |
| Latent Tuberculosis Screening | All Adults | Per USPSTF:<br>• Screen in those at high risk, such as:<br>  • Nursing home patients<br>  • Individuals who lived in high-risk countries (e.g., Mexico, Vietnam, Haiti)<br>  • Those with immunodeficiencies (i.e., HIV, receiving immunosuppressants)[1,18] |

| Topic | Sex/Age | Recommendation |
|---|---|---|
| | | • Screening tests: Mantoux tuberculin skin test and interferon-gamma release test.[1]<br>• Optimal screening interval unknown; consider yearly screening in those who are high risk.[1] |
| Obesity Screening | All Adults | Per USPSTF:<br>• Screen for individuals with body mass index (BMI) of ≥ 30 kg/m$^2$ and refer to weight reduction programs.[1]<br>• Optimal screening interval unknown.[1] |
| Osteoporosis | Women ≥ 65 | Per USPSTF:<br>• Initial bone mineral density testing with dual energy x-ray absorptiometry (DEXA).[1]<br>• Evidence is not sufficient to screen in men.[1]<br>• Optimal interval time unknown.[1,12] |
| Sensory Impairment – Hearing | Adults ≥ 50 | USPSTF recommends against routine screening in asymptomatic patients.[1]<br>The American Speech-Language Hearing Association recommends screening and referral to audiologist every 3 years.[15] |
| Sensory Impairment – Vision | Adults ≥ 65 | USPSTF recommends against routine screening in asymptomatic patients.[1]<br>The American Academy of Ophthalmology recommends eye exam every 1 to 2 years.[14] |

| Topic | Sex/Age | Recommendation |
|---|---|---|
| Sexually Transmitted Infections (STI) – Chlamydia and Gonorrhea Screening | Women > 24 | Per USPSTF:[1]<br>• Screening is recommended in older women with risk factors, such as:<br>  ◦ More than one sex partner<br>  ◦ Unprotected sex<br>• Evidence is not sufficient to screen in men.[1]<br>• Screening test: nucleic acid amplification tests.[1]<br>• Interval time depends on new or persistent risk factors. |
| STI – HIV Screening | Adults ≥ 65 | Per USPSTF:[1]<br>• Screen those who are sexually active with risk factors, such as:[1,7]<br>  ◦ Unprotected sex (mostly anal and/or vaginal)<br>  ◦ More than one sex partner<br>  ◦ Positive HIV sexual partner<br>  ◦ Sharing syringes with someone who has HIV<br>• Screening tests: reactive immunoassay, followed by confirmatory Western blot or immunofluorescent assay.<br>• Screen annually in adults at very high risk. |
| STI – Syphilis Screening | All Adults | Per USPSTF:[1]<br>• Screening is recommended in those who are sexually active for risk factors, such as:[1,8]<br>  ◦ Men who have sex with men<br>  ◦ Men and women with HIV<br>  ◦ History of incarceration<br>  ◦ Risky sexual behavior |

| Topic | Sex/Age | Recommendation |
|---|---|---|
| | | • Screening test: initial nontreponemal test, serum Venereal Disease Research Laboratory (VDRL) or serum rapid plasma reagin (RPR).<br>• Screening interval not determined.[1,8] |
| Thyroid Impairment | All Adults | USPSTF recommends against routine screening in asymptomatic patients.[1] |
| Tobacco Use | All Adults | Per USPSTF:[1]<br>• Encourage smoking cessation.<br>• Recommend behavioral interventions.<br>  • Counseling in person or over the phone<br>  • Self-help material<br>• Recommend pharmacotherapy.<br>  • Nicotine replacement (i.e., patches, gum)<br>  • Varenicline (Chantix)<br>  • Bupropion SR (Zyban) [*Caution use; is a Beers-listed item and lowers seizure threshold.*][36]<br>The Centers for Disease Control and Prevention (CDC) recommends to ask about tobacco use at every visit.[26] |

## Vaccinations

| Vaccine | Sex/Age | Recommendation |
|---|---|---|
| **Haemophilus Influenzae Type B Vaccine** Haemophilus Influenzae Type B Conjugate Vaccine (Hib) | **All Adults** | **One to three doses are recommended** (depending on certain risk factors). Those with hematopoietic stem cell transplant need three doses. |
| **Hepatitis A Vaccine** Antigen Hepatitis A Vaccine (HepA) or Hepatitis A and Hepatitis B Vaccine (HepA-HepB) | **All Adults** | **Two to three doses are recommended if not already received;** screen and provide vaccination if traveling to endemic areas and/or have chronic liver disease (*not required for most older adults*).[16,17] |
| **Hepatitis B Vaccine** Single-Antigen Hepatitis B Vaccine (HepB) or Hepatitis A and Hepatitis B Vaccine (HepA-HepB) | **All Adults** | **Three doses are recommended, if not already received.** Recommended in those with comorbidities that place them at risk: kidney disease, HIV, chronic liver disease (i.e., alcoholic or fatty liver disease, cirrhosis, hepatitis C virus infection, cirrhosis, autoimmune hepatitis and/or alanine transaminase [ALT] or aspartate aminotransferase [AST] more than double the normal).[16,23] |

| Vaccine | Sex/Age | Recommendation |
|---|---|---|
| **Herpes Zoster Vaccine (Shingles)** Zoster Vaccine Live (ZVL) Zostavax -OR- Recombinant Zoster vaccine (RZV) Shingrix | **Adults ≥ 60** | **Zostavax: one vaccination** (even if the patient has had shingles). Contraindications: severe immunodeficiency.[16] **Shingrix: requires two doses** (at 0 and 2–6 months). Recommended in adults ≥ 50 years old; for adults ≥ 60 years old RZV or ZVL can be administered (RZV preferred).[16,28,29] |
| **Influenza Vaccine (Flu)** Inactivated Influenza Vaccine (IIV) or Recombinant Influenza Vacccine (RIV) | **All Adults** | **Recommend yearly vaccine.** Contraindication: severe egg allergy.[16] |
| **Meningococcal Vaccine** Serogroups A,C,W, and Y Meningococcal Conjugate Vaccine (MenACWY) or Serogroup B Meningococcal Vaccine (MenB) | **All Adults** | **Recommend one or more doses** (depending on certain risk factors). Recommended in those with asplenia and/or at risk of the disease (i.e., traveling/live in countries with the disease); newly included are those with HIV.[16,23] |
| **Pneumococcal Vaccine** Pneumococcal Conjugate Vaccine (PCV13) and 23-Valent Pneumococcal Polysaccharide Vaccine (PPSV23) | **Adults ≥ 65** | **One vaccination of both PCV13 and PPSV23.**[16] (Administer PPSV23 a year following the PCV13.) |

| Vaccine | Sex/Age | Recommendation |
| --- | --- | --- |
| **Td/Tdap**<br>Tetanus and Diphtheria Toxoids (TD) booster; Tetanus Toxoid, Reduced Diphtheria Toxoid, and Acellular Pertussis Vaccine (Tdap) | **All Adults** | **Need Td booster every 10 years. If Tdap vaccine was not administered in the past, will need a one-time dose.**[16] |
| **Varicella Vaccine (Chickenpox)**<br>Single-Antigen Varicella Vaccine (VAR) | **All Adults** | **Two doses are recommended if the individual is without evidence of immunity to varicella.**<br>Almost all of Americans (99%) have had chickenpox, even if they can't recall having the disease.[24] |

## CLINICAL PEARLS

- Do not order screening tests in patients with end-stage diseases, advanced age, and/or multiple comorbidities, which could potentially prevent the patient from receiving treatment for the condition being screened. This practice could cause unnecessary testing and patient/family anxiety.
- Although the new ACC/AHA guideline lowers the blood pressure goal to < 130/80 mm Hg, this may not be realistic for some older adults when treated aggressively due to poor vascular compliance. Dizziness can occur in individuals with systolic pressures around 140 mm Hg.[34]
- For information on who should or should not receive vaccines based on medical conditions, visit the Centers for Disease Control and Prevention (CDC) at www.cdc.gov/vaccines/vpd/vaccines-age.html.

# References


1. US Preventive Services Task Force. (n.d.). Published Recommendations. Retrieved from https://www.uspreventiveservicestaskforce.org/BrowseRec/Index/browse-recommendations. Accessed September 17, 2017.
2. McNellis, R. J., & Beswick-Escanlar, V. (2016, October 15). Aspirin Use for the Primary Prevention of Cardiovascular Disease and Colorectal Cancer. American Academy of Family Physicians. Retrieved from http://www.aafp.org/afp/2016/1015/p661.html. Accessed September 17, 2017.
3. Ngo-Metzger, Q., & Blitz, J. (2016, March 15). Screening for High Blood Pressure in Adults. American Academy of Family Physicians. Retrieved from http://www.aafp.org/afp/2016/0315/p511.html. Accessed September 17, 2017.
4. Rosensen, R. S. (2016). Patient Education: High Cholesterol and Lipids (Hyperlipidemia) (Beyond the Basics). UpToDate. Retrieved from https://www.uptodate.com/contents/high-cholesterol-and-lipids-hyperlipidemia-beyond-the-basics. Accessed September 17, 2017.
5. Tuohy, C. V., & Dodson, J. A. (2015, March 10). Statins for Primary Prevention in Older Adults. American College of Cardiology. Retrieved from http://www.acc.org/latest-in-cardiology/articles/2015/03/10/07/46/statins-for-primary-prevention-in-older-adults. Accessed September 17, 2017.
6. Prevention and screening. In *Hazzard's Geriatric Medicine and Gerontology* (7th ed.). New York, NY: McGraw-Hill. Retrieved from http://accessmedicine.mhmedical.com/content.aspx?bookid=1923&sectionid=144518165. Accessed September 12, 2017.
7. Centers for Disease Control and Prevention (CDC). (2014, February 25). Sexually Transmitted Diseases. Retrieved from https://www.cdc.gov/std/general/default.htm. Accessed September 17, 2017.
8. Bibbins-Domingo, K. (2016). Screening for syphilis infection in nonpregnant adults and adolescents: US Preventive Services Task Force recommendation statement. *JAMA, 315*(21), 2321–2327. doi:10.1001/jama.2016.5824
9. National Institute on Alcohol Abuse and Alcoholism. (2017). Alcohol Facts and Statistics. Retrieved from https://www.niaaa.nih.gov/alcohol-health/overview-alcohol-consumption/alcohol-facts-and-statistics. Accessed September 17, 2017.
10. Ngo-Metzger, Q. (2016, June 15). Screening for abnormal blood glucose and type 2 diabetes mellitus. *American Family Physician*, 93(12), 1025–1026. Retrieved from http://www.aafp.org/afp/2016/0615/p1025.html. Accessed September 17, 2017.
11. Tucker, M. E. (2014). USPSTF: Screen Everyone 45 and Older for Abnormal Glucose. Medscape. Retrieved from http://www.medscape.com/viewarticle/832850. Accessed September 17, 2017.
12. Armstrong, K., & Martin, G. J. (2015). Screening and prevention of disease. In Kasper, D., Fauci, A., Hauser, S., Longo, D., Jameson, J., & Loscalzo, J. *Harrison's Principles of Internal Medicine* (19th ed.). New York, NY: McGraw-Hill. Retrieved from http://accessmedicine.mhmedical.com/content.aspx?bookid=1130&sectionid=63651647. Accessed September 13, 2017.
13. Cordell, C. B., Borson, S., Boustani, M., Chodosh, J., Reuben, D., & Verghese, J., . . . Fried, L. B. (2013). Alzheimers Association recommendations for operationalizing the detection of cognitive impairment during the Medicare Annual Wellness Visit in a primary care setting. *Alzheimers & Dementia,* 9(2), 141–150. doi:10.1016/j.jalz.2012.09.011

14. American Academy of Ophthalmology (AAO). (2017, February 14). Eye Exams 101. Retrieved from https://www.aao.org/eye-health/tips-prevention/eye-exams-101. Accessed September 17, 2017.
15. American Speech-Language-Hearing Association (ASHA). (n.d.). Who Should Be Screened for Hearing Loss. Retrieved from http://www.asha.org/public/hearing/Who-Should-be-Screened/. Accessed September 17, 2017.
16. Centers for Disease Control and Prevention. (2016, November 22). Vaccines and Preventable Diseases. Retrieved from https://www.cdc.gov/vaccines/vpd/vaccines-age.html. Accessed September 17, 2017.
17. Kelly, S. G., Barancin, C., & Lucey, M. R. (2017). Hepatic disease. In *Hazzard's Geriatric Medicine and Gerontology* (7th ed.). New York, NY: McGraw-Hill. Retrieved from http://accessmedicine.mhmedical.com/content.aspx?bookid=1923&sectionid=144526298. Accessed September 17, 2017.
18. Jin, J. (2016, September 6). Screening for latent tuberculosis. *JAMA, 316*(9), 1004. Retrieved from http://jamanetwork.com/journals/jama/fullarticle/2547757. Accessed September 17, 2017.
19. American Geriatric Society (AGS). (2010). *Prevention of falls in older persons.* AGS BGS Clinical Practice Guideline 2010. Retrieved from https://geriatricscareonline.org/FullText/CL014/CL014_BOOK003. Accessed September 23, 2017.
20. Bigelow, A., & Freeland, B. (2017). Type 2 diabetes care in the elderly. *Journal for Nurse Practitioners, 13*(3), 181–186. doi:10.1016/j.nurpra.2016.08.010
21. Enderlin, C., Rooker, J., Ball, S., Hippensteel, D., Alderman, J., & Fisher, S. J., . . . Jordan, K. (2015). Summary of factors contributing to falls in older adults and nursing implications. *Geriatric Nursing, 36*(5), 397–406. doi:10.1016/j.gerinurse.2015.08.006
22. Sandhya, G. (2015, October 4). Active Surveillance Encouraged for Prostate Cancer Screening. Clinical Advisor. Retrieved from http://www.clinicaladvisor.com/newsline/active-surveillance-encouraged-for-prostate-cancer-screening/article/441716/. Accessed September 23, 2017.
23. Campos-Outcalt, D. (2017, March). ACIP vaccine update, 2017. *Journal of Family Practice, 66*(3), 166–169. Retrieved from http://www.mdedge.com/jfponline/article/132250/vaccines/acip-vaccine-update-2017. Accessed September 24, 2017.
24. Centers for Disease Control and Prevention. (2016, November 22). What Everyone Should Know about Shingles Vaccine. Retrieved from https://www.cdc.gov/vaccines/vpd/shingles/public/index.html. Accessed September 29, 2017.
25. Walter, C., Edwards, N. E., Griggs, R., & Yehle, K. (2014). Differentiating Alzheimer Disease, Lewy body, and Parkinson dementia Using *DSM-5*. *The Journal for Nurse Practitioners, 10*(4), 262–270. doi:10.1016/j.nurpra.2014.01.002
26. Centers for Disease Control and Prevention. (2016). Identifying and Treating Patients Who Use Tobacco: Action Steps for Clinicians. Atlanta, GA: Centers for Disease Control and Prevention, US Department of Health and Human Services.
27. Last, A. R., Ference, J. D., & Menzel, E. R. (2017, January 15). Hyperlipidemia: Drugs for cardiovascular risk reduction in adults. *American Family Physician, 95*(2), 78–87.
28. Shingrix. (n.d.). Be One of the First to Get Information about Shingrix. Retrieved from https://www.shingrix.com/. Accessed January 19, 2018.
29. GlaxoSmithKline. (2017, October 25). CDC's Advisory Committee on Immunization Practices Recommends Shingrix as the Preferred Vaccine for the Prevention of Shingles for Adults Aged 50 and Up. Retrieved from https://www.gsk.com/en-gb/media/press-releases/cdc-s-advisory-committee-on-immunization-practices-recommends-shingrix-as-the-preferred-vaccine-for-the-prevention-of-shingles-for-adults-aged-50-and-up/. Accessed January 19, 2018.

30. Maurer, D. M., & Darnall, C. R. (2012). Screening for depression. *American Family Physician, 85*(2), 139–144. Retrieved from https://www.aafp.org/afp/2012/0115/p139.html#afp201201156p139-c1. Accessed February 5, 2018.
31. American Cancer Society (ACS). (2016, April 14). Recommendations for Prostate Cancer Early Detection. Retrieved from https://www.cancer.org/cancer/prostate-cancer/early-detection/acs-recommendations.html. Accessed February 17, 2018.
32. American Urological Association (AUA). (2015). Early Detection of Prostate Cancer. Retrieved from http://www.auanet.org/guidelines/early-detection-of-prostate-cancer-(2013-reviewed-and-validity-confirmed-2015). Accessed February 17, 2018.
33. James, P. A., Oparil, S., Carter, B. L., Cushman, W. C., Dennison-Himmelfarb, C., & Handler, J., . . . Ortiz, E. (2014). 2014 evidence-based guideline for the management of high blood pressure in adults. *JAMA, 311*(5), 507–520. doi:10.1001/jama.2013.284427
34. Bakris, G., & Sorrentino, M. (2018). Redefining hypertension—assessing the new blood-pressure guidelines. *New England Journal of Medicine,* 378(6), 497–499. doi:10.1056/nejmp1716193
35. American College of Cardiology. (2017, November 13). New ACC/AHA High Blood Pressure Guidelines Lower Definition of Hypertension. Retrieved from http://www.acc.org/latest-in-cardiology/articles/2017/11/08/11/47/mon-5pm-bp-guideline-aha-2017. Accessed February 17, 2018.
36. American Geriatrics Society 2015 Beers Criteria Update Expert Panel, Fick, D. M., Semla, T. P., Beizer, J., Brandt, N., & Dombrowski, R., . . . Steinman, M. (2015, October 8). American Geriatrics Society 2015 updated Beers criteria for potentially inappropriate medication use in older adults. *Journal of the American Geriatrics Society, 63*(11), 2227–2246. Retrieved from http://onlinelibrary.wiley.com/doi/10.1111/jgs.13702/abstract. Accessed October 3, 2017.
37. American Diabetes Association (ADA). (2016). Standards of medical care in diabetes – 2016. *Diabetes Care,* 39, S1–S81. Retrieved from http://care.diabetesjournals.org/content/suppl/2015/12/21/39.Supplement_1.DC2/2016-Standards-of-Care.pdf. Accessed January 13, 2018.
38. American Geriatrics Society Expert Panel on Care of Older Adults with Diabetes Mellitus, Moreno, G., Mangione, C. M., Kimbro, L., & Vaisberg, E. (2013, November). Guidelines abstracted from the American Geriatrics Society Guidelines for Improving the Care of Older Adults with Diabetes Mellitus: 2013 update. *Journal of the American Geriatrics Society, 61*(11), 2020–2026. doi:10.1111/jgs.12514

SECTION II

# Neurology and Psychiatry

## Cerebrovascular Accident

### Definition[1,2,3,6,7]

A cerebrovascular accident is a sudden disruption of cerebral perfusion, leading to brain ischemia; classified as either an ischemic stroke (thrombotic or embolic), which is most common, or hemorrhagic stroke (intracerebral and/or subarachnoid hemorrhage).

### Causes[2,3,4,7,9]

- Cardioembolic source (e.g., atrial fibrillation)
- Large-artery atherosclerosis (e.g., carotid stenosis, intracranial atherosclerosis)
- Hemorrhage from hypertension, anticoagulation use, aneurysm, arteriovenous malformation

### Risk Factors[1,2,3,4,6,7,8,9]

- Advanced age
- Male sex
- African-American or Hispanic ancestry
- Family history of stroke
- Hypertension
- Smoking
- Diabetes mellitus
- Atrial fibrillation
- Carotid artery stenosis
- Anticoagulation use
- Vascular malformations
- Hypercoagulable state

## Signs & Symptoms[1,2,3,5,6,7,9]

- Sudden onset of focal neurologic deficits
- Symptoms persisting past 24 hours
- Unilateral weakness
  - Muscular weakness in face, arm, and/or leg.
- Speech impairment
  - Can be expressive or receptive aphasia, dysarthria.
- Visual changes
  - Can present as unilateral vision loss, diplopia.
- Sensory defect (e.g., numbness)
  - On the same side of the hemiparesis.
- Severe headache
  - *(Seen with subarachnoid hemorrhage.)*

## Tests[1,2,3,5,7,8]

- Neurological exam
  - National Institutes of Health Stroke Scale (NIHSS)
    - www.mdcalc.com/nih-stroke-scale-score-nihss/
    - Used to quantify stroke severity and prognosis.
  - Quick prehospital screening tool: Cincinnati Stroke scale
    - Evaluate for arm drift, speech difficulties, and facial paresis.
- Prehospital interventions: check glucose and oxygen saturation
  - Evaluate for hypoglycemia, which can cause stroke-like symptoms.
  - Recommended to maintain oxygen level > 94%.

## Treatment & Management[1,2,3,4,5,7,8,9,10,11,12,13,14]

- **Send patient to the appropriate hospital/stroke center.**
  - Will need a head computed tomography (CT) scan without contrast or magnetic resonance imaging (MRI) and thrombolytic therapy (*if patient is a candidate and absence of hemorrhagic stroke on imaging*) within **3–4.5** hours of stroke onset.

- New guidelines from the American Heart Association and American Stroke Association have increased the time for an acute ischemic stroke eligible for mechanical thrombectomy from 6 hours to 24 hours.
- Admission to hospital for stroke management (i.e., further work-up of underlying cause, medication administration, and/or surgical intervention).

## Management Following Stroke

- **Nonpharmacological and nursing interventions:**
  - Encourage nutrition and fluids.
    - Volume depletion is a potential cause of deep vein thrombosis and can prolong recovery time following a stroke.
  - Be aware of and manage sensory impairments (e.g., vision, hearing).
  - Encourage self-care; set realistic goals.
  - Emotional support to prevent discouragement.
- **Pharmacological and other interventions:**
  - If stroke was from a ***noncardioembolic*** cause, consider aspirin, clopidogrel (Plavix), or aspirin and dipyridamole (Aggrenox). Taking both aspirin and Plavix is not recommended for secondary stroke prevention due to risk of major bleeding.
    - If stroke was from ***cardioembolic*** source (e.g., atrial fibrillation), warfarin (Coumadin) is appropriate (if unable to tolerate, switch to aspirin 75 to 325 mg/day).
      - Rivaroxaban (Xarelto), dabigatran (Pradaxa), or apixaban (Eliquis) are effective alternatives to warfarin. They are associated with lower risk of brain hemorrhage, however there is higher risk of gastrointestinal bleeding compared to warfarin.
  - Hold anticoagulants following intracerebral hemorrhage for approximately four weeks.
    - Exception: artificial heart valve.
    - Consider risks (bleeding) vs. benefits (stroke prevention) before restarting anticoagulation.

- Identify and treat stroke risk factors, such as:
  - Hypertension management.
  - Counseling on smoking cessation.
  - Diabetes management.
  - Dyslipidemia (statin therapy reduces future strokes).
  - Carotid artery stenosis, symptomatic: carotid endarterectomy (CEA) recommended with severe stenosis (> 70%) within 2 weeks.
- Assess for depression and consider medications, counseling, and/or psychiatry consultation/referral.
  - Selective serotonin reuptake inhibitors (SSRIs) are an option for post-stroke depression.
  - Some SSRIs are associated with fewer adverse effects (e.g., citalopram, escitalopram, sertraline).
- Speech, physical, and/or occupational therapy consultation/referral
  - To aid in returning to the highest level of function the patient can achieve.
- Palliative care referral
  - To improve quality of life and provide relief of symptoms; as patient declines consider transition to hospice services.

Note: Beers listed items, as mentioned above, include: SSRIs, aspirin in doses above 325 mg/day, short-acting dipyridamole, and the above anticoagulants.

## Differential Diagnosis[1,2,3,4,5,7,9]

- Transient ischemic attack: symptoms are brief, lasting a few minutes to 60 minutes and there will be no evidence of infarction. In comparison to stroke, symptoms persist, lasting more than 24 hours, and diagnosis is confirmed with imaging.
- Hypoglycemia: history of diabetes, may have impaired level of consciousness that improves with correction of glucose.

- Seizure: patient will likely have a history of seizures; there may be a loss of consciousness, a postictal state, symptoms will be temporary, and scans are negative.

### CLINICAL PEARLS[2,3,5,9]

- Use a stroke assessment tool, such as the NIHSS, to aid in identifying a true stroke versus a stroke mimic (e.g., hypoglycemia) evaluate stroke severity, and predict prognosis.
- It is paramount to determine the cause of a stroke to guide clinicians in the medical management following a stroke.
- Emphasize early mobility to reduce complications following stroke, such as pneumonia (significant cause of death), deep vein thrombosis, pulmonary embolism, and pressure injuries.

## References

1. Epocrates. (2017, February 6). Overview of Stroke. Retrieved from https://online.epocrates.com/diseases/1080/Overview-of-stroke. Accessed September 25, 2017.
2. Yew, K. S., & Cheng, E. M. (2015, April 15). Diagnosis of Acute Stroke. Retrieved from http://www.aafp.org/afp/2015/0415/p528.html. Accessed September 27, 2017.
3. Antoniello, D. (2014). Cerebrovascular disease. In *Current Diagnosis & Treatment: Geriatrics* (2nd ed.). New York, NY: McGraw-Hill. Retrieved from http://accessmedicine.mhmedical.com/content.aspx?bookid=953&sectionid=53375647. Accessed September 25, 2017.
4. Iyer, S., Roubin, G., & Olin, J. W. (2017). In Fuster, V., Harrington, R. A., Narula, J., & Eapen, Z. J. (Eds.). *Hurst's The Heart* (14th ed.). New York, NY: McGraw-Hill. Retrieved from http://accessmedicine.mhmedical.com/content.aspx?bookid=2046&sectionid=155643266. Accessed September 25, 2017.
5. Jauch, E. C., Saver, J. L., Adams, H. P., Bruno, A., Connors, J. J., & Demaerschalk, B. M., . . . Yonas, H., and on behalf of the American Heart Association Stroke Council, Council on Cardiovascular Nursing, Council on Peripheral Vascular Disease, & Council on Clinical Cardiology. (2013). Guidelines for the early management of patients with acute ischemic stroke: a guideline for healthcare professionals from the American Heart Association/American Stroke Association. *Stroke, 44*(3), 870–947. Retrieved from http://stroke.ahajournals.org/content/44/3/870.
6. Caplan, L. R., Kasner, S. E., & Dashe, J. F. (2017, July 7). Patient Education: Stroke Symptoms and Diagnosis (Beyond the Basics). UpToDate. Retrieved from https://www.uptodate.com/contents/stroke-symptoms-and-diagnosis-beyond-the

-basics?source=search_result&search=stroke&selectedTitle=1~100#H1. Accessed September 25, 2017.
7. National Institute of Neurological Disorders and Stroke. (n.d.). Stroke Information Page. Retrieved from https://www.ninds.nih.gov/Disorders/All-Disorders/Stroke-Information-Page#disorders-r1. Accessed September 26, 2017.
8. Burggraf, V., Kim, K. Y., & Knight, A. L. (2015). *Healthy Aging: Principles and Clinical Practice for Clinicians*. Philadelphia, PA: Wolters Kluwer Health.
9. Camargo, E., Ding, M., Zimmerman, E., & Silverman, S. (2017). Cerebrovascular disease. In *Hazzard's Geriatric Medicine and Gerontology* (7th ed.). New York, NY: McGraw-Hill. Retrieved from http://accessmedicine.mhmedical.com/content.aspx?bookid=1923&sectionid=144523594. Accessed September 25, 2017.
10. Belleza, M. (2016, November 8). Cerebrovascular Accident (Stroke) Nursing Care and Management: A Study Guide. Retrieved from https://nurseslabs.com/cerebrovascular-accident-stroke/. Accessed October 29, 2017.
11. American Heart Association. (2018, January 24). More Stroke Patients May Receive Crucial Treatments Under New Guideline. Retrieved from https://newsroom.heart.org/news/more-stroke-patients-may-receive-crucial-treatments-under-new-guideline. Accessed February 20, 2018.
12. American Geriatrics Society 2015 Beers Criteria Update Expert Panel, Fick, D. M., Semla, T. P., Beizer, J., Brandt, N., & Dombrowski, R., … Steinman, M. (2015, October 8). American Geriatrics Society 2015 updated Beers criteria for potentially inappropriate medication use in older adults. *Journal of the American Geriatrics Society, 63*(11), 2227–2246. Retrieved from http://onlinelibrary.wiley.com/doi/10.1111/jgs.13702/abstract. Accessed October 8, 2017.
13. Bamiou, D. E. (2015). Hearing disorders in stroke. *The Human Auditory System - Fundamental Organization and Clinical Disorders Handbook of Clinical Neurology,* 633–647. doi:10.1016/b978-0-444-62630-1.00035-4
14. Holloway, R. G., Arnold, R. M., Creutzfeldt, C. J., Lewis, E. F., Lutz, B. J., McCann, R. M., . . . Zorowitz, R. D. (2014). Palliative and End-of-Life Care in Stroke. A statement for healthcare professionals from the American Heart Association/American Stroke Association. *Stroke, 49*(5). doi:https://doi.org/10.1161/STR.0000000000000015

# Delirium

## Definition[1,4,6]

Delirium is a syndrome characterized by an acute, sudden change in mentation that occurs over hours to days; considered a medical emergency.

## Causes[1,2,3,4,5]

- Dehydration, malnutrition

- Medications (e.g., opiates, antihistamines, psychoactive, Parkinson's medications)
    - *(Mental change occurs as a result of anticholinergic or sedative properties.)*
- Infections (e.g., urinary tract infection, pneumonia)
- Metabolic disturbance (e.g., fluid and electrolyte imbalance, hepatic and/or renal failure, hypoxia, hypoglycemia)
- Anemia
- Prolonged sleep deprivation
- Sensory impairment (e.g., visual or hearing)
- Alcohol or drug abuse or withdrawal
- Immobilization (e.g., restraints, catheter)
- Surgery *(Occurs postoperatively due to anesthetics and stress.)*
- Uncontrolled pain
- Acute distress (e.g., loss of spouse)
- Fecal impaction
- Urinary retention

Note: Causes are multifactorial; not typically just one single cause.

## Risk Factors[1,2,4,5]

*Risk factors coincide with causes of delirium.*

- Prior or current cognitive impairment
- Age > 65 years

## Signs & Symptoms[1,2,3,4,5]

- Inattention (i.e., unable to direct or focus attention)
- Fluctuating cognitive changes (e.g., agitation, lethargy)
- Disoriented
- Hallucinations (usually visual)
- Paranoia
- Delusions (e.g., perceived persecution or threat)
- Sleep-wake cycle disturbance
- Caregiver reporting patient not acting like themselves

- Signs of infection (e.g., fever, tachypnea, hypoxia, pulmonary consolidation)
- Signs of volume depletion (e.g., dry mucous membranes, poor skin turgor)

## Tests[1,2,4,5,6,7]

*Diagnosis is made clinically based on history and exam.*

- Screening tests (e.g., confusion assessment method [CAM])
- Comprehensive metabolic panel (CMP), complete blood counts (CBC), glucose, thyroid-stimulating hormone (TSH), vitamin B12, folate, urine and serum drug levels, oxygen saturation, ammonia, blood cultures
  - Assess for electrolyte abnormalities, renal and/or hepatic failure, infection, anemia, hypo- or hyperglycemia, thyroid disorder, vitamin deficiency, drug toxicity, hypoxia, hepatic encephalopathy.
  - Testing for syphilis, human immunodeficiency virus (HIV).
    - Screening for neurosyphilis, HIV recommended in appropriate cases (e.g., multiple sex partners).
- Urinalysis and culture
  - Used to diagnose urinary tract infection.
- Electrocardiogram
  - Check for cardiac arrhythmias, myocardial infarction.
- Chest radiograph
  - Useful to diagnose pneumonia or heart failure.
- CT and/or MRI of brain
  - Not typically helpful unless evidence of focal neurologic signs, head trauma; order if concern for existing mass.
  - MRI gives better perspective on the underlying etiology of delirium; can pick up on infectious, inflammatory, and malignant conditions.

## Treatment & Management[1,2,4,6,7,8,9,10, 11, 12]

- **Identify and treat the underlying issue(s),** such as:

- Correct the metabolic derangement.
- Stop or reduce the medication triggering the delirium.
- Treat the underlying infection.

- **Nonpharmacological and nursing interventions**:
  - Frequent monitoring (e.g., place patient at nurse's station).
  - Provide frequent reorientation.
  - Give visual cues for orientation purposes (e.g., family photos, clocks).
  - Offer fluids and nutrition.
  - Avoid using restraints and/or catheters (if possible).
  - Promote sleep (i.e., encourage daytime activities; encourage calm, quiet environment).
  - Encourage use of eyeglasses and hearing aids.
  - Encourage mobility to the extent allowed.
- **Pharmacological and other interventions:**
  - Use of multivitamins and thiamine in those with alcohol toxicity or withdrawal.
  - First-generation antipsychotic (i.e., haloperidol [Haldol]) or a second-generation antipsychotic (i.e., risperidone [Risperdal]) for short-term use, at low doses *(to avoid adverse effects)*.
    - Example: haloperidol 2–5 mg PO/IM q1hr PRN acute psychosis.
    - Use antipsychotics only if nondrug measures were unsuccessful and patient is a danger to self or others.
    - Some have significant anticholinergic properties; are associated with increased mortaility, strokes, falls, and fractures. Second-generation antipsychotics have fewer extrapyramidal adverse effects.
  - Avoid benzodiazepines (e.g., lorazepam [Ativan]).
    - Causes paradoxical excitation; does not improve symptoms.
    - The exception is if the delirium is due to alcohol or benzodiazepine withdrawal.

- Increased risk of central nervous system (CNS) adverse effects, falls, and fractures.
- Physical and occupational therapy consultation/referral (to improve mobility)
- Psychiatry consultation/referral (Consider if the above interventions fail and/or for management of behaviors.)

Note: Beers listed items, as mentioned above, include benzodiazepines and antipsychotics.

## Differential Diagnosis[2,4,7]

- Dementia is irreversible, progressive, has a gradual onset, and memory is mostly affected. Delirium is, however, usually reversible (when underlying cause is identified and treated quickly), has an abrupt onset, and affects attention mostly.
- Depression is characterized by having normal speech, memory, and level of consciousness. In delirium, the level of consciousness waxes and wanes; speech and memory are impaired.

**CONFUSION ASSESSMENT METHOD (CAM) ALGORITHM**

(1) acute onset and fluctuating course

-and-

(2) inattention

-and either-

(3) disorganized thinking

-or-

(4) altered level of consciousness



**Figure 2-1** Confusion Assessment Method (CAM) Tool Algorithm

Reproduced from Confusion Assessment Method. Copyright 2003, Hospital Elder Life Program, LLC. Not to be reproduced without permission. Data from Inouye SK, et al. *Ann Intern Med*. 1990; 113:941-8. Available at hospitalelderlifeprogram.org.

## CLINICAL PEARLS[1,5,6,7]

- A mnemonic to remember common causes of delirium in older adults:
  - **WILD**
    - W = Water depletion
    - I = Infection
    - L = Labs, abnormal
    - D = Drugs (toxicity, adverse effects)
- There is no specific algorithm for the workup of delirium given the many causes. If the etiology is uncertain, start with the complete blood count, complete metabolic panel, chest film, and urinalysis with culture (with or without electrocardiogram and blood cultures).
- Direct attention on the nonpharmacological interventions *(i.e., constant reorientation, promoting sleep)* for the treatment and prevention of delirium, which are highly efficacious. Antipsychotics are reserved for individuals who failed these interventions and have severe agitation that poses a threat to self/others.

# References


1. Josephson, S., & Miller, B. L. (2015). Confusion and delirium. In Kasper, D., Fauci, A., Hauser, S., Longo, D., Jamesom, J., & Loscalzo, J. (Eds.) *Harrison's Principles of Internal Medicine* (19th ed.). New York, NY: McGraw-Hill. Retrieved from http://accessmedicine.mhmedical.com/content.aspx?bookid=1130&sectionid=79724923. Accessed September 19, 2017.
2. Alagiakrishnan, K. (2017, August 28). Delirium. Medscape. Retrieved from http://emedicine.medscape.com/article/288890-overview. Accessed September 20, 2017.
3. Wang, S., & Nussbaum, A. M. (2017). *DSM-5 Pocket Guide for Elder Mental Health*. Arlington, VA: American Psychiatric Association Publishing.
4. Huang, J. (2016, February). *Delirium – Neurologic Disorders*. Merck Manuals: Professional. Retrieved from http://www.merckmanuals.com/professional/neurologic-disorders/delirium-and-dementia/delirium. Accessed September 20, 2017.
5. Pisani, M. (2016, December 21). Evaluation of Delirium. Epocrates. Retrieved from https://online.epocrates.com/diseases/241/Evaluation-of-delirium. Accessed September 24, 2017.
6. Harper, G., Johnston, C., & Landefeld, C. Geriatric disorders. (2018). In Papadakis, M. A., McPhee, S. J., & Rabow, M. W. (Eds.). *Current Medical Diagnosis & Treatment 2018*. New York, NY: McGraw-Hill. Retrieved from http://accessmedicine.mhmedical.com/content.aspx?bookid=2192&sectionid=168006449. Accessed September 21, 2017.
7. Inouye, S. K., Growdon, M., & Fong, T. Delirium. (2017). In *Hazzard's Geriatric Medicine and Gerontology* (7th ed.). New York, NY: McGraw-Hill. Retrieved from http://accessmedicine.mhmedical.com/content.aspx?bookid=1923&sectionid=144521671. Accessed September 21, 2017.

8. Stahl, S. M., & Muntner, N. (2013, May 27). *Stahl's Essential of Psychopharmacology: Neuroscientific Basis and Practical Applications.* (4th ed.). New York, NY: Cambridge University Press.
9. American Geriatrics Society 2015 Beers Criteria Update Expert Panel, Fick, D. M., Semla, T. P., Beizer, J., Brandt, N., Dombrowski, R., & Steinman, M. (2015, October 8). American Geriatrics Society 2015 updated Beers criteria for potentially inappropriate medication use in older adults. *Journal of the American Geriatrics Society, 63*(11), 2227–2246. Retrieved from http://onlinelibrary.wiley.com/doi/10.1111/jgs.13702/abstract. Accessed October 3, 2017.
10. Bull, M. J. (2015, October). Managing delirium in hospitalized older adults. *American Nurse Today, 10*(10). Retrieved from https://www.americannursetoday.com/managing-delirium-hospitalized-older-adults/. Accessed February 20, 2018.
11. Hanlon, J. T., Semla, T. P., & Schmader, K. E. (2015). Alternative Medications for Medications in the use of High-Risk Medications in the Elderly and Potentially Harmful Drug-Disease Interactions in the Elderly Quality Measures. Retrieved from http://micmrc.org/system/files/AGS%202015%20Beers%20Criteria%20Alternative%20Medications%20List.pdf. Accessed October 3, 2017.
12. Terrery, C. L., & Nicoteri, J. L. (2016, March). The 2015 American Geriatric Society Beers Criteria: Implications for Nurse Practitioners. Retrieved from http://www.npjournal.org/article/S1555-4155(15)01124-1/fulltext. Accessed October 7, 2017.

# Dementia

## Definition[1,2,3,4,6,7,10,11,12,14,15,17,20,21]

Dementia is a syndrome associated with deterioration in cognitive function that hinders daily living. Most dementia cases in individuals age 60 or above are due to Alzheimer's disease (AD), vascular cognitive impairment (VCI) or vascular dementia (VaD), and Lewy body dementia (LBD). Frontotemporal lobar degeneration or frontotemporal dementia (FTD) can be seen in older adults, however is usually diagnosed between the ages of 40 and 60. The first three will be mentioned below.

## Causes[8,10,11,12,13,15,16,17]

| AD | VCI/VaD | DLB |
|---|---|---|
| Not fully understood<br>Amyloid plaques, neurofibrillary tangles, tau protein | Hypoperfusion to the brain (e.g., infarcts)[13] | Unknown<br>Accumulation of Lewy bodies |

## Risk Factors[4,5,6,8,9,10,11,12,14,16,17, 22, 23]

| AD | VCI/VaD | DLB |
|---|---|---|
| Older age first-degree relative with AD, genetics, apolipoprotein E4, hyperlipidemia, hypertension, diabetes, obesity, sedentary lifestyle, depression, low educational attainment, head injury | Cerebrovascular disease, Older age, hyperlipidemia, hypertension, diabetes, smoking | Older age |

## Signs & Symptoms[2,4,6,7,8,11,14,16,17]

| AD | VCI/VaD | DLB |
|---|---|---|
| Memory loss (insidious), language impairment (e.g., word finding), visual–spatial deficits (getting lost); impaired reasoning, judgment, and/or problem solving | Sudden cognitive decline following a stroke, focal neurological deficits, apathy, aphasia | Visual hallucinations (typical), cognitive impairment Parkinsonism, fluctuating attention, REM sleep behavior disorder, visual–spatial deficits |

## Tests[2,4,6,7,8,11,12,14,16,17]

- Screening tools (also used to follow dementia progression):
  - Mini-Mental State Exam (MMSE)
  - Mini-Cognitive (Min-Cog)
  - Montreal Cognitive Assessment (MOCA)
- Depression screening tools: Geriatric Depression Scale (GDS) and Cornell Scale for Depression in Dementia (CSDD)

- Laboratory tests; reasonable to start with:
  - TSH, CMP, CBC, vitamin B12
    - Evaluate for thyroid disease, liver or renal impairment, electrolyte imbalance, anemia, leukocytosis, B12 deficiency (these can be associated with cognitive changes).
  - Brain CT or MRI
    - Imaging helps to determine if neoplasm or tumor present.
    - Specific findings are noted with the different types of dementias (e.g., hippocampal atrophy with AD).
    - Especially useful in atypical dementia presentations.

## Treatment & Management (for all dementias)[4,5,6,7,8,11,12,13,14,16,17,18,19,24]

- **Identify and treat reversible causes that impair cognition**, such as:
  - B12 deficiency
  - Thyroid disease
  - Medication toxicity and/or adverse effects
  - Constipation
  - Infection
  - Electrolyte derangement
  - Hearing or vision impairment
  - Uncontrolled pain
  - Alcohol abuse (cessation may improve cognition)
- **Nonpharmacological and nursing interventions**:
  - Continue with the same daily routines, use of calendars, engaging in physical exercise, being a part of activities.
  - Constant reassurance and reorientation.
  - Avoidance of physical restraints.
  - Promote sleep; offer fluid and nutrition.
  - Assess the caregivers' stress.
    - Tools: Zarit Burden Interview (ZBI) or Caregiver Strain Index (CSI).
    - Encourage respite care to caregivers to reduce burden.

- The Alzheimer's Association is a useful resource for caregivers.
  - www.alz.org/
- **Pharmacological interventions:**
  - Cholinesterase inhibitors for mild to severe dementia.
    - Also used for visual hallucinations and depression symptoms.
    - Start low with dosing and titration (e.g., donepezil (Aricept) 2.5–5 mg daily, increase every 4 weeks to goal of 10 mg daily).
    - Can be taken with memantine (Namenda), which is approved for moderate to severe AD; may reduce nursing home placement.
  - When nonpharmacological interventions fail and patient is a potential harm to themselves or others:
    - Second-generation antipsychotics for agitation, hallucinations, aggression, uncooperative behavior; use short term.
      - Start low dose such as 12.5 mg daily of quetiapine (Seroquel).
      - Other examples: aripiprazole (Abilify), clozapine (Clozaril), risperidone (Risperdal).
      - Associated with increased risk of stroke and death in older individuals with dementia.
    - Use benzodiazepines for anxiety or restlessness
      - Use with caution; may cause paradoxical agitation.
      - Increased risk of CNS adverse effects, falls, and fractures.
  - Treat the depression (often coexists with dementia).
    - Use low-dose SSRI, such as escitalopram (Lexapro) 5 mg daily.
    - Citalopram (Celexa) improves not only depression but moderate agitation.
- Vascular risk factor management in VCI/VaD.
- Antiparkinson medication in LBD.
- Avoid first-generation antipsychotics in LBD (worsens tremor and confusion).

- Psychiatry consultation/referral.
- Palliative care referral.
  - To improve quality of life and provide relief of symptoms; as patient declines consider transition to hospice services.

Note: Beers listed items, as mentioned above, include benzodiazepines and antipsychotics.

## Differential Diagnosis

- Delirium is usually reversible, has an abrupt onset, and affects mostly attention. Dementia however is irreversible, has a gradual onset, and memory is mostly affected.
- Depression can present abruptly, there will be no changes on neuroimaging, and main symptoms will be depression related. Dementia, however, has a gradual onset, will have positive findings on neuroimaging, and memory impairment is the main symptom.

### CLINICAL PEARLS[4,7,17,19]

- Early diagnosis is key to jump-start discussions regarding future planning (establishing advance directives, appointing a durable power of attorney) and to initiate medications (e.g., cholinesterase inhibitors +/– memantine) to improve quality of life, prolong function, and reduce nursing facility placement.
- In regards to driving, check with your state's law on reporting dementia to the Department of Motor Vehicles, even if patient has a mild dementia.
- Antipsychotics (first and second generation) are potentially dangerous and can be used in behavioral problems of dementia if nondrug measures fail and patient is a harm to self or others.

## References

1. Alzheimer's Association. (n.d.). What Is Dementia? Signs, Symptoms, & Diagnosis. Retrieved from http://www.alz.org/what-is-dementia.asp. Accessed September 27, 2017.
2. Tampi, R. (2017, November 13). Evaluation of Dementia. Epocrates. Retrieved from https://online.epocrates.com/diseases/242/Evaluation-of-dementia. Accessed February 20, 2017.

3. National Institute on Aging. (2017, May 17). What Is Dementia? Retrieved from https://www.nia.nih.gov/health/what-dementia. Accessed September 27, 2017.
4. Dementia. In Kasper, D., Fauci, A., Hauser, S., Longo, D., Jameson, J., & Loscalzo, J. *Harrison's Principles of Internal Medicine* (19th ed.). New York, NY: McGraw-Hill. Retrieved from http://accessmedicine.mhmedical.com/content.aspx?bookid=1130&sectionid=79724950. Accessed September 27, 2017.
5. Alzheimer's Association. (n.d.). Alzheimer's Disease & Dementia: What Is Alzheimer's? Retrieved from http://www.alz.org/alzheimers_disease_what_is_alzheimers.asp. Accessed September 27, 2017.
6. Carlsson, C. M., Gleason, C. E., Puglielli, L., & Asthana, S. (2017). Dementia including Alzheimer disease. In *Hazzard's Geriatric Medicine and Gerontology* (7th ed.). New York, NY: McGraw-Hill. Retrieved from http://accessmedicine.mhmedical.com/content.aspx?bookid=1923&sectionid=144523735. Accessed September 27, 2017.
7. Sink, K. M., & Yaffe, K. (2014). Cognitive impairment and dementia. In *Current Diagnosis & Treatment: Geriatrics* (2nd ed.). New York, NY: McGraw-Hill. Retrieved from http://accessmedicine.mhmedical.com/content.aspx?bookid=953&sectionid=53375646. Accessed September 27, 2017.
8. Epocrates. (2017, August 7). Alzheimer Dementia: Risk Factors. Retrieved from https://online.epocrates.com/diseases/31732/Alzheimer-dementia/Risk-Factors. Accessed September 27, 2017.
9. Sandhya, G. (2015). Modifiable risk factors for Alzheimer's disease. *The Clinical Advisor,* 22.
10. *Ganong's Medical Physiology Examination & Board Review.* New York, NY: McGraw-Hill; Chapter 15: Learning, memory, language, & speech. Retrieved from http://accessmedicine.mhmedical.com/content.aspx?bookid=2139&sectionid=160312527. Accessed September 29, 2017.
11. Burggraf, V., Kim, K. Y., & Knight, A. L. (2015). *Healthy Aging: Principles and Clinical Practice for Clinicians.* Philadelphia, PA: Wolters Kluwer Health.
12. Fletcher, K. (2016, January 14). Dementia. ConsultGeri Topic. Retrieved from https://consultgeri.org/geriatric-topics/dementia. Accessed September 29, 2017.
13. Passmore, P. (2017, July 3). Vascular Dementia. Epocrates. Retrieved from https://online.epocrates.com/diseases/31924/Vascular-dementia/Etiology. Accessed September 29, 2017.
14. Alzheimer's Association. (n.d.). Vascular Dementia: Signs, Symptoms, & Diagnosis. Retrieved from http://www.alz.org/dementia/vascular-dementia-symptoms.asp#causes. Accessed September 29, 2017.
15. Alzheimer's Association. (n.d.). Dementia with Lewy Bodies Symptoms: Signs, Symptoms, & Diagnosis. Retrieved from http://www.alz.org/dementia/dementia-with-lewy-bodies-symptoms.asp. Accessed September 29, 2017.
16. Mayo Clinic. (2017, August 9). Lewy Body Dementia. Retrieved from http://www.mayoclinic.org/diseases-conditions/lewy-body-dementia/symptoms-causes/dxc-20200348. Accessed September 29, 2017.
17. Walter, C., Edwards, N. E., Griggs, R., & Yehle, K. (2014). Differentiating Alzheimer disease, Lewy body, and Parkinson dementia Using *DSM-5*. *Journal for Nurse Practitioners, 10*(4), 262–270. doi:10.1016/j.nurpra.2014.01.002
18. Williams, J. R., & Marsh, L. (2009). Validity of the Cornell scale for depression in dementia in Parkinsons disease with and without cognitive impairment. *Movement Disorders, 24*(3), 433–437. doi:10.1002/mds.22421
19. American Geriatrics Society 2015 Beers Criteria Update Expert Panel, Fick, D. M., Semla, T. P., Beizer, J., Brandt, N., & Dombrowski, R., . . . Steinman, M. (2015, October 8).

American Geriatrics Society 2015 updated Beers criteria for potentially inappropriate medication use in older adults. *Journal of the American Geriatrics Society, 63*(11), 2227–2246. Retrieved from http://onlinelibrary.wiley.com/doi/10.1111/jgs.13702/abstract. Accessed October 3, 2017.

20. Kverno, K. S., & Velez, R. (2018, March 1). Comorbid dementia and depression: The case for integrated care. *Journal for Nurse Practitioners, 14*(3), 196–201. doi:10.1016/j.nurpra.2017.12.032
21. Baborie, A., Griffiths, T. D., Jaros, E., Momeni, P., McKeith, I. G., & Burn, D. J., . . . Perry, R. (2012). Frontotemporal dementia in elderly individuals. *Arch Neurol, 69*(8), 1052–1060. doi:10.1001/archneurol.2011.3323
22. Katzel, L. I., Blumenthal, J. B., & Goldberg, A. P. (2017). Dyslipoproteinemia. In *Hazzard's Geriatric Medicine and Gerontology* (7th ed.). New York, NY: McGraw-Hill;. http://accessmedicine.mhmedical.com/content.aspx?bookid=1923&sectionid=144561473. Accessed April 30, 2018.
23. Chia-Chen, L., Takahisa, K., Huaxi, X., & Guojun, B. (2013). Apolipoprotein E and Alzheimer disease: Risk, mechanisms, and therapy. *Nature Reviews Neurology, 9*(2), 106-118. doi:10.1038/nrneurol.2012.263
24. What Are Palliative Care and Hospice Care? (2017, May 17). Retrieved from https://www.nia.nih.gov/health/what-are-palliative-care-and-hospice-care#palliative-vs-hospice. Accessed May 8, 2018

# Depression

## Definition[1,2,3,4,7]

Depression is a common mood disorder experienced by older adults, which can interfere with daily living and function.

Note: Depression oftentimes presents atypically in older adults and is underrecognized and undertreated. It affects about 15 out of every 100 Americans over the age of 65.

## Causes[1,2,3,4,7,10]

- Biological factors
  - Genetics, history of depression or suicide attempt, age changes in neurotransmitter concentrations
- Physical factors
  - Medical conditions that includes loss of function, loss of vision or hearing, chronic pain

- Psychological factors
  - Dementia or memory loss, substance abuse, unresolved conflicts (e.g., anger, guilt)
- Social factors
  - Loss of spouse/relative/close friends, loss of job or income, living alone, stressful life events

## Risk Factors[1,2,3,4,5,6,7,10]

*Risk factors of depression coincides with causes:*

- Female sex.
- Personal or family history of depression.
- Coexisting medical condition (e.g., cancer, stroke, dementia, diabetes).
- Have a disability.
- Socially isolated.
- Use of certain medications.
- Alcohol or drug misuse.
- Major life changes (e.g., moving to a retirement facility).
- Stressful life or traumatic events.

## Signs & Symptoms[1,2,3,4,10]

- Fatigue.
- Weight and/or appetite changes.
- Difficulty sleeping.
- Loss of interest in hobbies or activities.
- Impaired concentration or memory, or indecisiveness.
- Restlessness or irritability.
- Feelings of guilt or worthlessness.
- Suicidal thoughts.
- Functional impairment.
- Somatic symptoms unexplained by physical findings.
- Less frequently will complain of depressed mood, feeling sad, or experience crying episodes.

- Physical signs of depression on exam are often lacking, especially in the presence of chronic conditions (e.g., Parkinson disease, malignancy, chronic obstructive pulmonary disease).

## Tests[1,4,5,6,7,10]

- Screening tools
  - Patient Health Questionnaire, the 2 or 9 item
  - Geriatric Depression Scale
  - Cornell Scale for Depression in Dementia
  - Stroke Aphasic Depression Questionnaire
- Serum TSH, CMP, CBC, vitamin B12, folate, glucose, urinalysis, vitamin D
  - The following can imitate depressive symptoms:
    - Hypo and hyperthyroidism.
    - Electrolyte imbalance (especially hypo- or hypernatremia and hypercalcemia).
    - Dehydration/uremia.
    - Anemia.
    - Nutritional deficiencies.
    - Diabetes mellitus.
    - Infection.
    - Vitamin D deficiency may be associated with depression.

## Treatment & Management[1,2,3,4,7,9,10]

- **Nonpharmacological and nursing interventions:**
  - Encourage avoidance of alcohol and sleep aids.
  - Encourage regular exercise.
  - Promote effective sleep habits.
  - Monitor for patients complaining of wanting to harm themselves or attempting suicide.
    - A starting point for assessing suicidality can be asking the patient, "Do you feel like hurting yourself?" and "Do you have a plan on how to carry it out?"
    - Adults age 65 and above account for 18% of all suicides.

    - Inform caregivers to take the patient to the nearest emergency room, call 911 and/or their doctor, and call the 24-hour hotline of the National Suicide Prevention Lifeline, toll-free, at 1-800-273-TALK.
  - Advise patients to not abruptly stop taking their antidepressant (to avoid withdrawal symptoms).
    - Advise patient that depressive symptoms can improve as early as 1–2 weeks with medication.
- **Pharmacological and other interventions:**
  - Treat the illness that may be causing the symptoms (e.g., hypothyroidism).
  - Avoid medications that are making the depression symptoms worse.
    - Examples include antipsychotics, hypnotics, anticonvulsants, statins, barbiturates.
  - Vitamin D supplementation.
    - 1,000–2,000 IU of vitamin D daily can be considered in older adults with depression. There is, however, no definitive recommendation on supplementation for depression treatment.
    - Consider this especially if the older patient is not interested in taking an antidepressant.
  - Selective serotonin reuptake inhibitors (SSRIs) (e.g., citalopram [Celexa], escitalopram [Lexapro], fluoxetine [Prozac], sertraline [Zoloft]).
    - Example: sertraline 25–50 mg PO daily (max: 200 mg/day).
    - Consider sertraline or escitalopram as first-line options in late-life depression.
    - If no response to an SSRI after 6–8 weeks, try a serotonin-norepinephrine reuptake inhibitor (SNRI).
    - Fluoxetine has the longest half-life of 7–9 days.
    - Use with caution especially in individuals with history of falls or fracture; may cause hyponatremia.
  - Serotonin-norepinephrine reuptake inhibitors (SNRIs) (e.g., duloxetine [Cymbalta], venlafaxine [Effexor]).

    - Example: duloxetine 30 mg PO daily (initial starting dose); no evidence to support doses above 60 mg/day.
    - Consider duloxetine in adults suffering from both depression and pain.
    - Avoid venlafaxine in adults with hypertension.
    - These may cause hyponatremia.
  - Tricyclic antidepressants (TCAs) (e.g., amitriptyline [Elavil], nortriptyline [Pamelor]).
    - These drugs are best avoided due to adverse effects.
  - Monamine oxidase inhibitors (MAOIs) (e.g., phenelzine [Nardil], tranylcypromine [Parnate]).
    - These are reserved for treatment failures.
    - Have fallen out of favor due to interactions with certain foods containing tyramine, which can lead to hypertensive crisis, stroke, or myocardial infarction.
  - Other antidepressant medication options: trazodone (Oleptro, Desyrel), mirtazapine (Remeron), bupropion (Wellbutrin).
    - In older adults who can't tolerate an SSRI or SNRI, consider mirtazapine as an initial alternative. It can be combined with an SSRI or SNRI.

Note: for all the above medications, start the dose at half the recommended dose and increase the dose every 2–4 weeks if little or no response noted.

- Other treatment options: psychotherapy, electroconvulsive therapy.
  - There is insufficient evidence to support acupuncture or music therapy.
- Psychiatry or psychologist consultation/referral (consider when there is no response to nonpharmacological or pharmacological interventions).

Note: Beers listed items, as mentioned above, include mirtazapine, bupropion, TCAs, SSRIs, and SNRIs.

## Differential Diagnosis[1,3]

- Dementia: Memory impairment is a prominent symptom, it is not treatable, has a gradual onset, and has positive findings on neuroimaging. Older adults with depression can have cognitive impairment; however, symptoms present abruptly, is treatable in most cases, and there would be no changes on neuroimaging.
- Medication adverse effects: The depressive symptoms would be associated with medication use.
- Hypothyroidism: Symptoms are similar to depression (e.g., weight gain, decreased appetite, fatigue); however, will have an elevated TSH.

### CLINICAL PEARLS[1,7,8,9,10]

- To be diagnosed with major depressive disorder, per *DSM-5* criteria, patients must have more than five of the following symptoms (as listed below), for a minimum of almost every day for at least 2 weeks and is a decline from previous functioning. Depressed mood or loss of pleasure in activities must be one of their symptoms. In addition, these symptoms cause functional impairment (e.g., social, occupational).
    - Depressed mood
    - Loss of pleasure in activities (i.e., anhedonia)
    - Weight change (gain or loss)
    - Insomnia or hypersomnia
    - Psychomotor agitation or retardation
    - Loss of energy or fatigue
    - Feelings of worthlessness or guilt
    - Diminished ability to think or concentrate
    - Recurrent thoughts of death, suicidal ideation with or without a plan, or suicide attempt
- Before diagnosing an individual with depression, ensure their symptoms are not due to the effects of a substance or medical conditions known to cause depressive symptoms, such as substance abuse, especially alcohol and medication side effects.

(*continues*)

**CLINICAL PEARLS[1,7,8,9,10]** ***(Continued)***

- Treating depression significantly improves the quality of life in older patients.
- When depression occurs with another medical problem (e.g., hip fracture, osteoarthritis), there will be an exacerbation of pain, along with reduced motivation and recovery of function.
- In all older patients, antidepressant dosages should be started low and titrated slowly. SSRIs, which are frequently first-line treatments (due to safety profile) can contribute to hyponatremia.

## References

1. Kane, R. L., Ouslander, J. G., Resnick, B., & Malone, M. L. (Eds.) *Essentials of Clinical Geriatrics* (8th ed.). New York, NY: McGraw-Hill; Diagnosis and management of depression. Retrieved from http://accessmedicine.mhmedical.com/content.aspx?bookid=2300&sectionid=178119619. Accessed February 25, 2018.
2. Berger, F. K. (2016, July 29). Depression: Older Adults. MedlinePlus. Retrieved from https://medlineplus.gov/ency/article/001521.htm. Accessed February 25, 2018.
3. National Institute of Mental Health. (n.d.). Older Adults and Depression. Retrieved from https://www.nimh.nih.gov/health/publications/older-adults-and-depression/index.shtml. Accessed February 25, 2018.
4. Farrington, E., & Moller, M. (2013). Relationship of vitamin D3 deficiency to depression in older adults: A systematic review of the literature from 2008–2013. *Journal for Nurse Practitioners, 9*(8), 506–515. doi:10.1016/j.nurpra.2013.05.011
5. Adam, J., & Folds, L. (2014). Depression, self-efficacy, and adherence in patients with type 2 diabetes. *Journal for Nurse Practitioners, 10*(9), 646–652. doi:10.1016/j.nurpra.2014.07.033
6. Gote, C., & Bruce, R. D. (2014). Effectiveness of a reminder prompt to screen for diabetes in individuals with depression. *Journal for Nurse Practitioners, 10*(7), 456–464. doi:10.1016/j.nurpra.2014.04.021
7. Scrandis, D. A., & Watt, M. (2013). Antidepressant medication management in primary care: Not just another pill. *Journal for Nurse Practitioners, 9*(7), 449–457. doi:10.1016/j.nurpra.2013.04.019
8. American Psychiatric Association. (2013). *Diagnostic and Statistical Manual of Mental Disorders* (5th ed.) (*DSM-5*). Washington, DC: American Psychiatric Publishing.
9. American Geriatrics Society 2015 Beers Criteria Update Expert Panel, Fick, D. M., Semla, T. P., Beizer, J., Brandt, N., & Dombrowski, R., . . . Steinman, M. (2015, October 8). American Geriatrics Society 2015 updated Beers criteria for potentially inappropriate medication use in older adults. *Journal of the American Geriatrics Society, 63*(11), 2227–2246. Retrieved http://onlinelibrary.wiley.com/doi/10.1111/jgs.13702/abstract. Accessed October 3, 2017.

10. Kverno, K. S., & Velez, R. (2018). Comorbid dementia and depression: The case for integrated care. *Journal for Nurse Practitioners*. doi:10.1016/j.nurpra.2017.12.032
11. RxList. (n.d.). Retrieved from https://www.rxlist.com/script/main/hp.asp (used for medication examples/max doses). Accessed February 25, 2018.

# Parkinson's Disease

## Definition[1,2,3,4,10]

Parkinson's disease (PD) is a progressive neurodegenerative disease associated with dopamine deficiency in the brain.

## Causes[1,2,4,5,10]

- Unknown.
- Possible causes:
  - Environmental factors (e.g., pesticide exposure, consumption of well water)
  - Genetics

## Risk Factors[1,2,5,6]

- Advanced age.
- Family history of Parkinson's disease.
  - About 10%–15% are familial, the rest are sporadic.

## Signs & Symptoms[1,2,3,4,5,6]

- Resting tremor, usually asymmetric.
  - Complete relaxation significantly improves the tremor.
  - The "pill rolling" tremor is present in about 50%.
- Bradykinesia (i.e., slow movements).
- Rigidity (i.e., muscular stiffness of limbs, neck, trunk).
- Postural instability (i.e., impaired balance).
- Other symptoms may include cognitive impairment, speech difficulties (i.e., monotonous, cluttered), hypomimia (i.e., masked facies), drooling (unable to swallow frequently), depression, constipation.

## Tests[1,4,5]

*Diagnosis is made clinically based on history and exam; no tests required unless diagnosis is unclear.*

- Dopaminergic agent trial (i.e., levodopa or others)
  - Validates the diagnosis; will see improvement in symptoms.
- Neurological exam
  - Pull test (checking for postural instability).

## Treatment & Management[1,2,3,4,5,6,8,9,12,13]

- **Nonpharmacological and nursing interventions:**
  - Educate patient and family on Antiparkinson medication.
    - Stress importance of taking medications as prescribed for maximum benefit.
    - Educate patient on adverse effects and contraindications.
  - Refer patients and caregivers to the Parkinson's Foundation.
    - www.Parkinson.org/
  - Encourage exercise.
    - Helps slows disease progression, reduces pain, prevents falls.
  - Evaluate for safety concerns.
    - Assess if patient can take their own medication, drive, and live independently.
- **Pharmacological interventions:**
  - Levodopa – first-line treatment
    - Typical to order the combination drug of carbidopa-levodopa (Sinemet).
      - Example: 50 mg PO TID (immediate release) as a starting dose
    - Considered definitive treatment; improves motor symptoms.
    - Over time, the drug can wear off and produce dyskinesias.

- Amantadine
    - Initially ordered at 100 mg PO daily (max: 400 mg/day).
    - Used as an adjunctive medication to improve mild symptoms; reduces levodopa-induced dyskinesias, however poorly tolerated due to mental adverse effects.
- Monoamine oxidase-B (MAO-B) inhibitor (e.g., rasagiline [Azilect], selegiline [Zelapar])
    - Example: selegiline 5 mg PO BID
    - Used in combo with Sinemet for mild to moderate parkinsonism.
- Dopamine agonist (e.g., pramipexole [Mirapex], ropinirole [Requip], rotigotine transdermal [Neupro])
    - Example: rotigotine transdermal 2 mg/24 hr patch applied initially (max: 8 mg/24 hrs).
    - Can be used as a first-line treatment in mild parkinsonism over carbidopa/levodopa; less likely to cause dyskinesia.
    - Used in conjunction with levodopa/carbidopa in moderate parkinsonism.
- COMT inhibitors (e.g., entacapone [Comtan] and tolcapone [Tasmar])
    - Can be used with carbidopa-levodopa in moderate parkinsonism; improves the effects of wearing off, in which levodopa effects are lessened.
- Anticholinergic agents such as benztropine (Cogentin), amantadine (Symmetrel), or trihexyphenidyl (Artane)
    - Example: Initially use trihexyphenidyl immediate release 1 mg PO daily, followed by 2 mg PO daily (max: 15 mg/day).
    - Added to regimen to control tremor.
    - These agents can cause dry mouth and confusion (use with caution in those with cognitive impairment).

- For all the above medications:
    - Start at low doses and slowly titrate upward.
    - Gradually wean to stop the medications, do not abruptly stop *(with the exception of the above-mentioned anticholinergics)*.

- Deep brain stimulation
  - Useful in controlling tremor and dyskinesias refractory to drug therapies.
- Neurology consultation/referral
  - Associated with reduced mortality.
- Physical, occupational, and speech therapy consultation/referral
  - Physical therapy (PT) to improve gait and balance.
  - Occupational therapy (OT) to improve activities of daily living (e.g., self-care, chores).
  - Speech therapy (ST) to improve speech and swallowing difficulties (high risk of aspiration pneumonia).
- Palliative care referral
  - To improve quality of life and provide relief of symptoms; as patient declines consider transition to hospice services.

Note: Beers listed items, as mentioned above, include benztropine and trihexyphenidyl.

## Differential Diagnosis[1,2,3,5,7]

- Dementia with Lewy bodies: Characterized by visual hallucinations, dementia, and lack of motor symptoms. The motor symptoms are the typical features in Parkinson's disease.
- Drug-induced parkinsonism (e.g., metoclopramide, haloperidol, lithium): Causes symmetric symptoms. In Parkinson's disease, the tremor is usually asymmetric; dopamine transporter SPECT imaging can tell the difference between the two diagnoses.
- Essential tremor: May have a family history, has specific tremor characteristics (e.g., tremor usually bilateral, affects the head), lacks neurological signs, and alcohol reduces symptoms. Parkinson's disease rarely occurs on a familial basis, has specific tremor characteristics (e.g., asymmetrical in early stages and not likely to see head tremor), and will have other neurological signs. Dopamine transporter SPECT imaging can tell the difference between the two diagnoses.

## CLINICAL PEARLS[1,2,3,4,5,6,7,11]

- Not every patient with Parkinson's disease presents the same. Rule out other causes (e.g., medications), and ask about other symptoms (slowness, stiffness, depression), other than primarily focusing on the tremor.
- Although medications do not stop the progression of Parkinson's disease, they do provide significant functional benefits. Referral to a neurologist is recommended to ensure appropriate treatment and to reduce mortality.
- Failure to respond to levodopa should make you question if the diagnosis is truly Parkinson's disease
- Exercise improves function and may have a neuroprotective effect in PD.

## References

1. Bega, D. (2017). Parkinson Disease. Epocrates. Retrieved from https://online.epocrates.com/diseases/14711/Parkinson-disease/Key-Highlights. Accessed August 18, 2017.
2. Olanow, C., Schapira, A. V., & Obeso, J. A. (2015). Parkinson's disease and other movement disorders. In Kasper, D., Fauci, A., Hauser, S., Longo, D., Jameson, J., & Loscalzo, J. (Eds.). *Harrison's Principles of Internal Medicine* (19th ed.). New York, NY: McGraw-Hill. Retrieved from http://accessmedicine.mhmedical.com/content.aspx?bookid=1130&sectionid=79755616. Accessed September 24, 2017.
3. Aminoff, M. J., & Douglas, V. C., Nervous system disorders. In *Current Medical Diagnosis & Treatment 2018*. New York, NY: McGraw-Hill. Retrieved from http://accessmedicine.mhmedical.com/content.aspx?bookid=2192&sectionid=168019736. Accessed September 24, 2017.
4. Parkinson's Disease Foundation (PDF). (n.d.). About Parkinson's Disease. Retrieved from http://www.pdf.org/about_pd. Accessed September 24, 2017.
5. Kotagal, V., & Bohnen, N. I. (2017). Parkinson disease and related disorders. In *Hazzard's Geriatric Medicine and Gerontology* (7th ed.). New York, NY: McGraw-Hill. Retrieved from http://accessmedicine.mhmedical.com/content.aspx?bookid=1923&sectionid=144523856. Accessed September 24, 2017.
6. *Adams & Victor's Principles of Neurology* (10th ed.). New York, NY: McGraw-Hill; Chapter 39. Degenerative diseases of the nervous system. Retrieved from http://accessmedicine.mhmedical.com/content.aspx?bookid=690&sectionid=50910890. Accessed September 24, 2017.
7. Rudolph, J., & Walker, R. H. (2016). Parkinson's disease and related disorders. In *Principles and Practice of Hospital Medicine* (2nd ed.). New York, NY: McGraw-Hill. Retreived from http://accessmedicine.mhmedical.com/content.aspx?bookid=1872&sectionid=146986776. Accessed September 25, 2017.
8. Lynn, S. (2012, December). Caring for patients with Parkinson's disease. *American Nurse Today*, 7(12), Retrieved from https://www.americannursetoday.com/caring-for-patients-with-parkinsons-disease/. Accessed October 29, 2017.

9. Bishop, B. S. (2010, June 9). Early Nursing Intervention in Parkinson's Disease. Medscape. Retrieved from https://www.medscape.org/viewarticle/722897. Accessed October 29, 2017.
10. Gulanick, M., & Myers, J. L. (2017). *Nursing Care Plans: Diagnoses, Interventions, & Outcomes*. St. Louis, MO: Elsevier.
11. Ahlskog, J. E. (2011). Does vigorous exercise have a neuroprotective effect in Parkinson disease? *Neurology,* 77(3), 288–294. doi:10.1212/wnl.0b013e318225ab66
12. American Geriatrics Society 2015 Beers Criteria Update Expert Panel, Fick, D. M., Semla, T. P., Beizer, J., Brandt, N., & Dombrowski, R., . . . Steinman, M. (2015, October 8). American Geriatrics Society 2015 updated Beers criteria for potentially inappropriate medication use in older adults. *Journal of the American Geriatrics Society,* 63(11), 2227–2246. Retrieved from http://onlinelibrary.wiley.com/doi/10.1111/jgs.13702/abstract. Accessed October 3, 2017.
13. Palliative and Hospice Care. Retrieved from http://parkinson.org/pd-library/fact-sheets/Palliative-and-Hospice-Care. Accessed May 8, 2018.

SECTION III

# Cardiovascular

## Acute Coronary Syndrome

### Definition[1,3]

Acute coronary syndrome (ACS) occurs when a coronary artery becomes acutely obstructed, which can be fatal. It occurs as a result of coronary heart disease (CHD).

### Classification[1,2]

ST elevation myocardial infarction (STEMI) **OR** non-ST elevation acute coronary syndrome (NSTE-ACS), which includes unstable angina.

### Causes[1,3,4,5,8]

- Coronary heart disease
  - Thrombus forms, leading to an acute occlusion (partial or complete) of a coronary artery.

### Risk Factors[2,3,4,5,6,9]

- Advanced age > 65 years
- Male sex
- Family history of heart disease
- Hypertension
- Physical inactivity
- Diabetes
- Obesity
- Dyslipidemia
- Cigarette smoking
- Chronic kidney disease

## Signs & Symptoms[1,2,3,4,6,7,8,9]

- Atypical features: abdominal pain, nausea or vomiting, fatigue, confusion, dizziness
- Dyspneic
- Chest pain/discomfort
- Diaphoresis
- Anxiety
- Acute heart failure signs (e.g., pulmonary rales or increased jugular venous pressure)

## Tests[1,2,7]

- Electrocardiogram (EKG)
  - Guides decision making; fibrinolytics benefit patients with STEMI. No ST elevation will be seen with NSTE-ACS; look instead for ST depression and/or T-wave inversion. High prevalence of NSTE-ACS in older adults.
- Cardiac biomarkers (troponin I or T)
  - Gold standard in diagnosis over creatinine kinase-MB.
- Cardiac catheterization
  - Reserved in older adults who have ischemic symptoms despite medical treatment; order in those who are candidates for coronary revascularization.

## Treatment & Management[1,2,3,4,6,7,8,9,10]

- **Send patient to the appropriate hospital setting.** Percutaneous coronary intervention (PCI)-capable hospital recommended in patients with STEMI.
  - Reperfusion with PCI (preferred) or fibrinolytic therapy is recommended within the first **12 hours** with STEMI.
  - In patients with NSTE-ACS, fibrinolytic therapy is contraindicated, due to complications (e.g., risk of reinfarction).
  - ACS acute management includes *(prehospital care)*
    - A one-time dose of a nonenteric-coated aspirin 162–325 mg, chewable.

- Supplemental oxygen, if saturation < 90% and in respiratory distress.
- Nitroglycerin 0.4 mg sublingual q5min (max of three tablets in 15 minutes); hold for systolic blood pressure (BP) < 90 mm Hg.
- Intravenous morphine (4–8 mg q15min PRN) for ongoing chest pain.

## Management Following ACS

- **Nonpharmacological and nursing interventions:**
  - Reassess the patient's chest pain often, including the response to medications.
    - Ongoing chest pain despite optimal medication can indicate patient needs invasive management (e.g., coronary artery bypass graft).
  - Encourage lifestyle changes: physical activity, healthy eating, weight loss, stress control, and smoking cessation.
  - Monitor for signs of depression and anxiety.
  - Teach the patient to check their heart rate and blood pressure.
    - Multiple medications can reduce these.
  - Encourage the flu vaccine.
    - There is an association with influenza and ACS.
- **Pharmacological and other interventions:**
  - Treat and manage the potentially reversible risk factors of ACS, such as:
    - Hypertension, dyslipidemia, and diabetes
  - Beta blockers (e.g., metoprolol tartrate [Lopressor], atenolol [Tenormin])
    - Example: atenolol 50 mg PO daily (max: 100 mg/day).
    - Recommended indefinitely following ACS; they reduce mortality rates.

  - They improve coronary blood flow, thus ameliorating chronic angina.
  - Caution use in those with chronic obstructive pulmonary disease (COPD) and/or bradycardia or hypotension.
- Angiotensin-converting enzyme (ACE) inhibitors (ACEIs) or angiotensin receptor blockers (ARBs)
  - Example: enalapril 10 mg PO BID (max: 40 mg daily).
  - Used indefinitely following ACS; they prevent ventricular remodeling and reduce risk of another cardiovascular event.
  - Monitor for hyperkalemia, dry cough (ACE inhibitors), and renal impairment.
- Statin therapy (e.g., atorvastatin [Lipitor], rosuvastatin [Crestor])
  - Example: atorvastatin 10 mg PO daily (max: 80 mg/day).
  - Recommended indefinitely following ACS; they reduce recurrent cardiovascular events.
  - Statins can be combined with ezetimibe (Zetia), which is effective for secondary prevention.
  - Monitor for myopathy or myalgias (may improve with reduced dosage).
- Antiplatelet therapy (e.g., aspirin, clopidogrel)
  - Example: aspirin 81 mg PO daily, used indefinitely (use clopidogrel [Plavix] 75 mg PO daily if allergic to aspirin).
  - They reduce the risk of thrombosis formation and reinfarction.
  - Aspirin and clopidogrel combined are recommended following a myocardial infarction (MI) (includes ST and non-ST elevation), PCI, and coronary stents.
  - Monitor for upset stomach and bleeding.
- Calcium channel blockers (CCBs)
  - Although they do **not** improve mortality, they are used when beta blockers are contraindicated; effective at treating angina refractory to beta blockers.

    - Can be combined with a beta blocker.
    - Monitor for bradycardia (especially if nondihydropyridine CCB is combined with a beta blocker), pedal edema, and worsening heart failure.
- Referral to a cardiac rehabilitation program
- Cardiology consultation/referral
    - Assist with secondary prevention management.

Note: Beers listed items, as mentioned above, include aspirin (if dose > 325 mg/day) and nondihydropyridine CCBs. Avoid routine prescribing of an ACEI with a potassium-sparing diuretic.

## Differential Diagnosis[4,7,8]

- Arrhythmia, such as atrial fibrillation: Often asymptomatic unless heart rate goes above 100; EKG confirms rhythm type. Compared to ACS, the presenting symptom in older adults is typically dyspnea or atypical complaints (e.g., fatigue).
- Gastroesophageal reflux: Burning retrosternal pain will improve with antacids and biomarkers will be negative. Compared to ACS, cardiac biomarkers will be positive; chest pain would continue despite antacid.

### CLINICAL PEARLS[2,7]

- Following an ACS event, secondary prevention is essential to decrease the risk of morbidity and mortality.
- Monitor for known complications seen in older adults following a major myocardial infarction, such as heart failure and atrial fibrillation.

## References

1. Warnica, J. W. (2016, September). Overview of Acute Coronary Syndromes (ACS) – Cardiovascular Disorders. Merck Manuals: Professional. Retrieved from https://www.merckmanuals.com/professional/cardiovascular-disorders/coronary-artery-disease/overview-of-acute-coronary-syndromes-acs. Accessed November 10, 2017.
2. Switaj, T. L., Christensen, S. R., & Brewer, D. M. (2017). Acute coronary syndrome: Current treatment. *American Family Physician, 95*(4), 232–240.
3. Alexander, K. P., & Peterson, E D. (2017). Coronary heart disease. In *Hazzard's Geriatric Medicine and Gerontology* (7th ed.). New York, NY: McGraw-Hill. Retrieved

from http://accessmedicine.mhmedical.com/content.aspx?bookid=1923&sectionid=144524855. Accessed November 9, 2017.
4. Epocrates. (2017, February 6). Overview of Acute Coronary Syndrome. Retrieved from https://online.epocrates.com/diseases/152/Overview-of-acute-coronary-syndrome. Accessed November 10, 2017.
5. National Heart, Lung, and Blood Institute (NHBLI). (2011, June 1). What Is a Heart Attack? U.S. Department of Health and Human Services, National Institutes of Health. Retrieved from https://www.nhlbi.nih.gov/health/health-topics/topics/heartattack. Accessed November 10, 2017.
6. American Heart Association (AHA). (2017, April 26). Acute Coronary Syndrome. Retrieved from http://www.heart.org/HEARTORG/Conditions/HeartAttack/About-HeartAttacks/Acute-Coronary-Syndrome_UCM_428752_Article.jsp#.WgYWTbp-Fw2w. Accessed November 10, 2017.
7. Dhruva, S., & Cheitlin, M. Coronary disease. In *Current Diagnosis & Treatment: Geriatrics* (2nd ed.). New York, NY: McGraw-Hill. Retrieved from http://accessmedicine.mhmedical.com/content.aspx?bookid=953&sectionid=53375652. Accessed November 9, 2017.
8. Gulanick, M., & Myers, J. L. (2017). *Nursing Care Plans: Diagnoses, Interventions, & Outcomes*. St. Louis, MO: Elsevier.
9. Compton, D. (2014). Cardiovascular disease. In Burggraf, V., Kim, K. Y., & Knight, A. L. *Healthy Aging: Principles and Clinical Practice for Clinicians* (pp. 52–54). Philadelphia, PA: Lippincott Williams & Wilkins.
10. American Geriatrics Society 2015 Beers Criteria Update Expert Panel, Fick, D. M., Semla, T. P., Beizer, J., Brandt, N., & Dombrowski, R., . . . Steinman, M. (2015, October 8). American Geriatrics Society 2015 updated Beers criteria for potentially inappropriate medication use in older adults. *Journal of the American Geriatrics Society, 63*(11), 2227–2246. Retrieved from http://onlinelibrary.wiley.com/doi/10.1111/jgs.13702/abstract. Accessed October 8, 2017.

# Aortic Stenosis

## Definition[4,5]

Aortic stenosis (AS) is a narrowing of the aortic valve that obstructs blood flow, leading to impaired tissue perfusion and cardiac output.

## Causes[1,2,3,5,6,10]

- Aortic valve calcification
- Bicuspid aortic valve
- Rheumatic fever (*especially in developing nations*)

## Risk Factors[1,3,5,6]

- Advanced age
- Male sex
- Congenital heart defect

- Diabetes mellitus
- Dyslipidemia
- Hypertension
- Tobacco use
- Chronic kidney disease *(especially dialysis patients)*
- History of radiation therapy
- Rheumatic fever *(less common)*

## Signs & Symptoms[1,2,3,4,5,6,10,11]

*Many patients are asymptomatic until AS becomes severe.*

- Presyncope or syncope
- Angina
- Dyspnea
- Systolic ejection murmur
- Fatigue
- Palpitations
- Impaired exercise tolerance
- Heart failure symptoms (e.g., pedal edema, pulmonary congestion)

## Tests[1,2,3,4,5,6,8,10,11]

- Electrocardiogram (EKG)
  - Commonly demonstrates left ventricular (LV) hypertrophy.
- Echocardiogram, transthoracic
  - Confirms the diagnosis. Determines the degree of LV hypertrophy, along with thickening, calcification, and restricted opening of the valve leaflets.
- Exercise stress testing
  - Reserved in individuals who are asymptomatic; helps to determine severity of symptoms.
- Cardiac catheterization
  - Ordered if the echocardiogram is inconclusive.
  - Ordered with coronary angiography when aortic valve replacement is considered; many will have concomitant coronary artery disease (CAD), which requires bypass grafting.

## Treatment & Management[1,2,3,4,5,6,7,8,9,10,11,12]

- **Nonpharmacological and nursing interventions:**
  - Take measures to avoid volume depletion, such as offering fluids *(hypovolemia further decreases cardiac output)*.
  - Encourage lifestyle changes, such as:
    - Healthier eating practices (e.g., avoiding excess saturated fats, eating more fruits and vegetables).
    - Regular physical activity; however avoid strenuous activity in individuals with moderate to severe asymptomatic AS.
    - Stress reduction (e.g., meditation, relaxation).
    - Encourage tobacco cessation and target A1C of < 7% to reduce risk of postoperative infection.
  - Encourage optimal dental hygiene and routine dental care.
  - Education on warfarin (Coumadin, Jantoven) if used for mechanical prosthesis.
    - Take medication at the same time daily, never double up if a dose was missed. Monitor for bleeding or unusual bruising; keep the amount of vitamin K–rich foods (e.g., broccoli, spinach) consistent each day, and avoid alcohol.
- **Pharmacological and other interventions:**

  *No specific medication regimen exists for the treatment of AS; none have been shown to improve survival.*
  - Identify and treat cardiovascular risk factors, such as:
    - Hypertension, diabetes mellitus, dyslipidemia.
  - Antihypertensives (e.g., ACE inhibitors or ARBs, beta blockers)
    - Ordered in individuals with AS who are asymptomatic.
    - Important to treat comorbid hypertension because if left untreated, can lead to earlier onset of AS symptoms.
  - Nitroglycerin
    - Used to relieve angina associated with CAD (monitor for hypotension).

  - Statin therapy
    - Should be considered in individuals with coexisting conditions, such as CAD and dyslipidemia (to reduce cardiovascular events).
    - May slow the progression of leaflet calcification.
  - Diuretics, digoxin, ACE inhibitors (or ARB) can be used for heart failure symptoms in patients who are not surgical candidates.
  - Warfarin (Coumadin)
    - Reserved in individuals who undergo aortic valve replacement (AVR) with mechanical prostheses. However, most cardiac surgeons will implant a bioprosthetic valve, which does not require anticoagulation.
- Cardiology consultation/referral
  - To follow the progression of AS with frequent imaging.
- Surgical or transcatheter aortic valve replacement
  - Reserved in those with symptomatic severe AS and asymptomatic individuals with severe AS who plan on undergoing cardiac surgery, such as coronary artery bypass grafting (CABG).
  - AVR significantly improves symptoms and long-term survival.
  - In patients who are a high surgical risk, transcatheter aortic valve replacement (TAVR) is an alternative.

Note: Beers listed items, as mentioned above, include diuretics and digoxin (in doses > 125 mcg/day). If warfarin combined with NSAIDs or amiodarone, monitor INRs closely. Avoid routine prescribing of an ACEI with a potassium-sparing diuretic.

## Differential Diagnosis[1,8,11]

- CAD: Common to have Q waves; cardiac catheterization shows severity of plaque in the coronary arteries. Compared to AS, Q waves are not present and patient may have insignificant results upon cardiac catheterization (about half will have CAD).
- Aortic sclerosis: Murmur is not as intense compared to AS and echo will show insignificant pressure gradient across the

aortic valve; it can progress to AS. Compared to AS, there will be a systolic murmur usually ≥ 3/6; echo will show elevated gradient (at least 10mm Hg) across the aortic valve.

## CLINICAL PEARLS[1,2,3,4,11]

- It is important to refer symptomatic patients for AVR to improve longevity. The 10-year survival rate is about 60% in older adults following AVR. For those who have symptoms and do not undergo AVR, the average survival rate is about 2–3 years.
- Before referring individuals for AVR to improve symptoms, consider first if the surgery would provide meaningful benefit, especially in those with poor prognosis and advanced dementia (AVR not recommended).

# References


1. Kalra, G. L., Babaliaros, V., & Parker, R. M. (2017, October 12). Aortic stenosis. Retrieved from [ ]. Accessed November 21, 2017.
2. Aortic valve disease. In Kasper, D., Fauci, A., Hauser, S., Longo, D., Jameson, J., & Loscalzo, J. *Harrison's Principles of Internal Medicine* (19th ed.). New York, NY: McGraw-Hill. Retrieved from http://accessmedicine.mhmedical.com/content.aspx?bookid=1130&sectionid=79742791. Accessed November 21, 2017.
3. Valvular disease. In *Current Diagnosis & Treatment: Geriatrics* (2nd ed.). New York, NY: McGraw-Hill. Retrieved from http://accessmedicine.mhmedical.com/content.aspx?bookid=953&sectionid=53375655. Accessed November 21, 2017.
4. Valvular heart disease. In *Hazzard's Geriatric Medicine and Gerontology* (7th ed.). New York, NY: McGraw-Hill. Retrieved from http://accessmedicine.mhmedical.com/content.aspx?bookid=1923&sectionid=144524931. Accessed November 21, 2017.
5. American Heart Association (AHA). (2017, September 7). Problem: Aortic Valve Stenosis. Retrieved from http://www.heart.org/HEARTORG/Conditions/More/HeartValveProblemsandDisease/Problem-Aortic-Valve-Stenosis_UCM_450437_Article.jsp#.WhRw1bpFw2w. Accessed November 21, 2017.
6. Mayo Clinic. (2017, August 17). Aortic Valve Stenosis. Retrieved from https://www.mayoclinic.org/diseases-conditions/aortic-stenosis/symptoms-causes/syc-20353139. Accessed November 21, 2017.
7. Ren, M. (2017, October 23). Aortic Stenosis. Medscape. Retrieved from https://emedicine.medscape.com/article/150638-overview. Accessed November 22, 2017.
8. Novaro, G. M. (2014, July). Aortic Valve Disease. Cleveland Clinic Center for Continuing Education. Retrieved from http://www.clevelandclinicmeded.com/medicalpubs/diseasemanagement/cardiology/aortic-valve-disease/. Accessed November 22, 2017.
9. Lippincott Nursing Center. (2010, April). Taking Warfarin Safely. Retrieved from http://www.nursingcenter.com/Handlers/articleContent.pdf?key=pdf_00152193-201004000-00021. Accessed November 22, 2017.
10. Stoodley, L., & Keller, E. (2017). Valvular heart disease. *Journal for Nurse Practitioners, 13*(4), 195–198. doi: http://dx.doi.org/10.1016/j.nurpra.2016.10.011

11. Cary, T., & Pearce, J. (2013, April). Aortic stenosis: Pathophysiology, diagnosis, and medical management of nonsurgical patients. *Critical Care Nurse, 33*(2), 58–72. Retrieved from http://ccn.aacnjournals.org/content/33/2/58.full. Accessed November 22, 2017.
12. American Geriatrics Society 2015 Beers Criteria Update Expert Panel, Fick, D. M., Semla, T. P., Beizer, J., Brandt, N., & Dombrowski, R., . . . Steinman, M. (2015, October 8). American Geriatrics Society 2015 updated Beers criteria for potentially inappropriate medication use in older adults. *Journal of the American Geriatrics Society, 63*(11), 2227–2246. Retrieved http://onlinelibrary.wiley.com/doi/10.1111/jgs.13702/abstract. Accessed October 3, 2017.

# Atrial Fibrillation

## Definition[1,2,5,6,7,11]

Atrial fibrillation (AF) is a common arrhythmia, characterized as an irregularly irregular atrial rhythm, which increases the risk of stroke (*by at least 5 times*) and heart failure.

## Classification[1,5,6,9,10]

**Paroxysmal:** AF that lasts less than a week and converts to sinus rhythm without treatment; can re-occur and become permanent.
**Persistent:** AF lasting more than a week; requires treatment.
**Long-standing:** AF lasting more than a year; carries a possibility of converting over to sinus rhythm.
**Permanent:** AF that is permanent; no possibility of converting over to sinus rhythm.

## Causes[1,2,5,6,7,8,9,10,11,12]

*Most are idiopathic.*

- Hypertension
- Coronary artery disease
- Heart failure
- Cardiomyopathy (ischemic or nonischemic)
- Valvular diseases (e.g., mitral regurgitation, mitral stenosis)
- Hyperthyroidism
- Cardiac procedures or surgeries
- Alcohol abuse

- Sleep apnea
- Chronic lung disease
- Serious infections (e.g., pneumonia)

## Risk Factors[1,2,3,4,6,7,9,10,11]

*Risk factors coincide with the causes of AF.*

- Advanced age
- Male sex
- European ancestry
- Obesity
- Diabetes

## Signs & Symptoms[1,2,5,6,7,11]

*Often asymptomatic, especially with controlled ventricular response (60–100 beats per minute [bpm]).*

- Irregularly irregular rhythm
- Heart palpitations
- Dizziness
- Chest pain or pressure
- Dyspnea
- Anxiety
- Impaired exercise tolerance
- Fatigue
- Presyncope or syncope

## Tests[1,2,3,6,7,9,12,13]

- Electrocardiography (ECG)
  - Used to diagnosis AF (*i.e., no P waves, disorganized atrial activity, irregular R-R intervals). Fast ventricular response = rate > 100 bpm.*
- Holter monitor
  - Useful in diagnosing paroxysmal AF.
- Echocardiography
  - To assess atrial/ventricular size and function; evaluates for causes of AF, such as evidence of valvular disease.

Transesophageal echocardiography (TEE) is more specific over transthoracic in evaluating atrial thrombus (risk factor for stroke); performed prior to synchronized cardioversion.

- Comprehensive metabolic panel (CMP) (including magnesium), thyroid-stimulating hormone (TSH), hemoglobin and hemocrit (Hgb/Hct)
  - Important to determine renal and hepatic function as these influence treatment options; evaluate for hyperthyroidism. Electrolyte imbalances can exacerbate AF; anemia is important to monitor while on antithrombotic therapy.

## Treatment & Management[1,2,3,4,6,9,10,12,13,14]

- **Nonpharmacological and nursing interventions:**
  - Encourage lifestyle changes (e.g., avoid binge drinking, stress reduction, diet while on warfarin).
  - Encourage physical activity and weight reduction.
  - Educate patients on symptoms of rapid ventricular response: chest discomfort/pain, dyspnea, dizziness.
  - Monitor adverse effects of drug therapy associated with AF.
    - Monitor for bleeding with anticoagulants.
    - Bradycardia with AF rate control regimen.
- **Pharmacological and other interventions:**
  - Identify and treat the underlying cause(s), such as:
    - Treat the hyperthyroidism.
    - Treat the hypertension.
  - Rate control (goal of about < 100 bpm):
    - Beta blockers (e.g., metoprolol tartrate [Lopressor], atenolol [Tenormin])
      - Example: metoprolol tartrate at 12.5–100 mg PO BID.
      - Use in those with CAD and/or reduced systolic function.

- Nondihydropyridine calcium channel blockers (e.g., verapamil [Calan, Verelan], diltiazem [Cardizem])
  - Example: diltiazem (immediate release) 60–120 mg PO TID (max: 360 mg/day).
  - Avoid use in those with reduced systolic function.
  - Combo therapy with a beta blocker increases bradycardia.
- Digoxin *(least effective)*
  - Example: digoxin 125 mcg PO daily.
  - Can be taken with a beta blocker or calcium channel blocker.
- If the above agents are ineffective at controlling the rate, ablation of the atrioventricular (AV) node and permanent pacing are effective.

○ Rhythm control *(not as important if asymptomatic)*:
- Cardioversion: Reserved for those who are hemodynamically unstable; pharmacologic cardioversion is not as effective or safe as electrical cardioversion.
- Direct current cardioversion *(high risk of thromboembolism/stroke)*.
  - Recommended in nonvalvular AF that started within 48 hours and low risk of a thromboembolic event.
  - Not advised if AF present > 48 hours.
    - Will need to be anticoagulated for 3 weeks prior to cardioversion.
  - Need anticoagulation for a minimum of a month following cardioversion, possibly for lifetime.
  - Most effective in those with AF with an irreversible cause and/or short duration AF.
- Antiarrhythmic therapy for long-term maintenance of sinus rhythm:
  - Class 1a (e.g., quinidine)
    - Not used often due to limited efficacy.
  - Class 1c (e.g., flecainide, propafenone [Rhythmol])
  - Class III (e.g., amiodarone [Pacerone], dronedarone [Multaq], sotalol [Betapace])

        - Amiodarone is effective and is commonly prescribed.
      - Use antiarrhythmics once rate control has been maintained by a beta blocker or a nondihydropyridine calcium channel blocker.
      - There is currently no standard/optimal rhythm control drug therapy in older adults with symptomatic AF.
    - Catheter ablation: Success rate is high in paroxysmal AF.
    - Surgical Maze procedure: Success rate is high in refractory AF; reduces strokes.
  - Thromboembolism prevention (ordered based on CHA2DS2-VASc score):
    *Anticoagulation is recommended with score ≥ 2.*
    - Warfarin (e.g., Coumadin, Jantoven)
      - Used in patients with AF and mechanical heart valve (INR goal 2.5–3.5).
      - INR goal of 2.0–3.0 in those with nonvalvular AF.
      - Use fresh frozen plasma as emergent reversal with life-threatening bleeding; the antidote is vitamin K.
    - Newer anticoagulants (e.g., apixaban [Eliquis], dabigatran [Pradaxa], rivaroxaban [Xarelto])
      - Used in patients with nonvalvular AF.
      - **PROs:** not inferior to warfarin, alternative to warfarin when INRs are difficult to maintain; have short half-lives and fewer drug-drug interactions; do not require INR monitoring and no dietary restrictions.
      - **CONs:** avoid with creatinine clearance < 15 mL/min.
      - Dabigatran may cause life-threatening bleeding in patients > 80 years old. Idarucizumab (Praxbind) is the reversal agent.[15]
      - Apixaban is superior to warfarin and has reduced bleeding events.
    - Aspirin (75–325 mg/day)
      - Used in nonvalvular AF and CHA2DS2-VASc score of 1.
      - Use this when anticoagulants are contraindicated. It can be combined with clopidogrel (Plavix); however risk of bleeding is comparable to warfarin.

  - Factors that increase the risk of bleeding while taking antithrombotic therapy: uncontrolled hypertension, impaired liver or renal function, history of bleeding, concomitant use of an NSAID or antiplatelet, and age > 65–75 years.
- Cardiology consultation/referral
  - For appropriate selection of antiarrhythmic therapy and/or for procedures (ablation, pacemaker placement).

NOTE: Beers listed items, as mentioned above, include anticoagulants, amiodarone, dronedarone, digoxin, and nondihydropyridine calcium channel blockers.

## Differential Diagnosis[2,5]

- Myocardial infarction: Key symptoms are chest pain (characterized by squeezing or intolerable pressure) and/or dyspnea. Key symptoms are heart palpitations or fluttering in AF.
- Other supraventricular arrhythmias: Can present with similar symptoms as AF. 12-lead ECG can determine the correct arrhythmia.

### CLINICAL PEARLS[2,4,6,10]

- Treatment of AF focuses on rate control, rhythm control, and thromboembolism prevention. In older adults who are asymptomatic, rate control and thromboembolism prevention are preferred.

## References


1. National Heart Lung and Blood Institute (NHLBI). (2014, September 18). What Is Atrial Fibrillation? U.S. Department of Health and Human Services, National Institutes of Health, Retrieved from http://www.nhlbi.nih.gov/health/health-topics/topics/af/. Accessed November 4, 2017.
2. Heart failure and heart rhythm disorders. In *Current Diagnosis & Treatment: Geriatrics* (2nd ed.). New York, NY: McGraw-Hill. Retrieved from http://accessmedicine.mhmedical.com/content.aspx?bookid=953&sectionid=53375653. Accessed November 4, 2017.
3. *Essentials of Clinical Geriatrics* (7th ed.). New York, NY: McGraw-Hill; Chapter 11: Cardiovascular disorders. Retrieved from http://accessmedicine.mhmedical.com/content.aspx?bookid=678&sectionid=44833890. Accessed November 4, 2017.

4. Tondato, F., & Shen, W. (2017). In *Hazzard's Geriatric Medicine and Gerontology* (7th ed.). New York, NY: McGraw-Hill. Retrieved from http://accessmedicine.mhmedical.com/content.aspx?bookid=1923&sectionid=144525291. Accessed November 4, 2017.
5. American Heart Association (AHA). (2016, February 6). What Is Atrial Fibrillation (Afib or AF)? Retrieved from http://www.heart.org/HEARTORG/Conditions/Arrhythmia/AboutArrhythmia/What-is-Atrial-Fibrillation-AFib-or-AF_UCM_423748_Article.jsp#.Wf3Iy7pFw2w. Accessed November 4, 2017.
6. Mitchell, L. B. (2017, September). Atrial Fibrillation (AF) – Cardiovascular Disorders. Merck Manuals: Professional. Retrieved from https://www.merckmanuals.com/professional/cardiovascular-disorders/arrhythmias-and-conduction-disorders/atrial-fibrillation-af. Accessed November 4, 2017.
7. Heart Rhythm Society. (n.d.). Risk Factors for Atrial Fibrillation (AFib). Retrieved from http://www.hrsonline.org/Patient-Resources/Heart-Diseases-Disorders/Atrial-Fibrillation-AFib/Risk-Factors-for-AFib. Accessed November 4, 2017.
8. Ganz, L. I. (2017, June 21). Patient Education: Atrial Fibrillation (Beyond the Basics) (Knight, B. P., & Saperia, G. M., Eds.). UpToDate. Retrieved from https://www.uptodate.com/contents/atrial-fibrillation-beyond-the-basics. Accessed November 4, 2017.
9. Epocrates. (n.d.). Chronic Atrial Fibrillation. Retrieved from https://online.epocrates.com/diseases/121/Chronic-atrial-fibrillation/Definition. Accessed November 4, 2017.
10. Davis, L. L. (2013, November-December). Contemporary Management of Atrial Fibrillation. Retrieved from http://www.npjournal.org/article/S1555-4155(13)00525-4/fulltext. Accessed November 5, 2017.
11. Mayo Clinic. (2017, August 12). Atrial Fibrillation. Retrieved from https://www.mayoclinic.org/diseases-conditions/atrial-fibrillation/symptoms-causes/syc-20350624. Accessed November 5, 2017.
12. Banga, S., & Chalfoun, N. T. (2017). Arrhythmias and antiarrhythmic drugs. In Elmoselhi, A. & *Cardiology: An Integrated Approach*. New York, NY: McGraw-Hill. Retrieved from http://accessmedicine.mhmedical.com/content.aspx?bookid=2224&sectionid=171660848. Accessed November 05, 2017.
13. Gulanick, M., & Myers, J. L. (2017). *Nursing Care Plans: Diagnoses, Interventions, & Outcomes* (9th ed.). St. Louis, MO: Elsevier.
14. American Geriatrics Society 2015 Beers Criteria Update Expert Panel, Fick, D. M., Semla, T. P., Beizer, J., Brandt, N., & Dombrowski, R., . . . Steinman, M. (2015, October 8). American Geriatrics Society 2015 updated Beers criteria for potentially inappropriate medication use in older adults. *Journal of the American Geriatrics Society, 63*(11), 2227–2246. Retrieved from http://onlinelibrary.wiley.com/doi/10.1111/jgs.13702/abstract. Accessed October 8, 2017.
15. Finks, S. W., & Rogers, K. C. (2017). Idarucizumab (Praxbind): The First Reversal Agent for a Direct Oral Anticoagulant. *The American Journal of Medicine, 130*(5), 195-197. doi:10.1016/j.amjmed.2016.11.029

# Dyslipidemia

## Definition[1,5,6]

Dyslipidemia is an increase in serum cholesterol, triglycerides, or a combination of the two, with a decreased high-density lipoprotein (HDL). This condition contributes to atherosclerotic cardiovascular disease (ASCVD).

## Classification[1]

**Isolated hypercholesterolemia:** elevated cholesterol levels only
**Isolated hypertriglyceridemia:** elevated triglyceride levels only
**Mixed hyperlipidemia:** elevated cholesterol and triglycerides levels

## Causes[1,2,3,5,10]

- Primary causes:
  - Genetics (e.g., familial combined hyperlipidemia)
- Secondary causes:
  - Sedentary lifestyle
  - Unhealthy eating habits (i.e., excessive caloric intake, saturated fat, cholesterol)
  - Obesity
  - Diabetes
  - Alcohol abuse
  - Cigarette smoking
  - Chronic kidney disease
  - Nephrotic syndrome
  - Hypothyroidism
  - Liver diseases
  - Medications
    - Thiazide diuretics, beta blockers, protease inhibitors, estrogens, some atypical antipsychotics, and corticosteroids

## Risk Factors

*Risk factors of dyslipidemia coincide with causes.*

## Signs & Symptoms[1,4]

*There are usually no signs or symptoms associated with dyslipidemia.*

- Arcus senilis.

- Xanthomas.
  - Can appear anywhere, especially on elbows, hands, feet, joints, or buttocks.
- They, however, lead to symptoms associated with CAD (e.g., angina, dyspnea), cerebrovascular accidents, and peripheral arterial disease.
- Triglyceride levels > 1,000 mg/dL leads to acute pancreatitis (i.e., abdominal pain, nausea).

## Tests[1,5,6,8,9]

- Lipid panel
  - Values are affected by acute illness, recent myocardial infarction, and/or eating 12 hours prior to the test being drawn.
  - Repeat lipid panels are ordered at least every 12 weeks after prescribing or changing dyslipidemia medication therapies (to evaluate anticipated response). Once levels have normalized, repeating a lipid panel quarterly to annually is reasonable.
- Reasonable to also order: fasting serum glucose, TSH, liver panel, serum creatinine, and urine protein
  - To evaluate for secondary causes of dyslipidemia, such as diabetes, hypothyroidism, and/or liver or renal disease.
  - Baseline liver function is recommended with statin therapy.
- Coronary artery calcium score (≥ 300), C-reactive protein (≥ 2 mg/ L or 19.05 nmol/L), or ankle-brachial index (< 0.9)
  - Useful when a treatment decision is uncertain.

## Treatment & Management[1,3,5,6,7,9,10]

- **Nonpharmacological and nursing interventions:**
  - Encourage lifestyle changes:
    - Increase physical activity.
    - Promote healthy eating habits.
      - Decrease intake of saturated fats and cholesterol.
      - Increase dietary fiber.

        - Weight loss.
        - Smoking cessation.
        - Glycemic control in diabetics.
    - Encouraging alcohol is not recommended, given its adverse effects.
    - Educate on the adverse effects of medications used in dyslipidemia.
- **Pharmacological and other interventions:**
    - Identify and treat secondary causes of dyslipidemia, such as:
        - Diabetes: Metformin (Glucophage, Fortamet, Glumetza) not only improves glycemic control, but lowers triglycerides.
        - Hypothyroidism: Dyslipidemia will eventually improve with treatment.
        - Reducing or discontinuing drugs contributing to dyslipidemia.
    - Statins (e.g., atorvastatin [Lipitor], rosuvastatin [Crestor])
        - Example: Start atorvastatin 20–40 mg PO QD (max: 80 mg/day).
        - Recommended for primary and secondary prevention of ASCVD events. They are the most effective at treating dyslipidemias, especially in lowering LDL levels.
        - Statins are recommended based on the cardiovascular risk. Risk calculators are available to get an idea of the estimated 10-year risk of ASCVD in those *without* ASCVD.
            - www.cvriskcalculator.com
            - www.qrisk.org/
        - Statin therapy in adults > age 75 years for primary prevention should be individualized (current evidence is insufficient). If > age 75 years old with known ASCVD, moderate-intensity therapy is recommended.
        - Statin therapy is beneficial in the following: high risk of ASCVD (10-year risk ≥ 7.5%–10%), known ASCVD (e.g., acute coronary syndrome, stroke, or transient

ischemic attack [TIA], peripheral artery disease), diabetes with LDL level of 70–189 mg/dL, LDL level ≥ 190 mg/dl, and chronic kidney disease (not requiring dialysis).
    - Musculoskeletal complaints can occur and is dose dependent; liver toxicity is uncommon.
    - It is reasonable to use the lowest dose of statin therapy to prevent complications in older adults.
- Consider the following nonstatin medications in those who do not tolerate or respond as expected to statin therapy (e.g., high-intensity statin not producing a ≥ 50% reduction in LDLs):
  - Ezetimibe (Zetia)
    - Example: Start ezetimibe 10 mg PO QD (max: 10 mg/day).
    - Decreases LDL levels; minimally increases HDL.
    - Commonly combined with a statin.
    - Usually well tolerated.
  - Bile acid sequestrants (e.g., cholestyramine [Questran, Prevalite], colesevelam [Welchol], colestipol [Colestid])
    - Example: cholestyramine 4 g PO QD-BID (max: 24 g/day).
    - Lowers LDL; increases triglycerides transiently.
    - Commonly prescribed with a statin.
    - Monitor for gastrointestinal (GI) disturbances (e.g., nausea, cramping, constipation).
  - PCSK9 inhibitors (e.g., evolocumab [Repatha], alirocumab [Praluent])
    - Example: evolocumab 140 mg SC q2weeks or 420 mg SC qmonth.
    - Used as adjunct to treat heterozygous familial hypercholesterolemia.
    - Expensive.
  - Nicotinic acid (niacin), fibrates, and omega-3 fatty acids
    - Although these medications reduce lipid levels, it is recommended to avoid routine prescribing of these agents (A evidence rating).

- To reduce the risk of pancreatitis in individuals with high triglycerides (>1,000 mg/dL), fibrate or fish oil are recommended.

- Dietitian consultation/referral
  - For nutritional guidance

## CLINICAL PEARLS[1,6]

- The goal of dyslipidemia treatment is to prevent future ASCVD events. In those with known ASCVD, treatment is recommended.
- Do not prescribe statins or nonstatins in older adults with limited life expectancy.
- If statin therapy does not produce the desired affect (e.g., atorvastatin 40–80 mg daily not reducing LDL level by more than 50%), consider a nonstatin medication such as ezetimibe *(try first)*, a bile acid sequestrant, or a PCSK9 inhibitor.

# References


1. Goldberg, A. G. (2015, August). Dyslipidemia – Endocrine and Metabolic Disorders. Merck Manuals: Professional. Retrieved from https://www.merckmanuals.com/professional/endocrine-and-metabolic-disorders/lipid-disorders/dyslipidemia. Accessed November 8, 2017.
2. Rosenson, R. S. (2017, September 26). Secondary Causes of Dyslipidemia (Freeman, M. W., & Gersh, B. J., Eds.). UpToDate. Retrieved from https://www.uptodate.com/contents/secondary-causes-of-dyslipidemia?source=search_result&search=dyslipidemia&selectedTitle=6%7E150. Accessed November 8, 2017.
3. Compton, D. (2014). Cardiovascular disease. In Burggraf, V., Kim, K. Y., & Knight, A. L. (Eds.) *Healthy Aging: Principles and Clinical Practice for Clinicians* (pp. 67–71). Philadelphia, PA: Lippincott Williams & Wilkins.
4. Swanson, D. L., & Zieve, D. (2017, May 2). Xanthoma (Conaway, B., Ed.). MedlinePlus. Retrieved from https://medlineplus.gov/ency/article/001447.htm. Accessed November 8, 2017.
5. Rader, D. J., & Hobbs, H. H. (2015). Disorders of lipoprotein metabolism. In Kasper, D., Fauci, A., Hauser, S., Longo, D., Jamesom, J., & Loscalzo, J. (Eds.) *Harrison's Principles of Internal Medicine* (19th ed.). New York, NY: McGraw-Hill. Retrieved from http://accessmedicine.mhmedical.com/content.aspx?bookid=1130&sectionid=79753265. Accessed November 8, 2017.
6. Last, A. R., Ference, J. D., & Menzel, E. R. (2017). Hyperlipidemia: Drugs for cardiovascular risk reduction in adults. *American Family Physician, 95*(2), 78–87. Retrieved November 8, 2017.
7. Epocrates. (n.d.). Retrieved from https://www.epocrates.com (used for brand names and dosing instructions).

8. Mayo Clinic. (2016, April 30). Heart Scan (Coronary Calcium Scan). Retrieved from https://www.mayoclinic.org/tests-procedures/heart-scan/details/why-its-done/icc-20201897. Accessed November 9, 2017.
9. American Academy of Family Physicians (AAFP). (2014, August 15). ACC/AHA Release Updated Guideline on the Treatment of Blood Cholesterol to Reduce ASCVD Risk. Retrieved from http://www.aafp.org/afp/2014/0815/p260.pdf. Accessed November 9, 2017.
10. Gurgle, H. E., & Blumenthal, D. K. (2017). Drug therapy for dyslipidemias. In *Goodman & Gilman's: The Pharmacological Basis of Therapeutics* (13th ed.). New York, NY: McGraw-Hill. Retrieved from http://accessmedicine.mhmedical.com/content.aspx?bookid=2189&sectionid=170107373. Accessed November 9, 2017.

# Heart Failure

## Definition[1,2,5,8]

Heart failure (HF) is a syndrome characterized by impaired pump performance, resulting in an inability to meet the metabolic demands of the body.

## Types[1,2,5,8,10]

**Heart failure with reduced ejection fraction (HFrEF) or systolic heart failure:** due to impaired cardiac contractility; ejection fraction (EF) $\leq$ 40%.
**Heart failure with preserved ejection fraction (HFpEF) or diastolic heart failure:** inability of the ventricles to relax; will have ejection fraction (EF) > 40%–50%.

## Causes[1,2,3,4,5,7,8]

*Multifactorial, not typically just one single cause.*

- Hypertension and coronary artery disease
  - *Most common causes*
- Valvular heart disease (e.g., aortic stenosis, mitral regurgitation)
- Cardiomyopathies
  - Includes stress induced, alcohol induced, hypertrophic
- Chemotherapy-induced cardiotoxicity (e.g., anthracyclines, trastuzumab)
- Precipitants of *acute exacerbation* include:
  - Noncompliance to diet (e.g., excess sodium or fluid intake) and/or medications

- Myocardial ischemia or infarction
- Arrhythmias
  - Especially new-onset atrial fibrillation or flutter
- Severe infections (e.g., sepsis, pneumonia)
  - *Heart failure exacerbation occurs as a result of the inability to compensate from the increased demands.*
- Medications
  - Includes NSAIDs, thiazolidinediones, corticosteroids, minoxidil, calcium channel blockers (especially nondihydropyridine)
- Anemia
- Hyperthyroidism

## Risk Factors[2,4,5,7,8,9]

*Risk factors coincide with the causes of heart failure.*

- Age > 65 years
- African-American ancestry
- Overweight or obese
- Diabetes
- Sleep apnea
- Alcohol abuse
- Tobacco use

## Signs & Symptoms[1,2,3,4,5,8,9]

- Dyspnea (exertional or at rest)
- Orthopnea
- Paroxysmal nocturnal dyspnea (PND)
- Cough
- Impaired exercise tolerance
- Pedal edema
- Weight gain
- Crackles or rales
- Jugular venous distention
- Abnormal vital signs (e.g., tachycardia, tachypnea)
- Atypical presentation (e.g., fatigue, weight loss, confusion)

**Table 3-1** New York Heart Association Functional Classification

Doctors usually classify patients' heart failure according to the severity of their symptoms. The table below describes the most commonly used classification system, the New York Heart Association (NYHA) Functional Classification.[a] It places patients in one of four categories based on how much they are limited during physical activity.

| Class | Patient Symptoms |
|---|---|
| I | No limitation of physical activity. Ordinary physical activity does not cause undue fatigue, palpitation, or dyspnea (shortness of breath). |
| II | Slight limitation of physical activity. Comfortable at rest. Ordinary physical activity results in fatigue, palpitation, or dyspnea (shortness of breath). |
| III | Marked limitation of physical activity. Comfortable at rest. Less than ordinary activity causes fatigue, palpitation, or dyspnea. |
| IV | Unable to carry on any physical activity without discomfort. Symptoms of heart failure at rest. If any physical activity is undertaken, discomfort increases. |
| **Class** | **Objective Assessment** |
| A | No objective evidence of cardiovascular disease. No symptoms and no limitation in ordinary physical activity. |
| B | Objective evidence of minimal cardiovascular disease. Mild symptoms and slight limitation during ordinary activity. Comfortable at rest. |
| C | Objective evidence of moderately severe cardiovascular disease. Marked limitation in activity due to symptoms, even during less-than-ordinary activity. Comfortable only at rest. |
| D | Objective evidence of severe cardiovascular disease. Severe limitations. Experiences symptoms even while at rest. |

(*continues*)

**Table 3-1** New York Heart Association Functional Classification (*Continued*)

**For example:**

- A patient with minimal or no symptoms but a large pressure gradient across the aortic valve or severe obstruction of the left main coronary artery is classified:
    - **Function Capacity I, Objective Assessment D**
- A patient with severe anginal syndrome but angiographically normal coronary arteries is classified:
    - **Functional Capacity IV, Objective Assessment A**

[a] Reproduced from Dolgin M, Association NYH, Fox AC, Gorlin R, Levin RI, New York Heart Association. *Criteria Committee. Nomenclature and criteria for diagnosis of diseases of the heart and great vessels*. 9th ed. Boston, MA: Lippincott Williams and Wilkins; March 1, 1994.

Original source: Criteria Committee, New York Heart Association , Inc. *Diseases of the Heart and Blood Vessels. Nomenclature and Criteria for diagnosis*, 6th edition Boston, Little, Brown and Co. 1964, p 114.

This content was last reviewed May 2017.

## Tests[1,2,3,4,5,8,10]

- Laboratory tests, reasonable to start with:
    - B-type natriuretic peptide (BNP) *most useful serum test.*
        - BNP (*affected by age and renal impairment*) supports the diagnosis and helps differentiate from other causes of dyspnea, such as from a pulmonary cause. Level < 100 unlikely to be heart failure.
    - Thyroid function, complete blood count (CBC), complete metabolic panel (CMP), magnesium, liver panel, urinalysis, fasting serum glucose.
        - Evaluate for hyperthyroidism, anemia, electrolytes (*due to medical management, such as diuretics*), and renal or liver impairment (*occurs from hypoperfusion*). Tests are indicated to rule out other comorbidities.
- Chest X-ray
    - Checks for other causes of dyspnea (e.g., pneumonia). Used to assess for pulmonary edema, cardiomegaly, and/or parenchymal edema (seen with moderate-severe heart failure).

- Electrocardiogram (EKG)
  - Checks for arrhythmias, left ventricular hypertrophy, and Q waves (*signifies prior myocardial infarction*).
- Echocardiography (transthoracic)
  - Estimates ejection fraction and is the preferred test for evaluating left ventricular function.
- Cardiac catheterization
  - Not done routinely; order if there's evidence of coronary disease and intervention would be warranted.

## Treatment & Management[1,3,4,5,8,9,11,12]

- **Nonpharmacological and nursing interventions:**
  - Monitor body weight.
  - Encourage lifestyle modification (e.g., reducing sodium to < 2,000 mg in moderate-severe HF; fluid restrictions < 2 L/d with severe symptoms).
  - Promote physical activity.
  - Encourage diet and medication compliance.
  - Encourage alcohol and tobacco cessation.
- **Pharmacological and other interventions:**
  - Identify and treat the underlying causes of heart failure, such as:
    - Treat the hypertension.
    - Treat the dyslipidemia (*may prevent a future myocardial infarction*).
    - Aortic stenosis (consider aortic valve replacement).
    - Myocardial ischemia (consider coronary revascularization and/or antianginal agents).
  - ACE inhibitors (ACEIs) (e.g., lisinopril [Prinivil, Zetril], captropril [Capoten], enalapril [Vasotec])
    - Example: Start enalapril 2.5–5 mg BID (max: 40 mg/day).
    - First-line therapy in individuals with systolic dysfunction. They prevent left ventricular remodeling. The significance of ACEIs and ARBs in those with diastolic heart failure is uncertain.

  - Use an ARB, such as valsartan (Diovan) 20–40 mg PO BID (max: 320 mg/day), if unable to tolerate an ACEI due to side effect, such as cough.
  - Monitor for cough (*excluding ARBs*), renal impairment, angioedema (*rare with ARBs*), and hyperpotassemia.
- Beta blockers (e.g., metoprolol succinate [Toprol-XL], carvedilol [Coreg])
  - Example: Start carvedilol at 3.125 mg BID (max: 50 mg/day).
  - Reduces mortality and improves left ventricular function.
  - They may improve symptoms in those with diastolic heart failure.
  - Monitor closely for bradycardia, hypotension, and fatigue
- Diuretics, initially loops (e.g., furosemide [Lasix], bumetanide [Bumex])
  - Example: bumetanide 0.5–5 mg PO QD-BID (max: 10 mg/day).
  - Effective at relieving pulmonary congestion and edema in systolic and diastolic heart failure.
  - If high doses are not controlling the fluid overload, add an aldosterone antagonist (e.g., spironolactone [Aldactone]).
    - Example: Start spironolactone at 12.5–50 mg PO QD.
    - Recommended with NYHA class II–IV heart failure symptoms and EF $\leq$ 35%; reduces mortality in severe heart failure. May be beneficial in those with diastolic heart failure.
  - If pulmonary congestion or pedal edema is severe, add metolazone (Zaroxlyn) 2.5–10 mg PO QD.
  - Monitor renal function and electrolytes closely.
- Hydralazine and nitrate (isosorbide dinitrate) combination

    - Example: Start hydralazine 12.5–25 mg TID-QID (max: 300 mg/day) and isosorbide dinitrate 10 mg TID-QID (max: 120 mg/day).
    - Especially beneficial in blacks. Use this combo when unable to tolerate an ACEI or an ARB.
    - Monitor for common symptoms: headache and dizziness.
  - Digoxin *(fallen out of favor)*
    - Example: Dose of 125 mcg QD is typical; therapeutic target range between 0.5–0.9 ng/mL.
    - Increases the force of myocardial contraction, which improves HF symptoms with reduced ejection fraction. Not recommended in diastolic heart failure (unless used to improve rate with atrial fibrillation).
    - Monitor for GI disturbances (nausea/vomiting, abdominal pain) and bradycardia.
    - Used when patient is symptomatic despite taking other therapy. Not recommended as first-line therapy in HF.
- Not recommended to use calcium channel blockers with HfrEJ.
- For all the above medications:
  - Start at low doses and slowly titrate upward.
- Treat the depression and anxiety (often coexist with HF).
- Cardiology consultation/referral (when symptoms are refractory to medical therapy).
- Palliative care referral
  - To improve quality of life and provide relief of symptoms; as patient declines consider transition to hospice services.

Note: Beers listed items, as mentioned above, include digoxin and diuretics. Avoid routine prescribing of an ACEI with a potassium-sparing diuretic.

## Differential Diagnosis[4,6,10]

- Chronic obstructive pulmonary disease (COPD): Precipitants commonly include infection, allergies, or environmental triggers. Will have absence of paroxysmal nocturnal dyspnea and low BNP, whereas HF will have paroxysmal nocturnal dyspnea and elevated BNP.

- Pneumonia: May have acute dyspnea, productive sputum, and/or fever. HF can be acute or chronic dyspnea, cough can be dry or productive, and absence of fever.

## CLINICAL PEARLS[3,4,8,9,10]

- Have discussions with the family and patient regarding end-of-life care (e.g., how aggressive to be with overall care/advanced directives) given the overall poor prognosis of patients with established heart failure, especially with NYHA class III or IV.
- Aggressive treatment of coronary artery disease and hypertension are essential in preventing heart failure from worsening, given these are the most common causes of heart failure in older adults.
- Although ACEIs, ARBs, mineralocorticoid antagonists, and beta blockers are not considered standard therapy in diastolic heart failure, it is reasonable to use these agents to improve symptoms.

# References


1. Khan, M. K., & Sanchez, A. (2017). Congestive heart failure and management drugs. In Elmoselhi, A. & *Cardiology: An Integrated Approach*. New York, NY: McGraw-Hill. Retrieved from http://accessmedicine.mhmedical.com/content.aspx?bookid=2224&sectionid=171661368. Accessed November 1, 2017.
2. National Heart, Lung, and Blood Institute (NHLBI). (2015, June 22). What Is Heart Failure? U.S. Department of Health and Human Services, National Institutes of Health. Retrieved from https://www.nhlbi.nih.gov/health/health-topics/topics/hf/. Accessed November 1, 2017.
3. *Essentials of Clinical Geriatrics* (7th ed.). New York, NY: McGraw-Hill; Chapter 11: Cardiovascular disorders. Retrieved from http://accessmedicine.mhmedical.com/content.aspx?bookid=678&sectionid=44833890. Accessed October 31, 2017.
4. Heart failure and heart rhythm disorders. In *Current Diagnosis & Treatment: Geriatrics* (2nd ed.). New York, NY: McGraw-Hill. Retrieved from http://accessmedicine.mhmedical.com/content.aspx?bookid=953&sectionid=53375653. Accessed October 31, 2017.
5. American Heart Association. (n.d.). Heart Failure. Retrieved from http://www.heart.org/HEARTORG/Conditions/HeartFailure/Heart-Failure_UCM_002019_SubHomePage.jsp. Accessed November 1, 2017.
6. Epocrates. (n.d.). Retrieved from https://www.epocrates.com (used for brand names and dosing instructions).
7. Mayo Clinic. (2017, March 7). Heart Failure: When Your Heart Doesn't Work Efficiently. Retrieved from https://www.mayoclinic.org/diseases-conditions/heart-failure/basics/risk-factors/con-20029801. Accessed November 1, 2017.

8. Rich, M. W. (2017). Heart failure. In *Hazzard's Geriatric Medicine and Gerontology* (7th ed.). New York, NY: McGraw-Hill. Retrieved from http://accessmedicine.mhmedical.com/content.aspx?bookid=1923&sectionid=144525099. Accessed November 1, 2017.
9. Ding, Q., Yehle, K. S., Edwards, N. E., & Griggs, R. R. (2014, January). Geriatric heart failure: Awareness, evaluation, and treatment in primary care. *Journal for Nurse Practioners, 10*(1), 49–54. Retrieved from http://www.npjournal.org/article/S1555-4155(13)00403-0/fulltext#tbl2. Accessed November 2, 2017.
10. Mann, D. L., & Chakinala, M. (2015). Heart failure: Pathophysiology and diagnosis. In Kasper, D., Fauci, A., Hauser, S., Longo, D., Jamesom, J., & Loscalzo, J. (Eds.). *Harrison's Principles of Internal Medicine* (19th ed.). New York, NY: McGraw-Hill. Retrieved from http://accessmedicine.mhmedical.com/content.aspx?bookid=1130&sectionid=79742466. Accessed November 3, 2017.
11. American Geriatrics Society 2015 Beers Criteria Update Expert Panel, Fick, D. M., Semla, T. P., Beizer, J., Brandt, N., & Dombrowski, R., . . . Steinman, M. (2015, October 8). American Geriatrics Society 2015 updated Beers criteria for potentially inappropriate medication use in older adults. *Journal of the American Geriatrics Society, 63*(11), 2227–2246. Retrieved from http://onlinelibrary.wiley.com/doi/10.1111/jgs.13702/abstract. Accessed October 8, 2017.
12. Planning Ahead: Advanced Heart Failure. (2017, March 9). Retrieved from http://www.heart.org/HEARTORG/Conditions/HeartFailure/Planning-Ahead-Advanced-Heart-Failure UCM 441935. Article.isp#WvLfHUxFy3A. Accessed May 9, 2018.

# Hypertension

## Definition[1,2,5,6,13,14]

Hypertension (HTN) is a disease characterized by an elevation of systemic arterial blood pressure, often leading to cardiovascular disease (CVD)-related events or death.

Primary hypertension: Hypertension develops gradually with no known cause.

Secondary hypertension: Hypertension develops from an underlying cause.

## Classification[2]

**Normal:** pressure < 120/80 mm Hg
**Elevated:** systolic 120–129 mm Hg *plus* diastolic < 80 mm Hg
**Stage I hypertension:** systolic 130–139 mm Hg *or* diastolic 80–89 mm Hg
**Stage 2 hypertension:** pressure ≥ 140/90 mm Hg

**Hypertensive crisis:** systolic > 180 mm Hg and/or diastolic > 120 mm Hg

Note: The above represents the new classification system from the 2017 American College of Cardiology/American Heart Association (ACC/AHA) guidelines.[15]

*Older adults are typically classified based on their systolic results given isolated diastolic hypertension is uncommon.*

## Causes[2,5,6,13]

- Primary (essential) hypertension
  - Cause unknown
- Secondary hypertension
  - Kidney disease *(most common)*
  - Medications (e.g., decongestants, corticosteroids, NSAIDs)
  - Sleep apnea
  - Hypo- or hyperthyroidism
  - Hypercalcemia (primary hyperparathyroidism)

## Risk Factors[2,5,6,11,13]

- Older age (> 60 years)
- African-American ancestry
- Family history of hypertension
- Overweight or obese
- Sedentary lifestyle
- Tobacco use
- Alcohol abuse
- Smoking
- Stress
- High sodium intake

## Signs & Symptoms[5,6,13]

*There are usually no signs or symptoms associated with hypertension.*

- Some may have blurry vision, chest pain, epistaxis, and/or headache.

## Tests[1,11,13,16]

- Screening tests: office blood pressure measurement, ambulatory and home blood pressure monitoring
  - Office blood pressure measurement should be performed while the patient is sitting, using a manual or automated sphygmomanometer. The mean of two measurements is taken with an appropriately sized arm cuff with the arm at the level of the right atrium.
  - Ambulatory and home blood pressure monitoring confirm the diagnosis of hypertension; ambulatory blood pressure monitoring is preferred for confirmation.
- Urine albumin, basic metabolic panel (BMP), fasting blood glucose, lipid panel, TSH
  - Ordered to evaluate for renal impairment; serum electrolytes ordered due to medication therapy monitoring (e.g., ACEI/ARB, diuretics), impaired glucose and dyslipidemia often seen with hypertension, and thyroid to evaluate for underlying thyroid disease.
- Electrocardiogram or echocardiography
  - Evaluate for cardiac abnormalities (e.g., left ventricular hypertrophy).
- Polysomnography
  - If suspected sleep apnea.

## Treatment & Management[1,2,3,4,5,6,7,8,9,10,11,13,14,16,18]

- **Nonpharmacological and nursing interventions:**
  - Educate on adverse effects of antihypertensives.
    - All antihypertensives associated with postural hypotension.
  - Educate importance of compliance with medications.
    - Uncontrolled hypertension leads to end organ damage (e.g., stroke, heart failure, myocardial infarction, renal insufficiency, retinopathy)
  - Stress the importance of blood pressure measurement techniques.

- Encourage lifestyle changes, such as:
  - Healthier eating practices; decrease intake of sodium (< 2,400 mg/day) and alcohol (< 1–2 drinks/day)
  - Smoking cessation
  - Stress management (e.g., yoga, meditating)
  - Increasing physical activity (e.g., walking 30 min/day)
- **Pharmacological and other interventions:**
  - Thiazide diuretics (e.g., hydrochlorothiazide [Microzide] or chlorthalidone)
    - Example: Start chlorthalidone 12.5–25 mg QD, which is the recommended agent in this class.
    - Thiazides can be used alone or in combo with other drug classes.
    - They are especially effective when combined with ACE inhibitor.
    - Can be used as monotherapy or in combo with a calcium channel blocker in blacks.
    - Monitor for electrolyte imbalance (e.g., hyponatremia, hypokalemia), urinary frequency, and hyperuricemia.
  - ACE inhibitor (ACEI) (e.g., lisinopril [Zestril, Prinvil]) **or** angiotensin receptor blocker (ARB) (e.g., valsartan [Diovan])
    - Example: Start Lisinopril 5–10 mg QD (max: 80 mg/day due to HTN; max: 40 mg/day due to HF) or valsartan 80–160 mg QD (max: 320 mg/day).
    - They can be used alone or in combo with other drug classes.
    - Do not combine an ACE inhibitor with an ARB.
    - Use an ACE inhibitor or ARB with chronic kidney disease, heart failure, following myocardial infarction, coronary artery disease, and/or diabetes.
    - Monitor for cough, angioedema, hyperkalemia, and renal insufficiency.
  - Calcium channel blockers (CCB) include dihydropyridines (e.g., amlodipine [Norvasc]) or nondihydropyridines (e.g., diltiazem [Cardizem] or verapamil [Calan, Verelan])

- Example: Start amlodipine 2.5–5 mg QD (max: 10 mg/day).
- Can be used alone or in combo with other drug classes.
- Caution prescribing a nondihydropyridine with a beta blocker; combo increases risk of bradycardia.
- In systolic heart failure, they provide no mortality benefit; nondihydropyridines may worsen outcome by depressing cardiac function.
- Monitor for peripheral edema; caution use in patients with heart failure.

- Beta blockers (e.g., metoprolol tartrate [Lopressor], carvedilol [Coreg])
  - Example: Start metoprolol tartrate at 50 mg BID (max: 450 mg/day).
  - They are most often used in combo with other drug classes; used alone for hypertension without compelling indication is controversial.
  - Beta blockers are beneficial in patients with heart failure and following myocardial infarction.
  - Monitor for fatigue, dizziness, sexual dysfunction, and decreased pulse; avoid in severe COPD or asthma.
- Other options (not typically used as initial management): aldosterone antagonist (e.g., spironolactone [Aldactone]), loop diuretic (e.g., furosemide [Lasix]), hydralazine, peripheral alpha blocker (e.g., terazosin [Hytrin]), or central alpha agonist (clonidine [Catapres])

- For all the above medications:
  - Start at low dose and slowly titrate upward.
  - If not at target blood pressure goal, increase medication(s) to the max dose or add another medication.
- Consultation/referral to appropriate specialists (e.g., ophthalmology to evaluate for hypertensive retinopathy, nephrology with presence of kidney disease).

NOTE: Beers listed items, as mentioned above, include clonidine, peripheral alpha blockers, diuretics, and nondihydropyridine calcium channel blockers. Avoid routine prescribing of an ACEI with a potassium-sparing diuretic.

## CLINICAL PEARLS[2,13,14,15,16,17]

- Determining appropriate blood pressure goals in older individuals is controversial.
  - Eighth Joint National Committee (JNC 8) guidelines recommend for adults ≥ age 60 a target blood pressure goal of less than 150/90 mm Hg. If diabetes or chronic renal disease present, will need to maintain pressure goal of less than 140/90 mm Hg.
  - The American College of Physicians (ACP) and American Academy of Family Physicians (AFFP) recommend treatment in adults age 60 years or above with blood pressures persistently at or above 150 mm Hg. In individuals with a history of stroke or transient ischemic attack, and/or increased cardiovascular risk, a systolic blood pressure goal of less than 140 mm Hg is reasonable.
  - US Preventive Services Task Force (USPSTF) recommends a target blood pressure of 150/90 mm Hg in older adults age 60 years or older.
  - The new guidelines issued by the American College of Cardiology/American Heart Association (ACC/AHA) aim for a target of under 130/80 mm Hg, suggesting older adults should have the same goal as younger adults.
    - This may not be realistic for some older adults when treated aggressively to the guidelines (due to poor vascular compliance).
- Deciding on which antihypertensive agent to prescribe is patient specific; consider comorbidities and simplicity of the medication (e.g., once daily dosing) to increase compliance.

# References


1. Pearson, T. (2015). Treating hypertension: Losing sight of the forest for the trees? *The Clinical Advisor,* 55–60. Retrieved October 30, 2017.
2. Hypertension. In *Hazzard's Geriatric Medicine and Gerontology* (7th ed.). New York, NY: McGraw-Hill. Retrieved from http://accessmedicine.mhmedical.com/content.aspx?bookid=1923&sectionid=144525442. Accessed October 30, 2017.
3. Eighth Joint National Committee (JNC 8) Hypertension Guideline Algorithm. (2014). Retrieved from http://www.nmhs.net/documents/27JNC8HTNGuidelinesBookBooklet.pdf.
4. Epocrates. (n.d.). Retrieved from https://www.epocrates.com (used for brand names and dosing instructions).
5. Mayo Clinic. (2016, September 9). High Blood Pressure (Hypertension): Controlling This Common Health Problem. Retrieved from https://www.mayoclinic.org/diseases-conditions/high-blood-pressure/basics/causes/CON-20019580. Accessed October 30, 2017.
6. National Heart, Lung, and Blood Institute (NHBLI). (2015, September 10). Description of High Blood Pressure. U.S. Department of Health and Human Services,

National Institutes of Health. Retrieved from https://www.nhlbi.nih.gov/health/health-topics/topics/hbp. Accessed October 30, 2017.

7. Heart Foundation. (2014, November). Resources. Retrieved from https://www.heartfoundation.org/au/resources. Accessed October 30, 2017.
8. Colucci, W. S. (2016, August 24). Calcium Channel Blockers in Heart Failure with Reduced Ejection Fraction (Gottlieb, S. S., & S. B. Yeon, S. B., Eds.). UpToDate. Retrieved from https://www.uptodate.com/contents/calcium-channel-blockers-in-heart-failure-with-reduced-ejection-fraction. Accessed October 30, 2017.
9. Rosenson, R. S., Reeder, G. S., & Kennedy, H. L. (2017, July 10). Acute Myocardial Infarction: Role of Beta Blocker Therapy (Cannon, C. P., & Saperia, G. M., Eds.). UpToDate. Retrieved from https://www.uptodate.com/contents/acute-myocardial-infarction-role-of-beta-blocker-therapy. Accessed October 30, 2017.
10. Bashore, T. M., Granger, C. B., Jackson, K. P., & Patel, M. R. (2018). Heart disease. In *Current Medical Diagnosis & Treatment 2018*. New York, NY: McGraw-Hill. Retrieved from http://accessmedicine.mhmedical.com/content.aspx?bookid=2192&sectionid=168190671. Accessed October 31, 2017.
11. Schmieder, R. E. (2010, December). End Organ Damage In Hypertension. National Heart, Lung, and Blood Institute (NHBLI). U.S. Department of Health and Human Services, National Institutes of Health. Retrieved from https://www.ncbi.nlm.nih.gov/pmc/articles/PMC3011179/. Accessed October 31, 2017.
12. Wiysonge, C. S., Bradley, H. A., Volmink, J., Mayosi, B. M., & Opie, L. H. (2017, January 20). Beta-blockers for hypertension. *Cochrane Database System Review, 1*, CD002003. Retrieved from https://www.ncbi.nlm.nih.gov/pmc/articles/PMC5369873/. Accessed October 30, 2017.
13. Kotchen, T. A. (2015). Hypertensive vascular disease. In Kasper, D., Fauci, A., Hauser, S., Longo, D., Jamesom, J., & Loscalzo, J. (Eds.) *Harrison's Principles of Internal Medicine* (19th ed.). New York, NY: McGraw-Hill. Retrieved from http://accessmedicine.mhmedical.com/content.aspx?bookid=1130&sectionid=79743947. Accessed October 30, 2017.
14. Qaseem, A., Wilt, T. J., Rich, R., Humphrey, L. L., Frost, J., & Forciea, M. A. (2017). Pharmacologic treatment of hypertension in adults aged 60 years or older to higher versus lower blood pressure targets: A clinical practice guideline from the American College of Physicians and the American Academy of Family Physicians. *Annals of Internal Medicine, 166*(6), 430–437. doi:10.7326/m16-1785
15. Bakris, G., & Sorrentino, M. (2018). Redefining hypertension: Assessing the new blood-pressure guidelines. *New England Journal of Medicine,* 378(6), 497–499. doi:10.1056/nejmp1716193
16. U.S. Preventive Services Task Force (USPSTF). (n.d.). Published Recommendations from the U.S. Preventive Services Task Force. Retrieved from https://www.uspreventiveservicestaskforce.org/BrowseRec/Index/browse-recommendations. Accessed September 17, 2017.
17. American College of Cardiology (ACC). (2017, November 13). New ACC/AHA High Blood Pressure Guidelines Lower Definition of Hypertension. Retrieved from http://www.acc.org/latest-in-cardiology/articles/2017/11/08/11/47/mon-5pm-bp-guideline-aha-2017. Accessed February 17, 2018.
18. American Geriatrics Society 2015 Beers Criteria Update Expert Panel, Fick, D. M., Semla, T. P., Beizer, J., Brandt, N., & Dombrowski, R., . . . Steinman, M. (2015, October 8). American Geriatrics Society 2015 updated Beers criteria for potentially inappropriate medication use in older adults. *Journal of the American Geriatrics Society, 63*(11), 2227–2246. Retrieved from http://onlinelibrary.wiley.com/doi/10.1111/jgs.13702/abstract. Accessed October 3, 2017.

# Peripheral Arterial Disease

## Definition[2,3,8,9]

Peripheral arterial disease (PAD) refers to atherosclerosis in the arteries that circulate the lower extremities.

## Cause[1,3,4,8,9]

- Atherosclerosis

## Risk Factors[1,2,3,4,8,9]

- Cigarette smoking
- Diabetes
- Advanced age
- Personal or family history of coronary heart disease (CHD)
- Dyslipidemia
- Hypertension
- Elevated homocysteine

## Signs & Symptoms[1,2,3,4,5,8,9]

- Asymptomatic
- Intermittent claudication (i.e., achy or painful leg exacerbated with walking, alleviated by rest)
- Decreased walking distance
- Thick, brittle nails
- Lower extremity cool to the touch
- Skin pallor or cyanosis
- Atrophic skin and hair loss
- Dependent rubor
- Erectile dysfunction
- Slow or nonhealing wounds (severe PAD)
- Absent or weak pedal pulses (severe PAD)
- Leg rest pain (severe PAD)
- Atypical complaints: impaired exercise tolerance, joint pain

## Tests[1,2,3,4,5,8,9]

- Lipid panel, fasting blood glucose or HbA1c
  - Assists in managing risk factors associated with PAD (e.g., dyslipidemia, diabetes).
- Doppler ultrasonography
  - Used when peripheral pulses aren't palpable.
- Ankle-brachial index (ABI)
  - Determines severity of circulation; abnormal is $\leq 0.9$, severe is $\leq 0.4$.
  - Factors that may cause inaccurate readings: older age, diabetes, and end stage renal disease.
- Toe-brachial index (TBI)
  - Order this test when ABI is inconclusive. Reading of $< 0.7$ is consistent with PAD.
- Arterial duplex ultrasound
  - Provides an overview of the location and severity of PAD.
- Exercise ABI testing
  - Reserved in individuals with symptoms consistent with PAD but with normal resting ABI.
- Computed tomography (CT) or magnetic resonance angiography (MRA)
  - Reserved in individuals who are planning for surgical or endovascular revascularization.

## Treatment & Management[1,2,3,5,6,7,8,9,10]

- **Nonpharmacological and nursing interventions:**
  - Encourage lifestyle changes.
    - Get involved in an exercise program (e.g., at least 3 walking sessions/week).
    - Healthy eating (low-fat diet).
    - Weight loss.
    - Advise smoking cessation (*nicotine is a vasoconstrictor*).

- Encourage daily foot inspections and provide foot care, especially diabetics.
  - Advise not to walk barefoot.
  - Important to stay clean to prevent infections.
- Reinforce measures to prevent pressure injury.
  - Look over bony prominences for ulcers; if not treated, can develop into gangrene, requiring amputation.
- Advise against using drugs that lead to vasoconstriction (e.g., pseudoephedrine).

- **Pharmacological and other interventions:**
  - Identify and treat reversible risk factors of PAD.
    - Treat the hypertension *(to improve tissue perfusion)*, dyslipidemia, and diabetes (goal HgA1c of 7%).
  - Antiplatelet therapy (i.e., aspirin [Bayer, Bufferin, Ecotrin] or clopidogrel [Plavix])
    - Example: aspirin 81 mg PO daily (max: 325 mg/day).
      - If allergic to aspirin, use clopidogrel 75 mg daily.
    - These do not improve claudication symptoms, however they reduce cardiovascular and cerebrovascular events.
    - Monitor for upset stomach and bleeding.
  - Agents used for claudication relief (lifestyle limiting)
    - Cilostazol (Pletal) or pentoxifylline.
      - *Cilostazol is more effective than pentoxifylline.*
    - Example: cilostazol 100 mg PO BID. It can be combined with an antiplatelet.
    - Cilostazol improves walking distance in those with intermittent claudication.
    - Cilostazol may promote fluid retention and exacerbate heart failure.
    - Discontinue if no clinical improvement (i.e., walking distance) seen in about 3 months.
  - Statin therapy (e.g., atorvastatin [Lipitor], rosuvastatin [Crestor])
    - Example: Start atorvastatin 20–40 mg daily (max: 80 mg/day).

    - These should be started on all patients with confirmed PAD.
    - Reduce cardiovascular or cerebrovascular events, improve claudication symptoms, and slow the advancement of PAD.
    - Musculoskeletal complaints can occur and are dose dependent; liver toxicity is uncommon.
  - ACE inhibitors (ACEI) (e.g., captopril [Capoten], lisinopril [Zestril, Prinivil], ramipril [Altace])
    - Example: ramipril (Altace) 10 mg PO daily.
    - Provides some relief with claudication symptoms.
    - Monitor for hyperkalemia, dry cough, renal impairment.
  - Beta blockers (e.g., atenolol [Tenormin], propranolol [Inderal])
    - These are used to reduce cardiovascular risk factors, especially in those with coronary artery disease or heart failure.
    - Avoid in severe PAD.
- Vascular consultation/referral
  - Refer patients with leg pain despite medical therapy and/or evidence of critical limb ischemia or gangrene (for consideration of surgical revascularization or amputation).
- Podiatry referral
  - Refer diabetic patients for routine nail care.

NOTE: Beers listed items, as mentioned above, include cilostazol and aspirin (if dose > 325 mg/day). Avoid routine prescribing of an ACEI with a potassium-sparing diuretic.

## Differential Diagnosis[1,9]

- Deep vein thrombosis: Unilateral leg will have swelling or tenderness; will have thromboembolic risk factors such as immobility, malignancy, recent major surgery. In comparison to PAD, most patients are asymptomatic; will not typically have leg swelling. Strong risk factors include diabetes and tobacco smoking.

- Peripheral neuropathy: Will have numbness or tingling sensation distally in an extremity. In comparison to PAD, patients will not typically have numbness or tingling sensation (most are asymptomatic).
- Musculoskeletal disorders (e.g., arthritic knees or hips): Achy pains will be noted with activity or exertion; ABI testing will be normal. In comparison to PAD, X-ray of affected joint would be negative. ABI testing would be abnormal $\leq 0.9$.

## CLINICAL PEARLS[1,3,8,9]

- Risk factor modification is key to slow the advancement of PAD and prevent future acute coronary syndrome or strokes.

## References

1. Armstrong, E. (2016, April 4). Peripheral Vascular Disease. Epocrates. Retrieved from https://online.epocrates.com/diseases/431/Peripheral-vascular-disease. Accessed November 11, 2017.
2. Hallett, J. W. (2014, May). Peripheral Arterial Disease – Cardiovascular Disorders. Merck Manuals: Professional. Retrieved from https://www.merckmanuals.com/professional/cardiovascular-disorders/peripheral-arterial-disorders/peripheral-arterial-disease. Accessed November 11, 2017.
3. Peripheral arterial disease and venous thromboembolism. In *Current Diagnosis & Treatment: Geriatrics* (2nd ed.). New York, NY: McGraw-Hill. Retrieved from http://accessmedicine.mhmedical.com/content.aspx?bookid=953&sectionid=53375656. Accessed November 11, 2017.
4. National Heart, Lung, and Blood Institute (NHBLI). (2016, June 22). What Is Peripheral Artery Disease? U.S. Department of Health and Human Services, National Institutes of Health. Retrieved from https://www.nhlbi.nih.gov/health/health-topics/topics/pad. Accessed November 11, 2017.
5. John Hopkins Medicine. (n.d.). What Is Peripheral Vascular Disease? Retrieved from https://www.hopkinsmedicine.org/healthlibrary/conditions/cardiovascular_diseases/peripheral_vascular_disease_85,P00236. Accessed November 11, 2017.
6. Paravastu, S. C. V., Mendonca, D. A., & Da Silva, A. (2013, September 11). Beta Blockers for Peripheral Arterial Disease. Cochrane Database of Systematic Reviews. Retrieved from http://onlinelibrary.wiley.com/doi/10.1002/14651858.CD005508.pub3/full. Accessed November 12, 2017.
7. Hunter, M. R., Cahoon, W. D., & Lowe, D. K. (2013, November). Angiotensin-converting enzyme inhibitors for intermittent claudication associated with

peripheral arterial disease. *Annals of Pharacotherapy*, 47(11), 1552–1557. Retrieved from https://www.ncbi.nlm.nih.gov/pubmed/24285767. Accessed November 12, 2017.
8. Gulanick, M., & Myers, J. L. (2017). *Nursing Care Plans: Diagnoses, Interventions, & Outcomes*. St. Louis, MO: Elsevier.
9. Hennion, D. R., & Siano, K. A. (2013, September 1). Diagnosis and Treatment of Peripheral Arterial Disease. *American Family Physician*, 88(5), 306–310. Retrieved from http://www.aafp.org/afp/2013/0901/p306.html. Accessed November 13, 2017.
10. American Geriatrics Society 2015 Beers Criteria Update Expert Panel, Fick, D. M., Semla, T. P., Beizer, J., Brandt, N., & Dombrowski, R., . . . Steinman, M. (2015, October 8). American Geriatrics Society 2015 updated Beers criteria for potentially inappropriate medication use in older adults. *Journal of the American Geriatrics Society*, 63(11), 2227–2246. Retrieved from http://onlinelibrary.wiley.com/doi/10.1111/jgs.13702/abstract. Accessed October 3, 2017.

# Venous Thromboembolism

## Definition[1,2,3,4,5,6,7]

Venous thromboembolism (VTE) is a thrombus that forms in the veins and includes two types: deep vein thrombosis (DVT) and pulmonary embolism (PE). DVT occurs when a thrombus arises in the deep veins, most commonly in the lower extremities. Thrombus in the lower extremity (*usually more proximal DVTs*) can dislodge and travel into the pulmonary arteries, which is a pulmonary embolus (PE).

## Causes[3,4,5,6,7]

- Virchow's triad
  - Vascular endothelial injury
    - Associated with some medications, surgery, trauma, smoking.
  - Venous stasis
    - Associated with prolonged immobility, heart failure.
  - Hypercoagulability
    - Associated with malignancies, smoking, volume depletion, sepsis.

## Risk Factors[1,2,3,4,5,6,7]

- Advanced age
- Recent hospitalization

- Major surgery (e.g., hip or knee arthroplasty)
- Immobility
- Trauma
- Malignancy
- Infection or sepsis
- Heart failure exacerbation
- Obesity
- Travel
- Prior VTE
- Presence of central venous catheter
- Some medications (e.g., hormone therapy, erythropoietin, tamoxifen,[3] chemotherapy treatment)
- Inherited (e.g., factor V Leiden, protein C or S deficiency)
- Antiphospholipid antibodies
- Myeloproliferative disorders
- Smoking

## Signs & Symptoms[1,2,3,4,5,6,7]

**Table 3-2** Comparing Signs & Symptoms of DVT and PE

| Deep Vein Thrombosis (DVT) | Pulmonary Embolism (PE) |
|---|---|
| Many are asymptomatic | Many are asymptomatic |
| Extremity or calf pain | Confusion |
| Extremity edema | Pleuritic chest pain |
| Extremity erythema and warmth | Dyspnea |
| Homans sign (lacks sensitivity and specificity) | Cough (usually nonproductive, however may have hemoptysis) |
| | Palpitations |
| | Prescynope or syncope |
| | Abnormal vital signs (tachycardia, tachypnea, hypoxemia) |

Data from Criteria Committee, New York Heart Association , Inc. Diseases of the Heart and Blood Vessels. Nomenclature and Criteria for diagnosis, 6th edition Boston, Little, Brown and Co. 1964, p 114.

**Table 3-3** Model for Determining Clinical Suspicion of Pulmonary Embolism (PE)

| VARIABLES | POINTS* |
|---|---|
| Clinical signs and symptoms of deep vein thrombosis (minimum of leg swelling and pain with palpitation of the deep veins) | 3.0 |
| An alternative diagnosis is less likely than pulmonary embolism (PE) | 3.0 |
| Heart rate > 100 beats/min | 1.5 |
| Immobilization of surgery in the previous 4 wk | 1.5 |
| Previous deep vein thrombosis/pulmonary embolism | 1.5 |
| Hemoptysis | 1.0 |
| Malignancy (treatment ongoing or within previous 6 mo or palliative) | 1.0 |
| **Total points** | |

*Total score <= 4 indicates PE unlikely; score > 4 indicates PE likely.

Reproduced from Jeffrey B. Halter, Joseph G. Ouslander, Stephanie Studenski, et al. 2017. *Hazzard's Geriatric Medicine and Gerontology, Seventh Edition*. Table 106-1, p. 1575. New York: McGraw-Hill Medical.

**Table 3-4** Model for Determining Clinical Suspicion of Deep Vein Thrombosis (DVT)

| VARIABLES | POINTS* |
|---|---|
| Active cancer (treatment ongoing or within previous 6 mo or palliative) | 1 |
| Paralysis, paresis, or recent plaster immobilization of the lower extremities | 1 |
| Recently bedridden >= 3 days or major surgery within the past 4 wk | 1 |
| Localized tenderness along the distribution of the deep venous system | 1 |

(*continues*)

**Table 3-4** Model for Determining Clinical Suspicion of Deep Vein Thrombosis (DVT) (*Continued*)

| VARIABLES | POINTS* |
|---|---|
| Entire leg swollen | 1 |
| Affected calf 3 cm greater than asymptomatic calf (measured 10 cm before tibial tuberosity) | 1 |
| Pitting edema confined to the symptomatic leg | 1 |
| Dilated superficial veins (nonvaricose) | 1 |
| Previous deep vein thrombosis (DVT)/pulmonary embolism | 1 |
| Alternative diagnosis is at least as likely as that of deep vein thrombosis | -2 |
| **Total points** | |

*Total score 2 < indicates DVT unlikely; score > 2 indicates DVT likely.

Reproduced from Jeffrey B. Halter, Joseph G. Ouslander, Stephanie Studenski, et al. 2017. *Hazzard's Geriatric Medicine and Gerontology, Seventh Edition*. Table 106-2, p. 1576. New York: McGraw-Hill Medical.

## Tests[1,2,3,5,6,7]

- No lab studies are specific enough to diagnose VTE.
  - Positive D-dimers aren't helpful; they are positive in older adults, infections, and recent surgery. A negative D-dimer (< 0.4 μg/mL) however excludes VTE.
- Duplex ultrasound, venous.
  - Test of choice to diagnose a DVT. If test is negative and clinical suspicion still remains high, repeat test in about a week.
- Computed tomography pulmonary angiogram (CTPA).
  - Most commonly ordered to diagnose an acute PE. Although pulmonary angiography is the gold standard for diagnosis, CTPA is less invasive.
- Ventilation-perfusion (V/Q) lung scanning.
  - Used to diagnose acute PE. Order this if CT contrast is contraindicated.
- Chest radiography.

  - Most will be normal in acute PE; used to identify other causes of dyspnea, such as pneumonia.
- Calculate Wells criteria.
  - Aids in assessing the possibility of DVT or PE presence.

## Treatment & Management[2,3,4,8,9,10,11,12,13,14]

- **Send patient to the hospital, if appropriate.**
  - Abnormal vital signs or presumed massive PE for workup and management (e.g., thrombolytic therapy, vasopressors, fluid resuscitation).
  - Most patients with VTE can be safely treated as outpatients, including those with low-risk PE.
- **Nonpharmacological and nursing interventions:**
  - Offer warm heat to the affected leg (DVT)..
    - Relieves pain and inflammation.
  - Encourage patient to not massage the calf region.
    - This helps to prevent thrombus from dislodging.
  - Monitor for bleeding (effects of anticoagulation therapy).
  - Encourage lifestyle changes, including:
    - Encourage smoking cessation (causes vasoconstriction, which promotes clotting).
    - Maintain healthy weight.
    - Maintain euvolemic status (dehydration is associated with hypercoagulability).
    - Encourage early ambulation given this is effective for postthrombotic syndrome (compression stockings have *not* been shown to prevent this).
  - Educate patient on anticoagulation therapy.
    - Stress the importance of taking medications as prescribed.
    - Explain the importance of having routine INRs checked, while on warfarin. Provide education on vitamin K-rich foods while taking warfarin.
    - Educate patients to monitor for complications, such as bleeding.

- **Pharmacological and other interventions:**
  - Direct-acting oral anticoagulant (DOAC) (e.g., apixaban [Eliquis], edoxaban [Savaysa], rivaroxaban [Xarelto], dabigatran [Pradaxa])
    - Example: apixaban 10 mg PO BID for a week, then 5 mg PO BID.
      - Dose is changed to 2.5 mg PO BID if 2 of the following are noted: if age is > 80 years, weight is < 132 lbs. or serum creatinine > 1.5.
    - These are recommended over warfarin in acute VTE *without* cancer.
    - Compared to warfarin, these agents require no regular monitoring, no dietary restrictions, have fewer drug interactions, and cause less bleeding.
    - Adjustment of dose may be required due to renal impairment. They are also more expensive.
  - Warfarin (Coumadin, Jantoven)
    - Example: warfarin 5 mg PO daily.
    - Can be used in VTE not associated with cancer, although the DOACs are preferred.
    - Monitor INR closely (goal of 2.0–3.0); bleeding risk increases with certain drugs such as antibiotics, antifungals, and NSAIDs. Consumption of foods with vitamin K should be kept consistent.
  - Low-molecular-weight heparin (LMWH) (e.g., dalteparin [Fragmin], enoxaparin [Lovenox]).
    - Example: enoxaparin 1 mg/kg subQ q12 hrs
      - Adjust dose if CrCl < 30/min (bleeding risk)
    - LMWH is preferred over warfarin and DOACs in the setting of cancer-related VTE.
    - Will need to be added with warfarin until INR has been therapeutic (> 2.0) for 24 hrs.
    - If unable to use a LMWH, switch to unfractionated heparin, which is preferred in the setting of severe renal impairment.
    - In patients with recurrent VTE who are already on an oral anticoagulant (i.e., warfarin or DOAC), LMWH

should be used instead. If another VTE occurs while on LMWH, increase the dose by at least 25%.

- Anticoagulation duration.
    - Therapy is individualized (while also considering bleeding risk); in circumstances such as cancer, long-term anticoagulation is appropriate.
    - Lifelong treatment recommended if VTE returns for a second time.
    - Three months is recommended for VTEs that are provoked. If unprovoked, extended or lifelong anticoagulation is recommended.
- Inferior vena cava filter.
    - Used when patient cannot tolerate anticoagulation (such as bleeding risk). Not to be used while taking an anticoagulant.
- **Patient scenarios:**
    - Distal DVT: Treated *only* if symptomatic. If no symptoms are present, monitor and repeat imaging in 2 weeks. Treat for 3 months (DOACs preferred), if repeat imaging shows DVT extension or with severe symptoms.
    - Superficial venous thrombosis: 4–6 weeks of fondaparinux (preferred) or LWMH should be considered, especially if is above the knee (close to the greater saphenous vein).
    - Subsegmental pulmonary embolism: No anticoagulation needed if recurrence unlikely and absence of a DVT. These patients should instead be closely monitored.
    - Arm DVT: If caused by central venous catheter, do not remove patent catheter if needed for further use. Continue anticoagulation until three months after catheter discontinued.

NOTE: Beers listed items, as mentioned above, include enoxaparin and oral anticoagulants. If taking warfarin plus amiodarone or an NSAID, monitor INRs closely.

## Differential Diagnosis[1,3,5,6]

- Baker cyst: Pain will be acute in the calf region and ultrasound will confirm cyst. Compared to a DVT, many will be asymptomatic and ultrasound would have different findings.
- Cellulitis: Fever and/or leukocytosis may be present. Compared to a DVT, clinical leg findings (e.g., swelling) are more pronounced and not typical to have infectious findings.
- Pneumonia: May have productive sputum with fever; will have a positive sputum culture and leukocytosis. Compared to a PE, cough is common, however usually nonproductive. White blood count (WBC) is not typically elevated.

### CLINICAL PEARLS[2,3,8,9,11]

- Anticoagulation duration is individualized; consider the risk of bleeding, risk of falls, cost of medication, life expectancy, risk of VTE recurrence, and patient adherence to medication.
- Factors that increase the risk of bleeding while taking anticoagulation therapy: frequent falls, impaired liver or renal function, history of bleeding, concomitant use of an NSAID or antiplatelet, and age > 65–75 years.
- Periodically (at least annually) reassess the risks versus benefits of anticoagulation. If anticoagulation is stopped, low-dose aspirin can be used for treatment of recurrent VTE (although not as effective).

## References

1. Peripheral arterial disease and venous thromboembolism. In *Current Diagnosis & Treatment: Geriatrics* (2nd ed.). New York, NY: McGraw-Hill. Retrieved from http://accessmedicine.mhmedical.com/content.aspx?bookid=953&sectionid=53375656. Accessed November 13, 2017.
2. Tapson, V. F. (2015, March). Pulmonary Embolism (PE) – Pulmonary Disorders. Merck Manuals: Professional. Retrieved from https://www.merckmanuals.com/professional/pulmonary-disorders/pulmonary-embolism-pe/pulmonary-embolism-pe#v915358. Accessed November 14, 2017.
3. Merli, G., Galanis, T., Eraso, L., & Ouma, G. (2016, September 08). Deep Vein Thrombosis. Epocrates. Retrieved from https://online.epocrates.com/diseases/70/Deep-vein-thrombosis. Accessed November 13, 2017.

4. Gulanick, M., & Myers, J. L. (2017). *Nursing Care Plans: Diagnoses, Interventions, & Outcomes*. St. Louis, MO: Elsevier.
5. Merli, G., Eraso, L. H., Galanis, T., & Ouma, G. (2016, September 12). Pulmonary Embolism. Epocrates. Retrieved from https://online.epocrates.com/diseases/116/PE-pulmonary-embolism. Accessed November 14, 2017.
6. Wong, W., & Chaudry, S. (2011, April). Venous Thromboembolism (VTE). McMaster Pathophysiology Review. Retrieved from http://www.pathophys.org/vte/. Accessed November 14, 2017.
7. Johnson, S. A., & Rondina, M, T. (2017). Coagulation disorders. In *Hazzard's Geriatric Medicine and Gerontology* (7th ed.). New York, NY: McGraw-Hill. Retrieved from. http://accessmedicine.mhmedical.com/content.aspx?bookid=1923&sectionid=144560586. Accessed November 14, 2017.
8. Wilbur, J., & Shian, B. (2017, March 1). Deep venous thrombosis and pulmonary embolism: Current therapy. *American Family Physician, 95*(5), 295–302. Retrieved from http://www.aafp.org/afp/2017/0301/p295.html. Accessed November 14, 2017.
9. Grant, P. J. (2016, November). Updated ACCP guideline for antithrombotic therapy for VTE disease. *The Hospitalist, 2016*(11). Retrieved from http://www.the-hospitalist.org/hospitalist/article/121399/updated-accp-guideline-antithrombotic-therapy-vte-disease. Accessed November 15, 2017.
10. Clot Connect. (2012, February 27). New ACCP Guidelines – DVT and PE: Highlights and Summary. Education Blog for Healthcare Professionals. Retrieved from http://professionalsblog.clotconnect.org/2012/02/27/new-accp-guidelines-dvt-and-pe-highlights-and-summary/. Accessed November 15, 2017.
11. Garcia, D. (2016, July-August). Management of venous thromboembolism: An update of the ACCP guidelines, *The Hematologist, 13*(4). Retrieved from http://www.hematology.org/Thehematologist/Mini-Review/5668.aspx. Accessed November 15, 2017.
12. Kearon, C., Akl, E. A., Omelas, J., Blaivas, A., Jimenez, D., & Bounameaux, H., . . . Moores, L. (2016, March 2). Antithrombotic Therapy for VTE disease: CHEST guideline and expert panel report. *Chest, 149*(2), 315–352. Retrieved from http://www.acc.org/latest-in-cardiology/ten-points-to-remember/2016/03/02/15/45/antithrombotic-therapy-for-vte-disease. Accessed November 15, 2017.
13. Mayo Clinic. (2015, January 06). Warfarin Side Effects: Watch for Interactions. Retrieved from https://www.mayoclinic.org/diseases-conditions/deep-vein-thrombosis/in-depth/warfarin-side-effects/ART-20047592?pg=2. Accessed November 15, 2017.
14. American Geriatrics Society 2015 Beers Criteria Update Expert Panel, Fick, D. M., Semla, T. P., Beizer, J., Brandt, N., & Dombrowski, R., . . . Steinman, M. (2015, October 8). American Geriatrics Society 2015 updated Beers criteria for potentially inappropriate medication use in older adults. *Journal of the American Geriatrics Society, 63*(11), 2227–2246. Retrieved from http://onlinelibrary.wiley.com/doi/10.1111/jgs.13702/abstract. Accessed October 3, 2017.

SECTION IV

# Pulmonary

## Asthma

### Definition[2,3,4,5,8]

Asthma is a chronic inflammatory airway disease characterized by the presence of airflow obstruction, which can be partially or completely reversible.

### Causes[2,3,5,7]

- Exact cause is unknown.
- Genetics and environmental factors.

### Risk Factors[1,2,3,4,5,6,7]

- Atopic history (e.g., allergic rhinitis, eczema)
- Family history of asthma
- Allergen exposure (includes outdoor and indoor)
- Smoking and passive smoking
- Childhood viral infections
- Comorbid disease
- Diet (low in antioxidants or excess sodium)
- Obesity
- Gastroesophageal reflux disease
- Perinatal factors (e.g., insufficient maternal nutrition, prematurity, lack of breast milk)
- Some medications (e.g., beta blockers, aspirin, NSAIDs, cholinergic agents, hormone replacement therapy)

Note: Common triggers include: allergens, recent viral infection, exercise, cold air, medications, strong emotions (e.g., laughing hard), air pollutants and irritants (e.g., cigarette smoke, perfumes).

## Signs & Symptoms[2,3,4,5,6,7]

*Symptoms are typically worse at night or early morning hours.*

- Episodic wheezing
- Dyspnea
- Cough
- Chest tightness
- Sputum production
- Eczema
- Nasal polyps

## Tests[2,3,4,5,6,7]

- Pulmonary function tests
  - Asthma is diagnosed before and after bronchodilator spirometry.
- Pulse oximetry
  - To establish the severity of acute exacerbation.
- Arterial blood gas
  - Reserved in individuals with respiratory distress.
  - Increased $PaCO_2$ and respiratory acidosis indicates potential need for intubation and ventilation.
- Skin prick allergy testing
  - To identify triggers.
- Peak expiratory flow rate
  - Helps determine asthma severity and guides therapeutic decisions.
- Chest X-ray
  - Findings are usually normal.
  - Excludes other causes of dyspnea (e.g., heart failure [HF], pneumonia).
- Complete blood count (CBC) with differential
  - Not usually helpful; may have elevated eosinophils.

## Treatment & Management[1,2,3,4,5,6,8,9,10]

- **Nonpharmacological and nursing interventions:**
  - Educate on avoiding environmental tobacco smoke, perfumes, and fragranced body products; removing pets and

carpets to reduce dust mites and animal dander; avoiding exposure to other patient with viral respiratory infections.
- Encourage flu and pneumonia vaccination.
- Educate patients on the proper use and benefits of a peak flow meter.
  - Outcomes are improved when a treatment plan is in place for specific peak flow zones.
- Ensure proper use of medications and delivery devices (e.g., metered-dose or dry-powdered inhalers).
  - Spacers increase accurate medication delivery of metered-dose inhalers.
  - Drug delivery in older patients is most likely optimally achieved with dry-powder inhalers.
  - Nebulized medications are preferred in select patients (e.g., arthritis).
- Assess the need for supplemental oxygen.
  - Oxygen therapy is warranted if levels drop $< 90\%$.
- Monitor closely for respiratory compromise.
  - This includes dyspnea during normal conversations, increased respiratory rate and rhythm changes, diminished wheezing and/or inaudible breath sounds, accessory muscle use, hypoxemia, hypercapnia.
- Implement therapeutic interventions.
  - Keep head of bed elevated.
  - Encourage slow, deep breathing and use of pursed-lip breathing to exhale.
  - Encourage rest and promote calm environment to reduce fatigue, which increases oxygen requirements.
  - Encourage hydration (if not contraindicated in setting of cardiac or renal disease) to decrease viscosity of secretions.
- Encourage alternative therapies: acupuncture, breathing control, and yoga.

- **Pharmacological and other interventions:**
  - Manage comorbid conditions that hinder asthma management (e.g., gastroesophageal reflux disease, obesity, obstructive sleep apnea).

- Rescue therapy: short-acting beta agonists, metered-dose inhaler, or nebulizer (e.g., albuterol [ProAir HFA, Ventolin HFA], levalbuterol [Xopenex]).
  - Example: albuterol 2 puffs q4–6 hr PRN.
  - Medication works quickly, reduces bronchoconstriction, making it easier to breath. Additional drugs are needed if used on a daily basis.
  - Monitor for hypokalemia, inability to sleep, tremor, arrhythmias, and palpitations.
- Maintenance therapy (not used by itself): long-acting beta-2 agonists (LABA) (e.g., formoterol [Perforomist], salmeterol [Serevent Diskus], arformoterol [Brovana]).
  - Example: salmeterol inhaled 50 mcg 1 puff twice daily.
  - LABAs should be combined with an inhaled corticosteroid (e.g., budesonide/formoterol [Symbicort]) to improve asthma symptoms and reduce exacerbations.
  - LABAs are initiated starting at moderate persistent asthma.
  - Side effects are similar as the above rescue therapy, however milder.
- Anticholinergic inhaled bronchodilators, short acting (e.g., ipratropium bromide [Atrovent HFA]) or long acting (e.g., tiotropium [Spiriva]).

*Long acting is used for maintenance therapy, whereas short acting is used for acute exacerbations.*

  - Example: ipratropium bromide 2 puffs inhaled q6 hr PRN.
  - For acute symptoms, ipratropium can be added in the same nebulizer as albuterol (Duoneb).
  - When tiotropium is used for maintenance therapy, the low-dose soft-mist inhaler at 1.25 mcg/puff is the only dose recommended (ordered as 2 puffs once daily). When added with an inhaled corticosteroid, it improves asthma symptoms and lung function in those with uncontrolled asthma.

    - Monitor for xerostomia, taste changes, urinary retention, glaucoma.
- Corticosteroids: oral (e.g., prednisone) and/or inhaled (e.g., beclomethasone [Qvar], ciclesonide [Alvesco])

*Inhaled corticosteroids are used for maintenance therapy, whereas oral is used for acute exacerbations.*

    - Example: ciclesonide 80 or 160 mcg per actuation twice daily.
    - Inhaled corticosteroids are the cornerstone of asthma therapy; low doses are added when asthma is not controlled with a short-acting beta agonist. Doses are increased as asthma symptoms progress.
    - Oral corticosteroids are recommended with severe persistent asthma; short course burst doses are effective (e.g., prednisone 30–60 mg once daily for 5–10 days). They may cause or worsen delirium.
    - Inhaled corticosteroids increase the risk of pneumonia; oral increases the risk of osteoporosis (long-term use), hyperglycemia, and delirium.
- Leukotriene-receptor antagonist (LTRA) (e.g., montelukast [Singulair], zariflukast [Accolate])
    - Example: montelukast 10 mg once daily in the evening.
    - Not to be used for acute attacks; used as add-on therapy to improve lung function and reduce asthma symptoms.
    - Monitor for headache, flu-like symptoms, and gastrointestinal (GI) disturbances.
- Cromolyn inhaled (a mast cell stabilizer)
    - Example: cromolyn inhaled 20 mg/2 mL, 20 mg nebulizer TID-QID.
    - Used as a long-term control to prevent asthma symptoms.
    - Administer prior to exercise or following allergen exposure.

    - Monitor for throat irritation, taste changes, and/or complaint of dry throat.
  - Theophylline (Theo-24, Elixophyllin, Uniphyl)
    - Example: Start theophylline 300 mg PO daily (divided doses q6–8 hours).
    - Serves as a bronchodilator and has modest anti-inflammatory activity.
    - Aim for a goal serum concentration of 5–15 mcg/mL.
    - Caution use in patients with insomnia; has central nervous system (CNS) stimulant effects. Monitor for headaches, heartburn, and potential arrhythmias or seizures.
  - Immunomodulators (e.g., omalizumab [Xolair])
    - Example: 150–375 mg subcutaneous q2–4 weeks.
    - Reduces frequent exacerbation in patients with severe asthma.
    - Consider in patients with a known allergy.
    - Usually well tolerated; however anaphylaxis may occur.
- Pulmonology and/or allergist referral
  - Consider if:
    - The patient had a life-threatening asthma exacerbation.
    - The patient has required more than two bursts of oral steroids in 12 months or an exacerbation requiring hospitalization.
    - Patient is not responding to treatment.
    - Signs and symptoms are atypical.
    - Additional diagnostic testing is indicated (e.g., pulmonary function tests, allergy skin testing).
    - Immunotherapy is considered.
    - Patient requires step 4 or higher.

Note: Beers listed items, as mentioned above, include theophylline and oral corticosteroids.

## Differential Diagnosis[1,3]

- Chronic obstructive pulmonary disorder (COPD): Characterized by the lack of identifiable triggers, is affected by cigarette smoking, does not have fully reversible airflow on pulmonary function tests, lacks nocturnal symptoms, and has daily symptoms.
  - Asthma, however, has identifiable triggers, is not as affected by cigarette smoke as COPD, has close to fully reversible airflow on pulmonary function tests, is associated with nocturnal symptoms, and symptoms are intermittent.
- Heart failure (HF): Symptoms are closely related to asthma; however will likely have a history of coronary artery disease (CAD) and/or hypertension. Exam findings consistent with fluid overload (e.g., increased jugular vein distention [JVD], pedal edema), brain-type natriuretic peptide (BNP) levels will be elevated and may have positive chest X-ray (CXR) findings. Asthma will lack the cardiac history as seen with HF. Exam findings will lack findings associated with fluid overload. BNP levels will not be elevated unless HF is a comorbidity; CXR is usually normal in asthma.

### CLINICAL PEARLS[1,2,4,5,6,10]

- Use the Stepwise approach to managing asthma (shown in diagram on next page) to guide medical decision making.
- Asthma should be considered as an underlying diagnosis in those with unexplained and constant cough, especially at night.
- There are more asthma-related deaths in older individuals compared to any other age group. It is necessary to educate patients on asthma triggers, use of short-acting beta agonist during an acute exacerbation, and an action plan based on peak flow meter to improve outcomes.

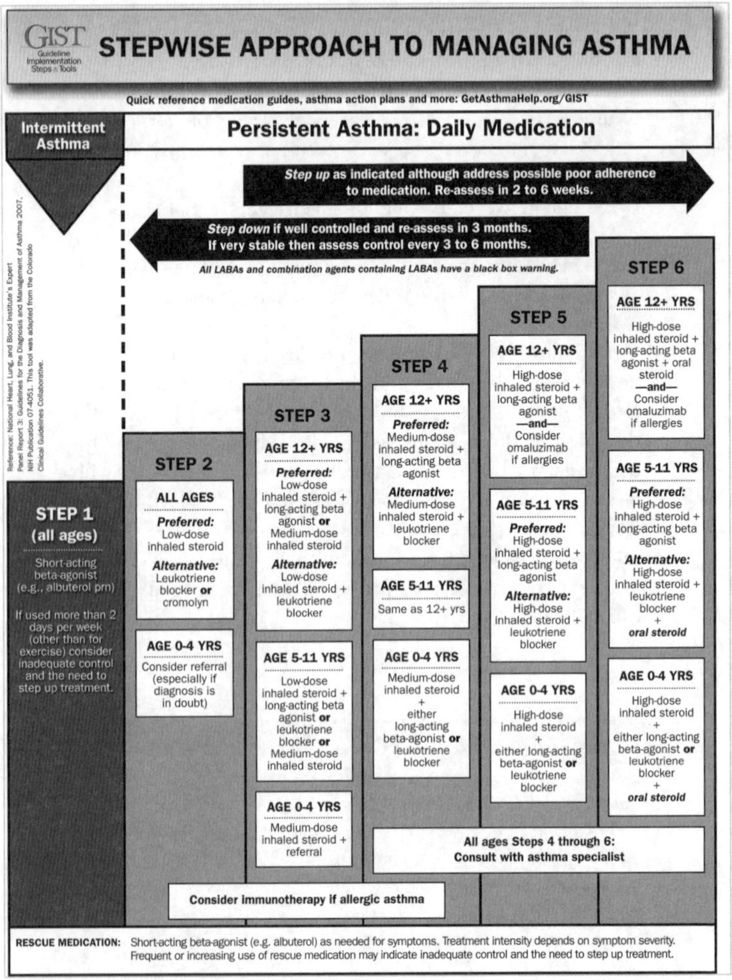


**Figure 4-1** GIST Stepwise Approach to Managing Asthma

Asthma Initiative of Michigan. Stepwise Approach to Managing Asthma. Retrieved from http://getasthmahelp.org/documents/gist-stepwise-approach.pdf.

## References

1. Akgün, K. M., Crothers, K., & Pisani, M. (2012, March). Epidemiology and management of common pulmonary diseases in older persons. *Journals of Gerontology Series A: Biological Sciences and Medical Sciences, 67A*(3), 276–291. Retrieved from https://www.ncbi.nlm.nih.gov/pmc/articles/PMC3297767/. Accessed November 25, 2017.
2. Ortega, V. E., & Pennington, E. J. (2017, March). Asthma – Pulmonary Disorders. Merck Manuals: Professional. Retrieved from http://www.merckmanuals.com/professional/pulmonary-disorders/asthma-and-related-disorders/asthma#v913553. Accessed November 30, 2017.
3. Ibrahim, I., & See, K. C. (2017, April 6). Asthma in Adults. Epocrates. Retrieved from https://online.epocrates.com/diseases/4411/Asthma-in-adults/Key-Highlights. Accessed November 30, 2017.
4. Rance, K., & O'Laughlen, M. (2014). Managing asthma in older adults. *Journal for Nurse Practitioners, 10*(1), 1–9. http://dx.doi.org/10.1016/j.nurpra.2013.11.009
5. Asthma. In Kasper, D., Fauci, A., Hauser, S., Longo, D., Jameson, J., & Loscalzo, J. *Harrison's Principles of Internal Medicine* (19th ed.). New York, NY: McGraw-Hill. Retrieved from http://accessmedicine.mhmedical.com/content.aspx?bookid=1130&sectionid=63653136. Accessed November 29, 2017.
6. Pulmonary disorders. In *Current Medical Diagnosis & Treatment 2018*. New York, NY: McGraw-Hill. Retrieved from http://accessmedicine.mhmedical.com/content.aspx?bookid=2192&sectionid=168189660. Accessed November 29, 2017.
7. National Heart, Lung, and Blood Institute. (2014, August 4). What Is Asthma? U.S. Department of Health and Human Services, National Institutes of Health. Retrieved from https://www.nhlbi.nih.gov/health/health-topics/topics/asthma. Accessed November 30, 2017.
8. Gulanick, M., & Myers, J. L. (2017). *Nursing Care Plans: Diagnoses, Interventions, & Outcomes*. St. Louis, MO: Elsevier.
9. American Geriatrics Society 2015 Beers Criteria Update Expert Panel, Fick, D. M., Semla, T. P., Beizer, J., Brandt, N., & Dombrowski, R., . . . Steinman, M. (2015, October 8). American Geriatrics Society 2015 updated Beers criteria for potentially inappropriate medication use in older adults. *Journal of the American Geriatrics Society, 63*(11), 2227–2246. Retrieved from http://onlinelibrary.wiley.com/doi/10.1111/jgs.13702/abstract. Accessed October 3, 2017.
10. National Heart, Lung, and Blood Institute. (n.d.). National Asthma Education and Prevention Program. Expert Panel Report 3: Guidelines for the Diagnosis and Management of Asthma. U.S. Department of Health and Human Services, National Institutes of Health. Retrieved from https://www.nhlbi.nih.gov/sites/default/files/media/docs/asthgdln_1.pdf. Accessed April 22, 2018.

# Chronic Obstructive Pulmonary Disease

## Definition[2,3,4,5]

Chronic obstructive pulmonary disease (COPD) is a progressive respiratory disease, characterized by the presence of airflow obstruction, which is partially reversible.

## Types[2,3,4,5]

*Main forms of COPD (can be both):*

- Emphysema: Alveoli are gradually destroyed (diagnosed pathologically).
- Chronic bronchitis: Inflamed bronchial tubes, leading to daily cough and sputum production for at least 3 months in 2 consecutive years (diagnosed clinically).

Note: The two forms of COPD are no longer distinguished between one another by the Global Initiative for Chronic Obstructive Lung Disease (GOLD).

## Causes[1,2,3,4,5,6,11]

- Cigarette smoke (e.g., pipe, cigar)
  - About 13 times more likely to die from COPD compared to nonsmokers.
- Secondhand smoke exposure
- Chronic environmental and/or occupational pollutants
  - Examples: chemical fumes and dusts, coal mine dusts, tunnel work, silica exposure.
- Alpha-1 antitrypsin deficiency
  - Rare; accounts for 2%–4% of cases.

## Risk Factors[1,2,4,5,11]

*Risk factors coincide with the causes of COPD.*

- Advanced age
- History of recurrent respiratory infections, asthma, or allergies
- Family history of COPD
- Low socioeconomic status

## Signs & Symptoms[1,2,4,5,11]

- Chronic cough
  - Worse in the morning.
- Sputum production
  - Suspect infectious exacerbation if sputum changes in color or amount.

- Dyspneic
  - Starts out being associated with exertion; with advanced disease, occurs at rest.
- Wheezing
- Impaired exercise tolerance
- Chest tightness
- Weight loss
- Diminished or distant breath sounds
- Hyperresonance on percussion
- Prolonged expiratory phase
- Increased anteroposterior chest diameter (barrel chest)
- Heart failure symptoms (e.g., jugular venous distention, pedal edema)
- Respiratory failure

## Tests[1,2,3,5,8,9,11,13]

- Pulmonary function test
  - Spirometry is the main test used to diagnose COPD.
- Pulse oximetry
  - In chronic COPD, oxygen saturation of 88%–90% is usually acceptable.
- Arterial blood gas
  - Shows severity of COPD and if oxygen therapy or intubation is warranted.
- Chest X-ray
  - Not required for diagnosis; findings are typically nonspecific; however can be ordered to evaluate for underlying conditions (e.g., lung mass, fibrotic changes, pulmonary edema, pneumonia).
- Complete blood count
  - May have elevated WBC. Can be ordered to evaluate for severe anemia, which can cause dyspnea.
- Chest computed tomography (CT) scan
  - More sensitive and specific for COPD than chest X-ray.
  - Not routinely ordered unless excluding other underlying pulmonary disease.

## Treatment & Management[1,2,3,4,5,8,9,11,14,15]

- **Nonpharmacological and nursing interventions:**
  - Identify and treat risk factors of COPD, such as:
    - Encouraging smoking cessation.
    - Avoiding secondhand smoke.
    - Inhaled toxic substances.
  - Encourage flu and pneumonia vaccination.
  - Assess the need for supplemental oxygen.
    - Oxygen therapy is warranted if levels drop below 88%–90%.
    - Start with low-flow oxygen therapy (e.g., nasal cannula 2 L/min) and titrate as indicated to avoid hypoxemia; monitor for oxygen-induced hypercapnia and apnea.
  - Assess the patient's hydration status (i.e., skin turgor, dry mouth).
    - Airway clearance is impaired when secretions are thickened; dehydration contributes to viscosity of secretions.
  - Encourage coughing to clear pulmonary secretions.
    - In individuals who are unable to clear secretions, perform nasotracheal suctioning with a lubricated catheter (reduces irritation).
    - To mobilize secretions, the following interventions can be done: Encourage fluid intake (at least 2 L/day unless contraindicated), use mucolytic agents, increase room humidification, encourage activity.
  - Caution administration of medications that lead to respiratory depression (e.g., opioids, benzodiazepines).
    - Monitor for decreased respiratory rate and hypoxemia.
    - Morphine is effective at reducing chronic dyspnea in severe COPD.
  - Monitor for infection and implement preventative measures.

    - Acute changes in sputum (e.g., production, color changes, and/or thickness) are signs of infection.
    - Encourage avoidance of crowds; ensure rest, optimal nutritional intake, and frequent handwashing to reduce infection.
  - Monitor closely for respiratory compromise.
    - Use of accessory muscles, tripod position, increased respiratory rate, rhythm changes, increasing $PaCO_2$ and decreased $PaO_2$.
    - Monitor patients closely for the following and anticipate potential intubation and mechanical ventilation: unable to maintain airway against aspiration (e.g., decreased consciousness and inability to handle secretions), inability to ventilate or oxygenate appropriately, or impending airway obstruction or failure.
- **Pharmacological and other interventions:**
  - Rescue therapy: short-acting beta-2 agonists, metered-dose inhaler or by nebulizer (e.g., albuterol [ProAir HFA, Ventolin HFA], levalbuterol [Xopenex])
    - Example: albuterol 1–2 puffs every 4–6 hr PRN.
    - These medications work quickly, reduce bronchoconstriction, making it easier to breath.
    - Recommended as needed in mild COPD and acute exacerbation.
    - Monitor for hypokalemia, inability to sleep, tremor, arrhythmias, and palpitations.
  - Maintenance therapy: long-acting beta-2 agonists (LABAs) (e.g., formoterol [Perforomist], salmeterol [Serevent Diskus], arformoterol [Brovana])
    - Example: formoterol inhaled 20 mcg nebulizer q12 hours.
    - These are recommended in moderate to severe COPD; they improve respiratory symptoms, nocturnal bronchospasms, exacerbations, exercise endurance, and quality of life and reduce hospital admissions.

- For additional improvement, they are combined with inhaled corticosteroids (e.g., budesonide/formoterol [Symbicort]) or long-acting anticholinergic bronchodilator (e.g., tiotropium [Spiriva]/formoterol [Perforomist]).
- Side effects are similar as the above rescue therapy; however milder.

- Maintenance therapy: anticholinergic inhaled bronchodilators, short acting (e.g., ipratropium bromide [Atrovent HFA]) or long acting (e.g., tiotropium [Spiriva])
  - Example: ipratropium bromide 2 puffs inhaled 4 times daily.
  - Short-acting anticholinergic works well with beta-2 agonists to further relieve bronchoconstriction (e.g., ipratropium bromide/albuterol inhaled [Duoneb]).
  - Longer-acting anticholinergics can be used by themselves for stable COPD and are superior to long-acting beta agonists.
  - Monitor for xerostomia, taste changes, urinary retention, glaucoma.
- Glucocorticosteroids, oral (e.g., prednisone [Deltasone]) or inhaled (e.g., beclomethasone [Qvar], ciclesonide [Alvesco])
  - Example: prednisone 40 mg daily PO for 5 days.
  - Oral is used for acute COPD exacerbations to reduce airway inflammation. Use lowest dose effective for short period; they may cause or worsen delirium.
  - Inhaled is indicated for long-term treatment in those with advanced COPD and frequent exacerbations not managed with a long-acting beta agonist or long-acting anticholinergic bronchodilator. It is not recommended as monotherapy in stable COPD; order in combination with long-acting beta agonist to improve lung function and reduce exacerbations.
  - Inhaled corticosteroids increase the risk of pneumonia, whereas oral increases the risk of osteoporosis (long-term use), hyperglycemia, and delirium.

- Maintenance therapy: theophylline, a nonspecific phosphodiesterase inhibitor
  - Example: Start theophylline 300 mg PO daily (divided doses q6–8 hours).
    - Avoid use if taking ciprofloxacin (Cipro) (increased risk of hospitalization).
  - Reduces COPD exacerbations; however does not improve lung function. Consider this medication in moderate to severe COPD when beta-2 agonist, inhaled anticholinergics, and steroids fail to achieve symptoms control.
  - Aim for a range of 8–13 mg/dL.
  - Caution use in patients with insomnia; has CNS stimulant effects. Monitor for headaches, heartburn, and potential arrhythmias or seizures.
- Maintenance therapy: phosphodiesterase-4 inhibitors (e.g., roflumilast [Daliresp])
  - Example: roflumilast 500 mcg PO daily.
    - Not to be given with theophylline.
  - Reduces inflammation and useful for frequent exacerbations in moderate to severe COPD.
  - Monitor for weight loss, gastrointestinal disturbances, insomnia, and headache.
- Mucolytic agents (e.g., guaifenesin [Mucinex])
  - Limited evidence supports its use.
  - Used during acute exacerbations to reduce sputum viscosity.
  - Usually well tolerated.
- Antibiotics (e.g., doxycycline [Vibramycin], cefprozil [Cefzil], azithromycin [Zmax, Zithromax], amoxicillin-clavulanate [Augmentin], or fluoroquinolone)
  - Azithromycin 250 mg PO daily or 3 times weekly can be used for maintenance therapy for frequent exacerbations (may cause QT prolongation or hearing loss).

    - Antibiotic depends upon local bacterial resistance patterns and risk of pseudomonas infection; 5 days is usually effective.
    - Antibiotics are recommended in those with COPD to treat the following: acute exacerbations (e.g., increase dyspnea, changes in sputum volume and purulence), acute bronchitis, and prophylactically to prevent exacerbation in chronic bronchitis.
  - Supplemental oxygen therapy
    - Titrate to keep oxygen saturation between 88%–92%.
- Palliative care referral
  - To improve quality of life and provide relief of symptoms; as patient declines consider transition to hospice services.
- Pulmonology consultation/referral
- Pulmonary rehabilitation
  - Improves exercise capacity, reduces depression and anxiety, and improves quality of life.

Note: Beers listed items, as mentioned above, include theophylline, oral corticosteroids.

## Differential Diagnosis[8,10,13]

- Asthma: This is typically diagnosed earlier on in childhood or adolescence; patients may have rhinitis or eczema and are typically nonsmokers. Flare-ups are caused by allergens, cold air, or exercise.
  - In comparison to COPD: Diagnosed later in life, patients typically have a history of tobacco smoke use or secondhand smoke exposure, and flare-ups are caused by respiratory tract infections.
- Heart failure (HF): Symptoms are similar to COPD; however, BNP levels may be elevated and chest X-ray positive for pulmonary edema or enlarged heart. Diagnosis is confirmed by echocardiogram. COPD risk factors are different (e.g., smoking) compared to HF (e.g., hypertension and CAD).

## CLINICAL PEARLS[2]

- Be sure to manage comorbidities that commonly coexist with COPD (e.g., CAD, HF, depression, anxiety) given these can worsen symptoms, cause acute COPD exacerbations, and impact prognosis.

# References


1. National Heart, Lung, and Blood Institute. (2017, April 28). What Is COPD? U.S. Department of Health and Human Services, National Institutes of Health. Retrieved from https://www.nhlbi.nih.gov/health/health-topics/topics/copd/. Accessed November 28, 2017.
2. Salzman, B., & Snyderman, D. Chronic obstructive pulmonary disease. In *Current Diagnosis & Treatment: Geriatrics* (2nd ed.). New York, NY: McGraw-Hill. Retrieved from http://accessmedicine.mhmedical.com/content.aspx?bookid=953&sectionid=53375658. Accessed November 28, 2017.
3. Fragoso, C., Akgün, K. M., Jeffery, S. M., Kapo, J. M., Possick, J. D., Rochester, C. L., & Lee, P. J. (2017). Chronic obstructive pulmonary disease. In *Hazzard's Geriatric Medicine and Gerontology* (7th ed.). New York, NY: McGraw-Hill. Retrieved from http://accessmedicine.mhmedical.com/content.aspx?bookid=1923&sectionid=144525549. Accessed November 28, 2017.
4. Goldwasser, J. (2014). Pulmonary disease. In Burggraf, V., Kim, K. Y., & Knight, A. L. (Eds.) *Healthy Aging: Principles and Clinical Practice for Clinicians* (pp. 161–176). Philadelphia, PA: Lippincott Williams & Wilkins.
5. Pulmonary disorders. In *Current Medical Diagnosis & Treatment 2018*. New York, NY: McGraw-Hill. Retrieved from http://accessmedicine.mhmedical.com/content.aspx?bookid=2192&sectionid=168189660. Accessed November 28, 2017.
6. Corbridge, S. J., & Nyenhuis, S. M. (2017). Promoting physical activity and exercise in patients with asthma and chronic obstructive pulmonary disease. *Journal for Nurse Practitioners, 13*(1), 41–46. http://dx.doi.org/10.1016/j.nurpra.2016.08.022
7. Boka, K. (2016, August 31). Emphysema (Mosenifar, Z., Ed.). Medscape. Retrieved from https://emedicine.medscape.com/article/298283-overview. Accessed November 28, 2017.
8. Sharifabad, M. A. (2017, June 15). COPD. Epocrates. Retrieved from https://online.epocrates.com/diseases/711/COPD/Key-Highlights. Accessed November 28, 2017.
9. Han, M. K. (2017, September 19). Patient Education: Chronic Obstructive Pulmonary Disease (COPD), Including Emphysema (Beyond the Basics) (Stoller, J. K., & Hollingsworth, H., Eds.). UpToDate. Retrieved from http://www.uptodate.com/contents/chronic-obstructive-pulmonary-disease-copd-including-emphysema-beyond-the-basics. Accessed November 28, 2017.
10. Is It Asthma or COPD? (2015, March 29). Lung Institute. Retrieved from https://lunginstitute.com/blog/is-it-asthma-or-copd/. Accessed November 28, 2017.
11. Gulanick, M., & Myers, J. L. (2017). *Nursing Care Plans: Diagnoses, Interventions, & Outcomes*. St. Louis, MO: Elsevier.
12. Lafferty, K. A. (2017, March 23). Rapid Sequence Intubation (Byrd, R. P., Ed.). Medscape. Retrieved from https://emedicine.medscape.com/article/80222-overview. Accessed November 29, 2017.

13. Wise, R.A. (2017, January). Chronic Obstructive Pulmonary Disease (COPD) – Pulmonary Disorders. Merck Manuals: Professional. Retrieved from http://www.merckmanuals.com/professional/pulmonary-disorders/chronic-obstructive-pulmonary-disease-and-related-disorders/chronic-obstructive-pulmonary-disease-copd#v8575629. Accessed November 29, 2017.
14. American Geriatrics Society 2015 Beers Criteria Update Expert Panel, Fick, D. M., Semla, T. P., Beizer, J., Brandt, N., & Dombrowski, R., . . . Steinman, M. (2015, October 8). American Geriatrics Society 2015 updated Beers criteria for potentially inappropriate medication use in older adults. *Journal of the American Geriatrics Society,* 63(11), 2227–2246. Retrieved from http://onlinelibrary.wiley.com/doi/10.1111/jgs.13702/abstract. Accessed October 8, 2017.
15. What Are Palliative Care and Hospice Care? (2017, May 17). https://www.nia.nih.gov/health/what-are-palliative-care-and-hospice-care#palliative-vs-hospice. Accessed May 8, 2018.

# Idiopathic Pulmonary Fibrosis

## Definition[1,2,3,4,5]

Idiopathic pulmonary fibrosis (IPF) is a rapidly progressive lung disease characterized by lung scar tissue.

## Causes[2,3,4,5]

- Unknown
- Possibly occupational, environmental, and/or genetic factors

## Risk Factors[1,2,3,4,5]

- Age > 60 years
- Male sex
- Family history of IPF
- Smoking cigarettes
- Chronic aspiration
- Exposure to organic and/or inorganic dust
  - Silica, metal dust, wood dust, bird proteins
- Some medications
  - Nitrofurantoin (Macrobid, Furadantin), amiodarone (Cordarone, Pacerone), methotrexate (Otrexup, Rasuov, Trexall)
- Gastroesophageal reflux disease *(possibly due to acid aspiration)*

- Acute and chronic viral infections
  - Epstein-Barr virus, hepatitis C, adenovirus, cytomegalovirus
- Diabetes

## Signs & Symptoms[1,2,3,4,5]

- Dyspnea (*most common symptom*).
- Cough (*nonproductive and intractable*).
- Bibasilar crackles.
- Fatigue.
- Clubbing.
- Weight loss.
- Hemoptysis.
- As IPF progresses, symptoms of heart failure and pulmonary hypertension will ensue.

## Tests[1,3,4,5,7]

*Serum laboratory testing offers little advantage in IPF diagnosis*

- Chest X-ray
  - Most will have abnormal findings (e.g., reticular opacities).
- CT, high-resolution
  - Should be ordered in all patients with presumed IPF.
  - Findings highly suggest IPF and can prevent the need for lung biopsy.
  - Findings in advanced IPF may reveal honeycombing and/or traction bronchiectasis.
- Lung function test
  - This test further supports the diagnosis; will show evidence of restriction and provides information regarding severity of disease.
- Pulse oximetry
  - Should be checked at rest and with ambulation to assess the need for oxygen therapy.
- Lung biopsy
  - Ordered when other tests do not support the diagnosis of IPF.

## Treatment & Management[1,2,3,4,5,6,7,8,9]

- **Nonpharmacological and nursing interventions:**
  - Encourage smoking cessation.
  - Encourage flu and pneumonia vaccination.
  - Educate patient and family members regarding the diagnosis and prognosis.
    - Most will not be familiar of IPF and are unaware of the poor survival rate.
  - Encourage involvement in support groups and offer coping strategies to reduce stress.
  - Monitor for acute exacerbations of IPF.
    - This includes worsening dyspnea (within a few days to a month), high-resolution CT findings that show ground-class opacities, and worsening hypoxemia in the absence of heart failure or infectious process.
- **Pharmacological and other interventions:**

  *There is no proven treatment for IPF.*
  - Prednisone (Rayos)
    - Example: prednisone 0.5 mg/kg PO daily for 4 weeks, followed by half the dose daily for 8 weeks, followed by half of that dose once daily.
    - Ordered for acute exacerbations.
    - Steroids increase the risk of osteoporosis (long-term use), hyperglycemia, and can worsen delirium.
  - Pirfenidone (Esbriet) or nintedanib (Ofev)
    - Example: pirfenidone 267 mg PO TID for a week, then gradually increased to 801 mg.
    - Slows disease progression and are recommended first-line treatment if not experiencing an exacerbation.
    - Pirfenidone may reduce IPF exacerbations.
      - May cause gastrointestinal disturbances, weight loss, and/or transaminitis.

- Proton-pump inhibitors (PPIs) (e.g., lansoprazole [Prevacid], omeprazole [Prilosec)
  - Example: omeprazole 20 mg PO QD-BID.
  - The use of these drugs is associated with longer survival time.
  - May cause diarrhea, vitamin B12 deficiency, or low magnesium levels if used long term.
- Benzonatate (Tessalon), guaifenesin (Mucinex), low-dose opiates (e.g., codeine), or thalidomide
  - Used to alleviate cough symptom.
- Manage comorbid conditions
  - Conditions such as heart failure can lead to acute deterioration.
- Oxygen therapy
  - Recommended when oxygen saturation drops < 90%.
- Pulmonary rehabilitation
  - This will improve function and quality of life.
- Lung transplant
  - Survival rate in older adults is lower following transplant; however is still offered to those > age 65 years, if no contraindications.
- Pulmonology, palliative or hospice care, and/or thoracic surgeon consultation/referral
  - Thoracic surgeon needed if planning for lung biopsy.
  - Palliative care improves quality of life and provides relief of symptoms; as patient declines consider transition to hospice services.

Note: Beers listed items, as mentioned above, include proton pump inhibitors (avoid use beyond 8 weeks) and oral corticosteroids.

## Differential Diagnosis[3,7]

- Sarcoidosis: This typically involves younger persons; involves the lungs, skin, and eyes. Lymphadenopathy is a key finding on chest imaging. IPF involves older adults and involves mainly lungs. Key finding on imaging are reticular opacities, honey-combing, and traction bronchiectasis.

- COPD: Symptoms are similar to IPF except wheezing and barrel chest are common with COPD; wheezing and barrel chest are not features seen with IPF. Spirometry is main test used to diagnose COPD. The main tests used in diagnosing IPF are a chest X-ray and high-resolution CT.

## CLINICAL PEARLS[1,2,4,5,6,7]

- Given poor prognosis of IPF and median survival rate of about 2–3 years, it is important to have discussions regarding advanced care planning, given patients will eventually need palliative care.

## References


1. Akgün, K. M., Crothers, K., & Pisani, M. (2012, March). Epidemiology and management of common pulmonary diseases in older persons. *Journals of Gerontology Series A: Biological Sciences and Medical Sciences, 67A*(3), 276–291. Accessed November 25, 2017.
2. Lee, J. (2016, April). Idiopathic Pulmonary Fibrosis – Pulmonary Disorders. Retrieved from http://www.merckmanuals.com/professional/pulmonary-disorders/interstitial-lung-diseases/idiopathic-pulmonary-fibrosis. Accessed December 4, 2017.
3. Flesch, J. D., & Kreider, M. E. (2017, February 27). Idiopathic Pulmonary Fibrosis. Epocrates. Retrieved from https://online.epocrates.com/diseases/44611/Idiopathic-pulmonary-fibrosis/Key-Highlights. Accessed December 4, 2017.
4. Scholand, M., & Paine, R. (2017). Diffuse parenchymal lung disease. In *Hazzard's Geriatric Medicine and Gerontology* (7th ed.). New York, NY: McGraw-Hill. Retrieved from http://accessmedicine.mhmedical.com/content.aspx?bookid=1923&sectionid=144525711. Accessed December 3, 2017.
5. Idiopathic pulmonary fibrosis. In *Clinical Genomics: Practical Applications in Adult Patient Care* (1st ed.). New York, NY: McGraw-Hill. Retrieved from http://accessmedicine.mhmedical.com/content.aspx?bookid=1094&sectionid=61905489. Accessed December 4, 2017.
6. Interstitial lung diseases. In Kasper, D., Fauci, A., Hauser, S., Longo, D., Jamesom, J., & Loscalzo, J. (Eds.) *Harrison's Principles of Internal Medicine* (19th ed.). New York, NY: McGraw-Hill. Retrieved from http://accessmedicine.mhmedical.com/content.aspx?bookid=1130&sectionid=79745176. Accessed December 4, 2017.
7. Duck, A. (2014, April 11). Management of idiopathic pulmonary fibrosis. *Nursing Times, 110*(16), 16–17. Retrieved from https://www.nursingtimes.net/Journals/2014/04/11/p/n/x/160414-Management-of-idiopathic-pulmonary-fibrosis.pdf. Accessed December 4, 2017.

8. American Geriatrics Society 2015 Beers Criteria Update Expert Panel, Fick, D. M., Semla, T. P., Beizer, J., Brandt, N., & Dombrowski, R., . . . Steinman, M. (2015, October 8). American Geriatrics Society 2015 updated Beers criteria for potentially inappropriate medication use in older adults. *Journal of the American Geriatrics Society, 63*(11), 2227–2246. Retrieved http://onlinelibrary.wiley.com/doi/10.1111/jgs.13702/abstract. Accessed October 3, 2017.
9. Rajala, K., Lehto, J. T., Saarinen, M., Sutinen, E., Saarto, T., & Myllärniemi, M. (2016). End-of-life care of patients with idiopathic pulmonary fibrosis. *BMC Palliative Care, 15*(85). doi:10.1186/s12904-016-0158-8

# Lung Cancer

## Definition[2,9]

Lung cancer is a malignant neoplasm that emerges from the lining of the lower respiratory tract (e.g., bronchioles, alveoli).

## Types[1,5,6,7]

**Non-small cell lung cancer (NSCLC):** This is the most common and accounts for ~85% of lung cancers. The subtypes include adenocarcinoma, squamous cell carcinoma, and large cell carcinoma.

Note: These subtypes are grouped under NSCLC due to corresponding diagnostic, staging, and treatment approaches.

**Small cell lung cancer (SCLC):** Also known as oat cell cancer; occurs mainly in heavy smokers, spreads rapidly, and accounts for ~10%–15% of lung cancers. About 80% will have metastatic disease by the time it is diagnosed.

**Lung carcinoid tumor:** Also known as lung neuroendocrine tumor; it accounts for less than 5% of lung cancers, grows at a slow pace, and rarely spreads.

## Causes[1,2,3,6,8,10]

- Smoking (leading cause).
- Genetic factors.
- Not all cases have a clear cause.

## Risk Factors[1,2,3,4,6,8]

- Smoking (e.g., cigarette, cigar, pipe)
- Secondhand smoke
- Radon gas exposure
- Asbestos exposure
- Outdoor air pollution
- Workplace exposure (e.g., diesel exhaust, coal products, mustard gas)
- Prior chest radiation therapy
- Comorbidities (pulmonary fibrosis, COPD, sarcoidosis, HIV)
- Personal or family history of lung cancer
- Advanced age
- Arsenic water (especially Southeast Asia and South America)
- Beta carotene supplementation

## Signs & Symptoms[1,3,6,7,8,10]

*Varies depending upon the type and location of primary tumor, the degree of local spread, and/or accompanying metastases.*

- Asymptomatic (25%)
- Persistent cough
- Chest or rib discomfort (description of this may be vague)
- Unintentional weight loss
- Dyspnea (*may be seen with development of a pleural effusion*)
- Hemoptysis
- Hoarseness (*may be seen due to laryngeal nerve involvement*)
- Bone pain or fractures (*may be seen with bone metastasis*)
- Headache, seizure, and/or dizziness (*may be seen with brain metastasis*)
- Lymphadenopathy
- Superior vena cava syndrome
  - Obstructed superior vena cava leading to facial swelling, dyspnea especially when supine, and dilated veins in the neck or face
  - Medical emergency
- Digital clubbing (*may be seen as a result of paraneoplastic syndrome; more common with NSCLC*)

## Tests[1,2,3,4,6,7,8,9,10]

- Serum CBC, ionized calcium, sodium, liver function tests (LFTs), and creatinine
  - CBC may show anemia (chemotherapy impairs hematopoiesis).
  - Paraneoplastic syndrome (i.e., how the body reacts to hormones secreted by tumor cells) can lead to hypercalcemia and syndrome of inappropriate diuretic hormone (SIADH).
  - Bone metastases can present with elevated liver enzymes.
  - Assessment of renal function is necessary prior to treatment (some chemotherapy agents impair renal function).
- Chest X-ray
  - Usually the first imaging test. Findings suggestive of lung cancer may include abnormal mass or nodule, enlarged hilum, infiltrate(s), widened mediastinum, or pleural effusion.
- Chest CT, contrast-enhanced
  - Ordered when suspicious for lung cancer and unremarkable chest radiograph.
  - Findings on CT can strongly suggest lung cancer and show the size, shape, and position of tumors.
  - Ordered to guide core needle biopsy.
- Cytology sputum
  - A simple and noninvasive test; indicated for central lesions. Recommended to obtain this in the early morning hours.
- Percutaneous biopsy
  - Useful for metastatic sites (e.g., peripheral lymph nodes).
- Bronchoscopy
  - Most often performed to diagnose lung cancer; works best for central lesions.
- Thoracentesis with cytology evaluation
  - Useful in diagnosing lung cancer in those with suspected malignant pleural effusions.

- Other tests: CT scan, magnetic resonance imaging (MRI), positive emission tomography (PET) scan, and/or bone scan
  - Used to check for metastatic disease.

## Treatment & Management[2,3,4,5,8,10,11,12,13,14,15]

- **Nonpharmacological and nursing interventions:**
  - Educate on avoiding tobacco use and/or exposure.
  - Provide supportive care to the patient and family members.
    - Varies depending upon severity of disease.
    - Offer psychological and spiritual assistance.
    - Some sources that offer advice on coping, understanding of lung cancer, and/or support system: www.cancer.org, www.lung.org, and www.nccn.org.
  - Anticipate treatment for paraneoplastic syndrome.
    - Limiting water intake with SIADH.
    - Encouraging fluid intake and use of bisphosphonates with hypercalcemia.
  - Monitor for oncological emergencies, such as superior vena cava syndrome.
    - Requires surgery, chemotherapy, and/or surgical intervention.
- **Pharmacological and other interventions:**

  *Treatment is individualized, complex, and involves a multidisciplinary approach.*
  - Provide adequate pain relief and monitor for common adverse effects, such as constipation.
    - NSAIDs: Treat muscle spasms associated with lung cancer.
      - Carries risk of gastrointestinal (GI) bleeding.
    - Opioids (short and/or long acting): Effective at relieving cancer pain, including bone metastases. Offer transdermal opioids if unable to take oral opioids.

## Non-Small Cell Lung Cancer

- Stage I and II disease
  - Surgical resection, preferably lobectomy or pneumonectomy.
    - In those with comorbidities and/or poor pulmonary reserve: wedge resection or segmentectomy.
    - If not a candidate for surgery, will need radiation therapy with adjuvant chemotherapy.
  - Chemotherapy and/or radiation.
- Stage III disease
  - Surgical resection, preferably lobectomy or pneumonectomy.
  - Chemotherapy, radiation therapy, and/or chemoradiation.
- Stage IV disease
  - Chemotherapy, palliative radiation therapy, and targeted drugs.
  - Goal at this stage is to relieve symptoms and reduce tumor burden.

## Small Cell Lung Cancer

- Limited stage and extensive stage: chemotherapy and/or radiation therapy
- Surgery
  - Rarely indicated.
- Cranial radiation
  - Warranted in some cases to prevent brain metastases.

## Lung Carcinoid Tumor

- Surgical resection (main treatment)
  - If unable to have surgery, radiation therapy is an option.
- Chemotherapy, radiation, somatostatin analogs (e.g., ocreotide [Sandostatin]), interferons, and targeted drugs

- Pulmonology, palliative or hospice care, oncology, radiation oncology, pathologist, radiology, and/or thoracic surgery consultation/referral
- Pain specialist consultation/referral
  - This would be appropriate if opioids are considered. Be aware of your state regulations and guidelines; some states require referral when going above specific dosage levels.

Note: Beers listed items, as mentioned above, include opioids and NSAIDs.

## Differential Diagnosis[11]

- COPD: Main symptoms are cough, sputum production, and dyspnea; imaging would not show a tumor. In comparison to lung cancer, some patients are asymptomatic whereas others have symptoms similar to COPD; however, imaging test (CT) will show a tumor.
- Pneumonia: May show infection symptoms such as fever and/or tachypnea; symptoms would improve with antibiotic therapy. In comparison to lung cancer, there would be a lack of infectious symptoms and symptoms would continue despite antibiotic therapy.

### CLINICAL PEARLS[4,5,8]

- Older individuals with lung cancer experience more side effects from chemotherapy and myelosuppression.
- Lung cancer prognosis is impacted by the stage of disease and performance status.
- Treatment is individualized; older adults with poor nutritional status and multiple comorbidities may not be able to undergo chemotherapy, radiation, or surgery. Palliative care, when implemented early on, can prolong longevity, improve mood, and improve quality of life.

# References


1. Mayo Clinic. (2015, September 25). Lung Cancer: Reduce Your Risk by Quitting Smoking. Retrieved from https://www.mayoclinic.org/diseases-conditions/lung-cancer/basics/definition/CON-20025531. Accessed December 1, 2017.
2. American Cancer Society. (n.d.). Lung Cancer. Retrieved from https://www.cancer.org/cancer/lung-cancer.html. Accessed December 1, 2017.
3. Tsao, A. S. (2016, March). Lung Carcinoma – Pulmonary Disorders. Merck Manuals: Professional. Retrieved from http://www.merckmanuals.com/professional/pulmonary-disorders/tumors-of-the-lungs/lung-carcinoma. Accessed December 1, 2017.
4. Presley, C., Maggiore, R., & Gajra, A. (2017). Lung cancer. In *Hazzard's Geriatric Medicine and Gerontology* (7th ed.). New York, NY: McGraw-Hill. Retrieved from http://accessmedicine.mhmedical.com/content.aspx?bookid=1923&sectionid=144527301. Accessed December 1, 2017.
5. Common cancers. In *Current Diagnosis & Treatment: Geriatrics* (2nd ed.). New York, NY: McGraw-Hill. Retrieved from http://accessmedicine.mhmedical.com/content.aspx?bookid=953&sectionid=53375668. Accessed December 1, 2017.
6. Cancer. In *Current Medical Diagnosis & Treatment 2018*. New York, NY: McGraw-Hill. Retrieved from http://accessmedicine.mhmedical.com/content.aspx?bookid=2192&sectionid=168004201. Accessed December 1, 2017.
7. Nickloes, T. A. (2017, May 15). Superior Vena Cava Syndrome (Rowe, V. L., Ed.). Medscape. Retrieved from https://emedicine.medscape.com/article/460865-overview?pa=009n7%2B42VkuAsxjmiDkbEB5xPA%2B%2BJ3uHqjqBLq6PMjX8BmQW1nK5ae3J12zaCk2JJyGvMX%2Fu%2BWdIXoARf%2FT0zw%3D%3D#a4. Accessed December 2, 2017.
8. Latimer, K. M., & Mott, T. F. (2015, February 15). Lung cancer: Diagnosis, treatment principles, and screening. *American Family Physician,* 91(4), 250–256. Retrieved from http://www.aafp.org/afp/2015/0215/p250.html. Accessed December 2, 2017.
9. Heist, R. S. (2016, October 10). Small Cell Lung Cancer. Epocrates. Retrieved from https://online.epocrates.com/diseases/108111/Small-cell-lung-cancer/Key-Highlights. Accessed December 1, 2017.
10. Gulanick, M., & Myers, J. L. (2017). *Nursing Care Plans: Diagnoses, Interventions, & Outcomes*. St. Louis, MO: Elsevier.
11. Baldwin, D. R., & Popat, S. (2016, October 10). Non-Small Cell Lung Cancer. Epocrates. Retrieved from https://online.epocrates.com/diseases/108211/Non-small-cell-lung-cancer/Key-Highlights. Accessed December 3, 2017.
12. American Geriatrics Society 2015 Beers Criteria Update Expert Panel, Fick, D. M., Semla, T. P., Beizer, J., Brandt, N., & Dombrowski, R., . . . Steinman, M. (2015, October 8). American Geriatrics Society 2015 updated Beers criteria for potentially inappropriate medication use in older adults. *Journal of the American Geriatrics Society,* 63(11), 2227–2246. Retrieved from http://onlinelibrary.wiley.com/doi/10.1111/jgs.13702/abstract. Accessed October 3, 2017.
13. Dowell, D., Haegerich, T. M., & Chou R. CDC Guideline for Prescribing Opioids for Chronic Pain — United States, 2016. MMWR Recomm Rep 2016;65(No. RR-1):1–49. DOI: http://dx.doi.org/10.15585/mmwr.rr6501e1
14. The American Academy of Pain Medicine. For the Primary Care Provider: When to Refer to a Pain specialist. (2016, December 1). Retrieved from http://www.painmed.org/files/when-to-refer-a-pain-specialist.pdf. Acccessed April 25, 2018.
15. What Are Palliative Care and Hospice Care? (2017, May 17). Retrieved from https://www.nia.nih.gov/health/what-are-palliative-care-and-hospice-care#palliative-vs-hospice. Accessed May 18, 2018.

# Pneumonia

## Definition[1,4,5]

Pneumonia is an infectious process involving the lung parenchyma.

## Types[1,4,8]

**Community-acquired pneumonia (CAP):** pneumonia occurring outside the hospital setting.
**Atypical pneumonia:** a type of CAP, which is a pneumonia caused by less common organisms.
**Aspiration pneumonia:** pneumonia caused from regurgitated food or liquid (includes saliva and vomit).
**Healthcare-associated pneumonia (HCAP):** pneumonia occurring with any one of the following:

- Residing in a nursing home or long-term care facility
- Hospitalized for ≥ 2 days in the past 3 months
- Undergone infusion therapy in the prior month
- Received dialysis in the prior month
- Receiving home wound care in the prior month
- Close relative who has infection due to multidrug-resistant organism

## Causes[1,2,4,5,6,8,9]

- Bacteria (most commonly the cause of pneumonia)
  - *Streptococcus pneumonia,* aka pneumococcus
    - Most common cause of CAP.
  - *Haemophilus influenzae*
  - *Staphylococcus aureus*
    - Seen among nursing home patients.
  - *Pseudomonas aeruginosa*
    - Seen in individuals with severe COPD ($FEV_1 < 35\%$).
  - *Enterobacteriaceae* and/or anaerobic organisms
    - Common in those who are institutionalized and with aspiration pneumonia, poor oral hygiene, and/or dysphagia.

  - Methicillin-resistant *Staphylococcus aureus* (MRSA)
    - Especially with HCAP.
  - Atypical bacteria: *Legionella pneumophila* (found in fresh water environments), *Chlamydophila pneumoniae*, *Mycoplasma pneumoniae*
- Viruses
  - Influenza (*most common*)
  - Respiratory syncytial virus (RSV)
  - Human metapneumovirus (HMPV)

Note: These listed viruses answer for ~8%–14% of pneumonias in older adults.

- Fungi (not as common)
  - *Aspergillus* spp.
  - *Pneumocystis jirovecii*
    - Seen in immunosuppressed states, such as HIV infection.

## Risk Factors[1,2,3,4,6,8]

- Advanced age
- Male sex
- Dysphagia and/or aspiration history
- Tobacco use
- Functional disability
- Malnutrition
- Cancer
- Lung disease (e.g., COPD, asthma)
- Neurological disorders (e.g., stroke, Parkinson's disease, dementia)
- Recent hospitalization or surgery
- Some medications (e.g., sedatives, antipsychotics)
- Feeding tube
- Cardiovascular disease
- Diabetes
- Heart failure
- Liver and/or renal disease
- Immunosuppressed state

## Signs & Symptoms[1,2,3,6,7,8,9]

*Most are asymptomatic or present atypically.*

- Lack of abnormal vital signs (e.g., fever, hypoxemia, tachycardia)
- Few respiratory symptoms (e.g., cough, expectoration)
- New onset dyspnea and bronchospasms (*especially viral pneumonia*)
- Chills, body aches, possible fever, sore throat, and cough with influenza
- Delirium
- Exacerbation of underlying conditions
- Fatigue
- Falls
- Impaired appetite
- Dizziness
- Volume depletion
- Incontinence

## Tests[1,3,4,5,6,8,9]

*Physical examination to establish pneumonia has poor sensitivity.*

- Chest X-ray
  - Establishes the diagnosis; radiologic signs are not as clear in those with volume depletion and/or neutropenia.
  - If chest X-ray is negative and clinical suspicion remains high, repeat test in 24–48 hours.
- Serum C-reactive protein (CRP), procalcitonin, WBC, lactate, blood cultures, blood urea nitrogen (BUN)/creatinine
  - Older adults may lack elevated CRP and/or WBC levels.
  - Procalcitonin can be used for severity assessment.
  - Lactate levels $\geq$ 2 mmol/L predicts mortality within a months' time in older adults.
  - Blood cultures are reserved in severe pneumonia; identifies causative pathogen if bacteremia is present and guides appropriate antibiotic regimen.
  - Checking renal function guides antimicrobial selection.

- Nasopharyngeal swab, polymerase chain reaction
  - If suspicious for influenza-related pneumonia.
- Computerized tomography (CT)
  - Very accurate; however, reserved in those who do not improve with pneumonia treatment. Can check for complications such as lung abscess or pleural effusion.
- Gram stain and culture of sputum
  - If is often difficult to obtain quality sputum specimens; about one-third will have adequate cultures. It is therefore not helpful in most older adults.
- Urine test to obtain bacterial antigen
  - Not routinely ordered in the outpatient setting.
  - Specific to pneumococcal and *L. pneumophila* bacteria.

## Treatment & Management[1,3,5,6,7,8,9,10,11,12]

- **Nonpharmacological and nursing interventions:**
  - Encourage flu and pneumonia vaccination in all patients age 65 and above (protective factor).
  - Wash hands frequently, cover coughs and sneezes, and do not share eating utensils to prevent the spread.
  - Encourage smoking cessation.
  - Encourage routine oral care.
    - Proper oral care in those with risk of aspiration pneumonia may reduce pneumonia.
  - Encourage activity.
    - Early mobility is linked to more favorable outcomes (e.g., decreased hospital days, mobilizes secretions, reduces atelectasis).
  - Encourage sufficient nutritional and fluid status.
    - Nutritional supplementation is associated with faster recovery.
    - Offering fluids reduces confusion and improves airway clearance by reducing viscosity of secretions; offer a minimum of 1–2 L daily.

- Offer oxygen in patients with hypoxemia (recommended to have saturation ≥ 90%).
- Use humidifier at bedside to reduce viscosity of secretions.
- Isolate patients with MRSA in a private room.
- Encourage coughing and deep breathing to remove secretions. Use bedside incentive spirometry to facilitate deep breathing. If not effective, nasotracheal suctioning may be required.

• **Pharmacological (empiric) interventions:**
  - Remove medications that can increase risk of aspiration such as sedatives and antipsychotics, especially in older adults with dysphagia.
  - Treat comorbidities.
    - Treatment of conditions such as hypertension and heart failure may include an angiotensin-converting-enzyme (ACE) inhibitor, which reduces the risk of pneumonia because it stimulates the cough reflex.

## Community-Acquired Pneumonia

- Macrolide (e.g., azithromycin [Zithromax], clarithromycin [Biaxin XL, Biaxin] **or** doxycycline [Vibramycin, Monodox, Acticlate])
  - Example: azithromycin 500 mg PO once, followed by 250 mg QD for 4 days.
  - Alternative (if allergic): doxycycline 100 mg PO BID (minimum 5 days).
  - The above regimen is used in older adults with **no** comorbidities.
- Fluoroquinolone (e.g., moxifloxacin [Avelox], levofloxacin [Levaquin]) **or** a beta lactam (e.g., amoxicillin/clavulanate [Augmentin], cefpodoxime proxetil, cefuroxime axetil [Ceftin], ceftriaxone [Rocephin]), including a macrolide
  - Example: levofloxacin 500–750 mg PO/IV daily for at least 5 days *(dosing depends upon renal function)*.

- The above regimen is used in older adults with comorbidities (e.g., chronic lung disease, renal failure, diabetes).

## Healthcare-Associated Pneumonia (Not Extensive)

- Common outpatient regimen includes fluoroquinolone (e.g., levofloxacin [Levaquin] or moxifloxacin [Avelox]) **or** ceftriaxone (Rocephin), ertapenem (Invanz), or ampicillin/sulbactam (each as monotherapy).

## Aspiration Pneumonia

- Anaerobic bacteria coverage with amoxicillin-clavulanate 875 mg PO BID *(dosing depends upon renal function)*.
- Alternative: metronidazole (PO or IV) plus amoxicillin or penicillin G.

- Duration of antibiotic treatment in older adults with bacterial pneumonia: 7 days. Longer duration recommended if infection caused by *Legionella*, resistant gram-negative bacilli, or MRSA, and/or fever beyond 3 days.
- If laboratory testing reveals a specific organism, switch antibiotic to cover the specific organism as directed by sensitivity report.
- If MRSA is suspected, add vancomycin (Vancocin) or linezolid (Zyvox).

## Viral Pneumonia

- Antiviral medication (e.g., oseltamivir [Tamiflu] or zanamivir [Relenza]).
  - Example: oseltamivir 75 mg PO BID for 5 days.
  - Recommended within the first 48 hours for treating influenza.
  - Has few adverse effects.

- Other medications to consider: bronchodilators, expectorants, chlorhexidine gluconate (in cases of gingivitis), saliva substitutes (dry mouth), and analgesics.

## Differential Diagnosis[9,13]

- Heart failure: Will have other symptoms other than respiratory related, such as fluid overload (e.g., pedal edema, weight gain, and/or jugular vein distention [JVD]). Pneumonia will lack the symptoms associated with fluid overload.
- COPD exacerbation: Will exhibit more of a respiratory disease severity and oxygen therapy need compared to pneumonia. In patients with pneumonia who also have COPD, the following will be more prominent: fever, hypotension, and/or lab abnormalities (e.g., leukocytosis, elevated CRP).
- Pulmonary embolism: Will lack systemic symptoms, will have minimal to no sputum production, and will have risk factors consistent with venous thromboembolism (VTE). Pneumonia will have more of an infectious component (e.g., possible fever, elevated WBC) and is typically associated with productive cough.

### CLINICAL PEARLS[1,3,6,8,9]

- Be alert to the possibility of pneumonia when patients present with confusion, falls, and/or worsening of underlying diseases. It is not uncommon for older adults to present atypically with pneumonia, including lack of fever.
- Use the CURB-65 score to determine pneumonia severity. With a score ≥ 2, it is reasonable to send to hospital for management.
  - 1 point for each of the following:
    - **C**onfusion
    - **U**remia
    - **R**espiratory rate above 30 breaths/min
    - **B**lood pressure (systolic < 90 mm Hg or diastolic ≤ 60 mm Hg)
    - Age ≥ **65** years
- Pneumonia is often the final cause of death in patients with poor prognosis and advanced dementia. Intravenous antibiotic therapy has not been proven effective; it is therefore reasonable in select patients to not administer antibiotic therapy.

# References


1. del Castillo, J., & Martín Sánchez, F. (2017). Pneumonia. In *Hazzard's Geriatric Medicine and Gerontology* (7th ed.). New York, NY: McGraw-Hill. Retrieved from http://accessmedicine.mhmedical.com/content.aspx?bookid=1923&sectionid=144563755. Accessed November 25, 2017.
2. Akgün, K. M., Crothers, K., & Pisani, M. (2012, March). Epidemiology and management of common pulmonary diseases in older persons. *Journals of Gerontology Series A: Biological Sciences and Medical Sciences, 67A*(3), 276–291. Retrieved from https://www.ncbi.nlm.nih.gov/pmc/articles/PMC3297767/. Accessed November 25, 2017.
3. Mody, L., Riddell, J., IV, Kaye, K. S., & Chopra, T. Common infections. In *Current Diagnosis & Treatment: Geriatrics* (2nd ed.). New York, NY: McGraw-Hill. Retrieved from http://accessmedicine.mhmedical.com/content.aspx?bookid=953&sectionid=53375671. Accessed November 25, 2017.
4. National Heart, Lung, and Blood Institute. (2016, September 26). Pneumonia. U.S. Department of Health and Human Services, National Institute of Health. Retrieved from https://www.nhlbi.nih.gov/health/health-topics/topics/pnu/. Accessed November 25, 2017.
5. Centers for Disease Control and Prevention (CDC). (2017, August 29). Pneumonia Retrieved from https://www.cdc.gov/pneumonia/index.html. Accessed November 25, 2017.
6. Simonetti, A. F., Viasus, D., Vidal, C. G., & Carratala, J. (2014, February). Management of community-acquired pneumonia in older adults. *Therapeutic Advances in Infectious Disease,* 2(1), 3–16. Retrieved from https://www.ncbi.nlm.nih.gov/pmc/articles/PMC4072047/. Accessed November 25, 2017.
7. Goldwasser, J. (2014). Pulmonary disease. In Burggraf, V., Kim, K. Y., & Knight, A. L. (Eds.) *Healthy Aging: Principles and Clinical Practice for Clinicians* (pp. 161–176). Philadelphia, PA: Lippincott Williams & Wilkins.
8. Sethi, S. (2017, March). Health Care–Associated Pneumonia – Pulmonary Disorders. Merck Manuals: Professional. Retrieved from http://www.merckmanuals.com/professional/pulmonary-disorders/pneumonia/health-care%E2%80%93associated-pneumonia. Accessed November 25, 2017.
9. Sethi, S. (2017, March). Community-Acquired Pneumonia – Pulmonary Disorders. Merck Manuals: Professional. Retrieved from http://www.merckmanuals.com/professional/pulmonary-disorders/pneumonia/community-acquired-pneumonia. Accessed November 25, 2017.
10. Cilloniz, C., & Torres, A. (2016, March 30). Community-Acquired Pneumonia. Epocrates. Retrieved from https://online.epocrates.com/noFrame/showPage?method=diseases&MonographId=17. Accessed November 26, 2017.
11. Gulanick, M., & Myers, J. L. (2017). *Nursing Care Plans: Diagnoses, Interventions, & Outcomes*. St. Louis, MO: Elsevier.
12. Bartlett, J. G. (2017, August 9). Aspiration Pneumonia in Adults (Sexton, D. J., & Bond, S., Eds.). UpToDate. Retrieved from https://www.uptodate.com/contents/aspiration-pneumonia-in-adults. Accessed November 26, 2017.
13. Boixeda, R., Bacca, S., Elias, L., Capdevila, J. A., Vilà, X., Mauri, M., & Almirall, J. (2014, December). Pneumonia as comorbidity in chronic obstructive pulmonary disease (COPD). Differences between acute exacerbation of COPD and pneumonia in patients with COPD. *Archivos de Bronconeumologia, 50*(12), 514–520. Retrieved from https://www.ncbi.nlm.nih.gov/pubmed/25443591. Accessed November 26, 2017.

# Upper Respiratory Illness

## Definition[1,2,5,7]

An upper respiratory illness (URI), also known as the common cold, is a benign self-limited viral infection.

Note: The average adult experiences two to three colds a year.

## Causes[1,6,7,9]

Over 200 subtypes of viruses associated with URI; common ones include:

- Rhinovirus (most common)
- Adenovirus
- Enterovirus
- Parainfluenza virus
- Coronavirus
- Respiratory syncytial virus

Note: incubation period for most common cold viruses is 24–72 hours.

## Risk Factors[1]

- Immunodeficiency disorders
- Underlying chronic disease
- Cigarette smoking
- Psychological stress
- Poor nutrition
- Lack of sleep
- Sick exposure

## Signs & Symptoms[1,2,5,6,7,9]

- Nasal discharge: usually clear.
  - Discolored nasal discharge may be seen (*does not always indicate bacterial infection*).
- Reduced ability to smell.
- Nasal congestion.
- Sore throat.

- Cough.
- Sneezing.
- Headache.
- General malaise.
- Duration of symptoms: typically, under 10 days, sometimes as long as 2 weeks in about 25% of patients.
- Physical exam findings: erythematous, engorged nasal mucosa; pharyngeal erythema; conjunctival injection; nasal watery discharge; lung examination is usually clear.

Note: fever is uncommon in adults; if present, tends to be low grade.

## Tests[1,5,6,11]

*The diagnosis of URI is made clinically; testing not routinely indicated.*

- Chest X-ray
  - Ordered if concerned over consolidation or other parenchymal disease.

## Treatment & Management[1,2,3,4,5,7,8,9,10,11]

- **Nonpharmacological and nursing interventions:**
  - Encourage rest, fluids, and aggressive handwashing.
    - Most URIs are transmitted through hand-to-hand contact (viruses remain viable on skin about 120 minutes).
    - The benefit of antibacterial versus nonbacterial soap is not significantly different.
  - Monitor for complications, such as acute bacterial rhinosinusitis.
    - Usually seen when symptoms persist beyond 10 days; may see purulent or yellow nasal secretions, including unilateral facial or dental discomfort.
- **Pharmacological interventions:**
  - OTC analgesics: acetaminophen (e.g., Tylenol) and/or NSAIDs (e.g., ibuprofen [Motrin, Advil], naproxen [Naprosyn])
    - Example: acetaminophen 325–1,000 mg PO q4–6 hr PRN.

  - Recommended short term to reduce pain.
  - Naproxen is effective in treating acute cough.
  - NSAIDs a risk of gastrointestinal bleeding (use of PPI decreases this risk), can exacerbate heart failure and worsen renal function. Cox-2 selective NSAIDs are associated with lower risk of adverse effects.
- Inhaled anticholinergic, ipratropium (Atrovent)
  - Treats cough caused by the common cold.
- Intranasal ipratropium bromide (Atrovent Nasal)
  - Example: 2 sprays/nostril 3–4 times/day PRN.
  - Improves rhinorrhea and sneezing but not nasal congestion.
  - May cause nasal dryness, epistaxis, or taste changes.
- Decongestant, nasal spray (e.g., oxymetazoline [Afrin], phenylephrine [Neo-Synephrine])
  - Example: oxymetazoline 2 sprays/nostril q10–12hr PRN.
  - For acute symptom management for 3 days only (to prevent rebound congestion).
  - May cause restlessness, insomnia, arrhythmias or hypertension.
- Decongestants, oral (e.g., pseudoephedrine [Sudafed], phenylephrine)
  - Example: pseudoephedrine 120 mg PO BID PRN.
  - Improves rhinorrhea and nasal obstruction (modest benefit).
  - Often given with an antihistamine to improve cold symptoms.
  - CNS stimulant effects; may cause insomnia.
- Antihistamines, first generation (e.g., diphenhydramine [Benadryl], doxylamine [Unisom], chlorpheniramine [Chlor-Trimeton])
  - Minimally improve symptoms (e.g., runny nose, sneezing).

    - These agents are sedating, can cause dizziness and dry mouth. Alternative (less sedating): second-generation antihistamine (e.g., cetirizine [Zyrtec]).
  - Saline nasal spray
    - May improve symptoms of the common cold.
  - Guaifenesin and/or dextromethorphan
    - Some studies demonstrate effective for cough and others not.
  - Codeine
    - Codeine is no more effective than placebo for acute cough due to URI.
  - Intranasal corticosteroids
    - No more effective than placebo; they do however reduce inflammation in the nasal mucosa.
  - Vitamin C (ascorbic acid) and echinacea
    - Evidence to support these are weak.
  - Zinc (use is controversial)
    - Doses of zinc acetate greater than 75 mg/day may reduce duration of symptoms.
  - Antibiotics should not be used to treat uncomplicated URI. URI are caused by viruses, not bacteria.

Note: Beers listed items, as mentioned above, include oral antihistamines, oral decongestants, and NSAIDs.

## Differential Diagnosis[1,2,4,5,11]

- Allergic rhinitis: Symptoms (e.g., sneezing, rhinorrhea) occur due to specific allergen(s) exposure; symptoms such as a sore throat would indicate URI more likely.
- Influenza: Will have more severe symptoms compared to URI; common features include high fever, headache, malaise, and myalgias.
- Acute bacterial rhinosinusitis (sinusitis): Will have facial pain over affected sinuses and purulent nasal discharge; associating symptoms may include malaise, fever, headache, and cough. Symptoms would not improve with topical or oral decongestant.

## CLINICAL PEARLS[1,2,5,7,11]

- Complications of the common cold may include bacterial sinusitis, asthma exacerbation, or pneumonia.
- Goal of URI treatment is to relieve symptoms, reduce complications, prevent the spread to others, and avoid adverse effects from medication used.
- Nasal drainage is usually clear with the common cold; however can also be purulent. The presence of discolored nasal drainage is not enough to distinguish between the common cold and sinusitis.

# References


1. Sexton, D. J. (2018, January 15). The Common Cold in Adults: Diagnosis and Clinical Features (Hirsch, M. S., & Libman, H., Eds.). UpToDate. Retrieved from https://www.uptodate.com/contents/the-common-cold-in-adults-diagnosis-and-clinical-features?search=The%20common%20cold%20in%20adults:%20Diagnosis%20and%20clinical%20features&source=search_result&selectedTitle=1~150&usage_type=default&display_rank=1. Accessed January 30, 2018.
2. Lustig, L. R., & Schindler, J. S. (2018). Ear, nose, and throat disorders. In *Current Medical Diagnosis & Treatment 2018*. New York, NY: McGraw-Hill. Retrieved from http://accessmedicine.mhmedical.com/content.aspx?bookid=2192&sectionid=168008266. Accessed January 30, 2018.
3. American Geriatrics Society 2015 Beers Criteria Update Expert Panel, Fick, D. M., Semla, T. P., Beizer, J., Brandt, N., & Dombrowski, R., . . . Steinman, M. (2015, October 8). American Geriatrics Society 2015 updated Beers criteria for potentially inappropriate medication use in older adults. *Journal of the American Geriatrics Society, 63*(11), 2227–2246. Retrieved from http://onlinelibrary.wiley.com/doi/10.1111/jgs.13702/abstract. Accessed October 3, 2017.
4. Broek, V. D., Gudden, C., Kluijfhout, W. P., Stam-Slob, S. C., Aarts, M. C., & Kaper, N. M. (2014). No evidence for distinguishing bacterial from viral acute rhinosinusitis using symptom duration and purulent rhinorrhea: systematic review of the evidence base. *Otolaryngoly—Head and Neck Surgery, 150*(4), 533–537. doi:10.1177/0194599814522595
5. Rhinosinusitis, Acute Viral (Common Cold). In Papadakis, M. A., & McPhee, S. J. (Eds.) *Quick Medical Diagnosis & Treatment 2017*. New York, NY: McGraw-Hill. http://accessmedicine.mhmedical.com/content.aspx?bookid=2033&sectionid=152416880. Accessed January 30, 2018.
6. Lefebvre, C. W. (2016). Acute bronchitis and upper respiratory tract infections. In Tintinalli, J. E., Stapczynski, J., Ma, O., Yealy, D. M., Meckler, G. D., & Cline, D. M. (Eds.) *Tintinalli's Emergency Medicine: A Comprehensive Study Guide* (8th ed.). New York, NY: McGraw-Hill. Retrieved from http://accessmedicine.mhmedical.com/content.aspx?bookid=1658&sectionid=109429323. Accessed January 30, 2018.
7. Arroll, B. (2008). Common cold. *BMJ Clinical Evidence*. Retrieved from https://www.ncbi.nlm.nih.gov/pmc/articles/PMC2907967/. Accessed January 31, 2018.

8. National Institutes of Health, Office of Dietary Supplements. (2011, June 24). Vitamin C Fact Sheet. Retrieved from https://ods.od.nih.gov/factsheets/VitaminC-Consumer/. Accessed January 31, 2018.
9. Fashner, J., Ericson, K., & Werner, S. (2012). Treatment of the common cold in children and adults. *American Family Physician,* 86(2), 153–159. Retrieved from https://www.aafp.org/afp/2012/0715/p153.html. Accessed January 31, 2018.
10. Li, S., Yue, J., Dong, B. R., Yang, M., Lin, X., & Wu, T. (2013). Acetaminophen (paracetamol) for the common cold in adults. *Cochrane Database of Systematic Reviews*. doi:10.1002/14651858.cd008800.pub2
11. Arroll, B., & Kenealy, T. (2018, January 23). Common Cold. Epocrates. Retrieved from https://online.epocrates.com/diseases/25211/Common-cold/Key-Highlights Accessed February 2, 2018.

SECTION V

# Gastroenterology

## Constipation

### Definition[1,2,3,4]

Constipation is a disturbance in bowel function, characterized by infrequent or difficult defecation.

### Causes[1,2,3,5,6,7]

- Functional disorders
  - Normal colonic transit, slow transit constipation, dyssynergic defecation (e.g., anismus or pelvic floor dysfunction)
- Medications
  - Opioids, anticholinergics, calcium channel blockers, iron supplementation, antacids
- Neurological disorders
  - Parkinson's disease, multiple sclerosis, spinal cord injury, dementia
- Metabolic disorders
  - Hypothyroid, diabetes, hypercalcemia
- Blockages of the colon
  - Colon cancer, stricture or narrowing
- Mood-related disorders
  - Depression, anxiety

### Risk Factors[1,2,3,6,7]

*Risk factors of constipation coincide with causes.*

- Advanced age
- Female sex
  - More than twice as common than men
- Reduced mobility
- Low-fluid intake

- Low-fiber diet
- Low socioeconomic status

## Signs & Symptoms[1,2,3,4,6]

- Have ≤ three stools/week.
- Rectal fullness or feeling of inadequate bowel emptying.
- Straining with defecation.
- Hard or lumpy stools.

## Tests[1,2,3,4,6,7]

*Tests are warranted if constipation has no clear etiology.*

- Complete blood count (CBC)
  - The presence of anemia suggests a secondary cause and should be investigated.
- Thyroid-stimulating hormone (TSH)
  - Checks for the presence of hypothyroidism (secondary cause of constipation).
- Basic metabolic panel (BMP), magnesium, and fasting glucose
  - Checks for electrolyte imbalance (hypercalcemia, low magnesium, and/or potassium) and hyperglycemia, which are secondary causes of constipation.
- Plain abdominal radiography
  - Checks for significant stool retention.
- Colonoscopy
  - Recommended if warning signs are present (e.g., anemia, unexplained weight loss, positive fecal occult blood, gastrointestinal [GI] bleeding, or constipation refractory to treatment).

## Treatment & Management[1,2,3,4,6,7]

- **Nonpharmacological and nursing interventions:**
  - Identify and treat potentially reversible causes of constipation.
    - Increase dietary fiber to 25–35 g per day.
    - Encourage adequate fluid intake (goal of 1.5–2 L/day).
    - Increase physical activity.

- Monitor for warning signs of possible malignancy.
  - Constipation presenting acutely, anemia, abdominal pain, unintentional weight loss, rectal bleeding, or a family history of colorectal cancer.
- Schedule bathroom time.
  - Make time to have a bowel movement and ensure privacy.
  - Remind patients that the best potential for a bowel movement is in the morning and about 45 minutes following a meal.
  - Do not postpone having a bowel movement if there is an urge to defecate.
- Educate patients on constipation.
  - If there are minimal to no constipation symptoms, instruct patient to stop taking laxatives.
  - Being obsessed over bowel movements is not good; having a daily bowel movement is not necessary.
  - Patients need to engage in exercise and increase their fiber intake.
- Biofeedback.
  - Effective treatment for dyssynergic defecation.

- **Pharmacological and other interventions:**
  *Consider discontinuing medications that have a side effect of constipation (if appropriate).*
  - Bulking agents (e.g., psyllium [Metamucil]).
    - Example: psyllium 1 tsp (3.4 g) QD-TID with fluids PRN.
    - Promotes softer stool by increasing the bulk of the stool. Will need to drink plenty of water for a better outcome.
    - Not recommended as first-line agent in patients on high-dose opioids or with dysphagia.
    - May cause bloating or flatulence.
  - Stool softeners (e.g., docusate sodium [Colace]).
    - Example: Colace 100 mg PO BID.
    - Not to be used as chronic treatment.
    - Well tolerated and can be combined with a bulking agent.

- Osmotic agents (e.g., lactulose [Kristalose], polyethylene glycol [Miralax], magnesium citrate).
  - Example: lactulose 15–30 mL PO QD-BID.
  - Lactulose recommended in those residing in nursing homes.
  - Consider when bulking agents and stool softeners are ineffective.
  - May cause bloating and/or flatulence. Magnesium citrate should be avoided with renal impairment.
- Stimulants (e.g., senna [Peri-Colace, Senokot], or bisacodyl [Dulcolax]).
  - Example: bisacodyl 5–15mg PO QD.
  - Should be used short term and avoided with bowel obstruction. Used when osmotic agents are ineffective.
  - Increases peristaltic contractions and can have unfavorable side effects such as abdominal cramping.
- Secretagogues (i.e., lubiprostone [Amitiza] and linaclotide [Linzess]).
  - Example: lubiprostone 24 mcg PO BID.
  - Recommended as monotherapy and not with other laxatives.
  - They are usually well-tolerated; however, may cause GI disturbances (e.g., diarrhea, nausea, abdominal distention).
- Alvimopan (Entereg) or methylnaltrexone (Relistor)
  - Treats opioid-induced constipation.
- Enemas (used when there is evidence of fecal impaction)
  - Soapsuds enemas should not be given to older adults.
  - Tap water enemas are the safest for regular use.
  - Phosphate enemas are associated with hyperphosphatemia and should be avoided in renal disease.

- Gastroenterology consultation/referral
  - To guide treatment when the above regimen is ineffective.
- Nutritionist consultation/referral
  - To aid in dietary changes

## Differential Diagnosis[1,3,4,7]

- Colon cancer: Will have warning signs such as weight loss, positive occult blood, hematochezia, and change in bowel habits (e.g., increased frequency of bowel movements, loose stools). If there are concerns for colon cancer, consider colonoscopy or other tests (e.g., computer tomography [CT] scan of abdomen/pelvis).
- Irritable bowel syndrome with constipation (IBS-C): More common in those ≤ age 50 years and will have recurrent abdominal pain, relieved by defecation. It can be difficult to differentiate between the two; however abdominal pain is not a feature of constipation by itself. Chronic constipation is exceptionally common in older adults, whereas there are lower rates of IBS diagnosed in individuals ≥ age 50 years.

### CLINICAL PEARLS[2]

- Consider the possibility of a bowel obstruction if constipation is severe or comes on suddenly.
- Some patients are obsessive–compulsive regarding their constipation and should be reminded that daily bowel movements are not required; the bowel needs a chance to work, and daily laxatives or enemas is not the answer.
- The Rome III Criteria is used to diagnose constipation (Table 5-1).

**Table 5-1** Rome III Diagnostic Criteria: Functional Constipation and IBS-C

- Symptoms ≥3 mo; onset ≥6 mo prior to diagnosis

| Functional Constipation | IBS-C |
|---|---|
| • Must include >2 of the following:<br>• Straining*<br>• Lumpy or hard stools*<br>• Sensation of incomplete evacuation* | • IBS: Recurrent abdominal pain/discomfort ≥3 d/mo for the past 3 mo, associated with ≥2 of the following:<br>• Improvement with defecation |

(*Continues*)

**Table 5-1** Rome III Diagnostic Criteria: Functional Constipation and IBS-C (*Continued*)

| Functional Constipation | IBS-C |
|---|---|
|     • Sensation of anorectal obstruction/blockage*<br>    • Manual maneuvers to facilitate defecation (eg, digital evacuation, support of the pelvic floor)*<br>    • <3 defecations/wk<br>• Loose stool rarely present w/o use of laxatives<br>• Insufficient criteria for IBS-C |     • Onset associated with change in stool frequency<br>    • Onset associated with change in stool form<br>• IBS is subtyped by predominant stool pattern<br>    • IBS-C: hard or lumpy stools[†] ≥ 25% of defecations; loose or watery stools[‡] <25% of defecations[§] |

*≥25% of defecations. †Bristol Stool Form Scale 1–2: separate, hard lumps like nuts (difficult to pass); or lumpy, sausage-shaped stool. ‡Bristol Stool Form Scale 6–7: fluffy pieces of stool with ragged edges; mushy stool; or watery w/out solid pieces (entirely liquid). §In the absence of use of antidiarrheals or laxatives.

Reproduced from Peura, D. A., and Shiller, L. (n.d.). *Overcoming Obstacles in the Management of Functional Chronic Constipation and Irritable Bowel Syndrome with Constipation*. Table 2. Retrieved from http://ww3.peerviewpress.com/gpimgs/fastcast/n165/n165.html.

# References


1. Rao, S., & Sharma, A. (2017, August 4). Constipation in Adults. Epocrates. Retrieved from https://online.epocrates.com/diseases/154/Constipation-in-adults. Accessed December 10, 2017.
2. Greenberger, N. J. (2016, March). Constipation – Gastrointestinal Disorders. Merck Manuals: Professional. Retrieved from https://www.merckmanuals.com/professional/gastrointestinal-disorders/symptoms-of-gi-disorders/constipation. Accessed December 10, 2017.
3. Acosta, A., Tangalos, E. G., & Harari, D. (2017). Constipation. In *Hazzard's Geriatric Medicine and Gerontology* (7th ed.). New York, NY: McGraw-Hill. Retrieved from http://accessmedicine.mhmedical.com/content.aspx?bookid=1923&sectionid=144526800. Accessed December 10, 2017.
4. Markland, A. (2014). Constipation. In *Current Diagnosis & Treatment: Geriatrics* (2nd ed.). New York, NY: McGraw-Hill. Retrieved from http://accessmedicine.mhmedical.com/content.aspx?bookid=953&sectionid=53375660. Accessed December 10, 2017.
5. Wald, A. (2017, February 1). Management of Chronic Constipation in Older Adults (Talley, N. J., & Grover, S., Eds.). UpToDate. Retrieved from https://www.uptodate.com/contents/management-of-chronic-constipation-in-adults?source=search_result&search=constipation&selectedTitle=1~150#H30890925. Accessed December 10, 2017.
6. Mayo Clinic. (2016, October 19). Constipation. Retrieved from https://www.mayoclinic.org/diseases-conditions/constipation/symptoms-causes/syc-20354253. Accessed December 10, 2017.
7. Moyer, D., & Tierney, A. (2015, May). Outpatient Management of Constipation in Older Adults. Elder Care. Tucson, AZ: University of Arizona. Retrieved from https://nursingandhealth.asu.edu/sites/default/files/constipation.pdf. Accessed December 10, 2017.

# Dysphagia

## Definition[1,3,5,6]

Dysphagia refers to swallowing difficulty.

## Types[2,5,7]

**Oropharyngeal dysphagia (transfer):** impaired movement of a food bolus or liquid from the oropharynx to upper esophagus
**Esophageal dysphagia (transit):** impaired movement of food bolus through the esophagus distal to the upper esophageal sphincter (most common)

## Causes[2,3,4,5,7]

| Oropharyngeal Dysphagia | Esophageal Dysphagia |
|---|---|
| Neurologic: stroke, Parkinson's disease, dementia, multiple sclerosis, mass lesion | Mechanical obstruction: esophageal cancer, esophageal stricture (commonly caused by gastroesophageal reflux), Schatzki ring |
| Muscular: myasthenia gravis, polymyositis | Motility disorders: diffuse esophageal spasms, achalasia |
| Metabolic: thyrotoxicosis, Cushing disease | Esophageal carcinoma (Consider squamous cell if there is a history of smoking or alcohol abuse.) |
| Infection: syphilis, oral mucositis | |
| Radiation to the oral cavity or neck | |
| Oropharyngeal tumors | |
| Xerostomia (e.g., anticholinergic drugs) | |
| Poor dentition or poor fitting dentures | |

## Risk Factors

*Risk factors coincide with the causes of dysphagia.*

- Advanced age

## Signs & Symptoms[2,3,4,5,7]

| Oropharyngeal Dysphagia | Esophageal Dysphagia |
|---|---|
| Dysphagia is noted within a second of attempting to swallow. | Dysphagia is noted several seconds after initiating a swallow. |
| Coughing during meals. | Feeling of food or liquids "catching" in the throat (usually worse with solids). |
| Gagging. | Regurgitation. |
| Aspiration. | Heartburn. |
| Odynophagia. | Chest pain (seen with esophageal spasm). |
| Change in voice (e.g., hoarseness). | |

- Unintentional weight loss and anemia
  - Needs to be investigated; sign of potential underlying malignancy.

## Tests[2,3,5,6,7]

- Modified barium swallow (MBS) or videofluoroscopy
  - MBS is typically the first test ordered in the workup of dysphagia.
  - An alternative to videofluoroscopy: Fiberoptic endoscopic evaluation of swallowing (FEES) commonly used in long-term care facilities.
- Esophagogastroduodenoscopy (EGD)
  - Can take biopsies and allows for dilation of strictures.
- Esophageal manometry
  - Used to identify neuromuscular disorders; ordered if the above tests are negative and dysphagia persistent.

## Management & Treatment[1,2,3,4,5,6,7,8]

- **Nonpharmacological and nursing interventions:**
  - Identify and treat the underlying cause of dysphagia.
    - Performing a full neurological examination can assist in determining the underlying cause of dysphagia (e.g., rigidity or shuffling gait can indicate Parkinson's disease).
  - Implement measures to prevent malnutrition and aspiration.
    - This includes diet modification, slowing the rate of eating, eating in an upright posture, and reducing bolus size.
    - Ensuring thickened-liquids and avoiding liquids to avoid aspiration pneumonia.
  - Teach the Heimlich maneuver.
    - This is crucial for staff and family members.
  - Medication modifications.
    - Consider switching PO meds to liquid form, if able. Teach patients if medications can be crushed to make administration easier.
    - Ensure adequate fluid intake when taking medications to avoid esophageal damage.
  - Encourage proper oral hygiene.
    - Poor oral care is a risk factor for pneumonia; encourage routine dental visits.
    - Encourage products that alleviate dry mouth.
- **Pharmacological and other interventions:**
  - Medications in select patients may include:
    - Botulinum toxin injection.
      - Reserved in individuals who are poor surgical candidates.
    - Nitrates, calcium channel blockers.
      - Reserved in individuals with motility disorders (achalasia, esophageal spasms).
  - Speech therapy consultation/referral
    - Certain tests are coordinated by a speech language pathologist, such as the MBS, which can identify which foods are better swallowed.

        - Will make suggestions regarding eating and drinking aids to improve swallowing safety.
    - Dietitian consultation/referral
        - To ensure patient is on the proper diet.
    - Rehabilitative exercises
        - To strengthen swallowing muscles.
    - Percutaneous endoscopic gastrostomy tube
        - Considered when nutritional status is poor and/or recurrent aspiration (risks vs benefits should first be discussed, especially in patients with advanced dementia).
    - Surgical intervention
        - Endoscopic dilatation recommended with strictures.

Note: Beers listed items, as mentioned above, include nondihydropyridine calcium channel blockers.

## CLINICAL PEARLS[1,2,6]

- If dysphagia is not treated, it can lead to pulmonary complications (e.g., silent aspiration, pneumonia), malnutrition, and death. It is the third leading cause of infection-related death in adults > age 85.
- Dysphagia is an independent risk factor for aspiration pneumonia and malnutrition.
- Dysphagia to liquids and solids is usually due to an underlying neuromuscular disorder. If due to solids alone, this is reflective of an underlying mechanical obstruction.

## References

1. Rogus-Pulia, N., Barczi, S., & Robbins, J. (2017). Disorders of swallowing. In *Hazzard's Geriatric Medicine and Gerontology* (7th ed.). New York, NY: McGraw-Hill. Retrieved from http://accessmedicine.mhmedical.com/content.aspx?bookid=1923&sectionid=144520375. Accessed December 16, 2017.
2. Gastrointestinal and abdominal complaints. In *Current Diagnosis & Treatment: Geriatrics* (2nd ed.). New York, NY: McGraw-Hill. Retrieved from http://accessmedicine.mhmedical.com/content.aspx?bookid=953&sectionid=53375659. Accessed December 16, 2017.
3. Gyawali, C. P. (2010, November). Dysphagia. American College of Gastroenterology. Retrieved from http://patients.gi.org/topics/dysphagia/. Accessed December 16, 2017.

4. Charous, S. J. (2016, September 12). Evaluation of Dysphagia. Epocrates. Retrieved from https://online.epocrates.com/diseases/226/Evaluation-of-dysphagia. Accessed December 16, 2017.
5. Gastrointestinal disorders. In *Current Medical Diagnosis & Treatment 2018*. New York, NY: McGraw-Hill. Retrieved from http://accessmedicine.mhmedical.com/content.aspx?bookid=2192&sectionid=168013478. Accessed December 16, 2017.
6. Azimi, E., Carnahan, J., Denson, K., & Kuester, J. (n.d.). Clinical Skills Workshop: Dysphagia Evaluation & Treatment. Milwaukee, WI: Medical College of Wisconsin. Retrieved from https://geriatricscareonline.org/application/content/products/M002/slide/day2/R1445_27_Kathryn_Denson.pdf
7. Lembo, A. J., & Robson, K. M. (2015, June 2). Oropharyngeal Dysphagia: Clinical Features, Diagnosis, and Management (Talley, N. J., Ed.). UpToDate. Retrieved from https://www.uptodate.com/contents/oropharyngeal-dysphagia-clinical-features-diagnosis-and-management?search=dysphagia risk factor&source=search_result&selectedTitle=2~150&usage_type=default&display_rank=2. Accessed December 20, 2017.
8. American Geriatrics Society 2015 Beers Criteria Update Expert Panel, Fick, D. M., Semla, T. P., Beizer, J., Brandt, N., & Dombrowski, R., . . . Steinman, M. (2015, October 8). American Geriatrics Society 2015 updated Beers criteria for potentially inappropriate medication use in older adults. *Journal of the American Geriatrics Society, 63*(11), 2227–2246. Retrieved from http://onlinelibrary.wiley.com/doi/10.1111/jgs.13702/abstract. Accessed October 8, 2017.

# Fecal Incontinence

## Definition[1,4,6]

Fecal incontinence (FI) is the loss of bowel control, resulting in the involuntary passage of feces.

Note: FI is the second leading cause of nursing home placement.

## Types[1,4,6]

**Passive incontinence:** unaware of passing small amount of stool.
**Urge incontinence:** aware of the need to defecate; however has leakage of stool due to inability to get to the restroom in time.
**Fecal leakage:** the leakage of stool following incomplete bowel movement.

## Causes[1,2,4,6]

- Idiopathic
- Neurological conditions (e.g., dementia, multiple sclerosis, stroke)

- Inflammatory conditions (e.g., inflammatory bowel disease, radiation proctitis)
- Infectious diarrhea
- Dysfunction of the anorectal sphincters
- Fecal impaction
- Excessive laxative use
- Diabetes

## Risk Factors[1,2,4,6]

- Advanced age
- Nursing home patient
- Female sex
- Immobility
- Rectal trauma
- History of pelvic radiation therapy
- Depression
- Renal disease
- Urinary incontinence

## Signs & Symptoms[1,2,4,5]

- Urinary incontinence
- Constipation
- Skin irritation
- Hemorrhoids
- Anal fissures
- Perineal scarring (can indicate prior trauma or surgery)
- Weakened sphincter tone
- Patulous anus

## Tests[1,2,4,5,6,7]

*Diagnosis is made clinically.*

- CBC, C-reactive protein (CRP)
  - Not ordered routinely, ordered if concern for underlying infection or inflammation.

- Abdominal plain film
  - Ordered if there is a concern for fecal impaction.
- Anorectal manometry
  - Ordered in select patients to determine rectal resting and squeeze pressures.
- Anal ultrasonography
  - Evaluates for damage of the anal sphincters.
- Colonoscopy or flexible sigmoidoscopy
  - To determine if a mechanical cause is present (e.g., colonic mass).

## Management & Treatment[1,2,4,5,6,7,8,9]

- **Nonpharmacological and nursing interventions:**
  - Investigate and treat the underlying reversible causes of fecal incontinence, such as:
    - Treat the infectious source.
    - Treat the fecal impaction.
    - Encourage mobility.
  - Biofeedback and pelvic floor exercises.
    - Patient must be cognitively intact and cooperative for biofeedback to be effective.
  - Encourage dietary changes.
    - Make one food change at a time and keep record of this in a food diary, with goal to determine if symptoms change.
      - Foods that are known to contribute to loose stools include, but not limited to: prunes, figs, artificial sweeteners, caffeine, and some vegetables. Remove any offending foods.
    - Encourage increased consumption of dietary fiber (this creates bulk and bulky stools stimulates peristalsis).
  - Schedule bathroom time.
    - Encourage using the bathroom following a meal, and ensure privacy.

- Offer emotional support (fecal incontinence can be socially embarrassing).
- Manual disimpaction.
  - An option in older adults with fecal impaction and laxative ineffective.
- Implement measures to prevent skin breakdown (FI can lead to pressure ulcers).
  - Frequent turning and use of barrier cream (e.g., zinc oxide).
- Use of a stool collection system.
  - Preferred over pads or diapers; use of pouches or rectal tubes prevent exposure of perianal skin to stool and reduces odor and embarrassment. These are a good option in bedbound older adults.

- **Pharmacological and other interventions:**
  - Rid of excessive laxative use.
  - Bulking agent (e.g., psyllium [Metamucil] or methylcellulose [Citrucel]).
    - Example: psyllium 1 tsp (3.4 g) QD-TID with fluids PRN.
    - Improves stool consistency and reduces the frequency of defecation; should be gradually introduced to avoid bloating.
  - Antidiarrheal agents (e.g., loperamide [Imodium], codeine).
    - Example: loperamide 2–4 mg PO following loose stools (max 16 mg/day).
    - *Rule out infection before starting medication.*
    - These agents slow down bowel motility. Can be used with radiation proctitis and inflammatory bowel disease.
    - Loperamide recommended as first-line treatment (may cause xerostomia, dizziness, or abdominal cramps). If not tolerated, switch to codeine or low-dose amitriptyline (Elavil) (10–25 mg QHS).

- Enemas and/or suppositories (e.g., phosphate enema, glycerin rectal, bisacodyl [Dulcolax]).
  - Example: glycerin rectal 2 g suppository once daily PRN.
  - Used if fecal impaction is the underlying cause of FI and in those with spinal injury.
  - Rectal preparation is used as first-line treatment but, if not effective, can switch to an oral laxative (e.g., lactulose [Generlac, Enulose] or sennosides [Senokot]).
  - Suppositories may cause perianal irritation whereas enemas used chronically can lead to fluid and electrolyte imbalance.
- Wound, ostomy continence (WOC) nurse consultation/referral
  - Enhances the care for patients suffering from FI; research has shown agencies with WOC nurses have significantly better outcomes than those without WOC nurses.
- Gastroenterology consultation/referral
  - Can guide medical decision making and determine if surgery is the right option, especially if fecal incontinence is refractory to medical therapy.

Note: Beers listed items, as mentioned above, include amitriptyline.

## Differential Diagnosis[1]

- Colorectal cancer: Will have warning signs, such as rectal bleeding and/or anemia, and/or family history of colon cancer. A colonoscopy can confirm colonic mass.
- Inflammatory bowel disease (IBD): May have rectal bleeding and abdominal pain; lab studies may reveal leukocytosis and/or elevated inflammatory markers.

### CLINICAL PEARLS[3]

- Fecal incontinence is distressing physically, psychologically, and socially, placing older adults at risk for nursing home placement and poor health.

## References

1. Brown, S. (2016, July 29). Fecal Incontinence in Adults. Epocrates. Retrieved from https://online.epocrates.com/diseases/840/Fecal-incontinence-in-adults. Accessed December 11, 2017.
2. Ansari, P. (2016, October). Fecal Incontinence – Gastrointestinal Disorders. Merck Manuals: Professional. Retrieved from http://www.merckmanuals.com/professional/gastrointestinal-disorders/anorectal-disorders/fecal-incontinence. Accessed December 11, 2017.
3. Acosta, A., Tangalos, E. G., & Harari, D. (2017). Constipation. In *Hazzard's Geriatric Medicine and Gerontology* (7th ed.). New York, NY: McGraw-Hill. Retrieved from http://accessmedicine.mhmedical.com/content.aspx?bookid=1923&sectionid=144526800. Accessed December 11, 2017.
4. Hall, K. E. (2014). Gastrointestinal and abdominal complaints. In *Current Diagnosis & Treatment: Geriatrics* (2nd ed.). New York, NY: McGraw-Hill. Retrieved from http://accessmedicine.mhmedical.com/content.aspx?bookid=953&sectionid=53375659. Accessed December 11, 2017.
5. Ferzandi, T. R. (2016, May 5). Fecal Incontinence (Talavero, F., Isaacs, C., & Strohbehn, K., Eds.). Medscape. Retrieved from https://emedicine.medscape.com/article/268674-overview. Accessed December 11, 2017.
6. Shah, B. J., Chokhavatia, S., & Rose, S. (2012, July 8). Fecal Incontinence in the Elderly: FAQ. *American Journal of Gastroenterology, 107*(11). Retrieved from http://gi.org/wp-content/uploads/2012/10/7-ajg2012284a.pdf. Accessed December 11, 2017.
7. Gulanick, M., & Myers, J. L. (2017). *Nursing Care Plans: Diagnoses, Interventions, & Outcomes*. St. Louis, MO: Elsevier.
8. American Geriatrics Society 2015 Beers Criteria Update Expert Panel, Fick, D. M., Semla, T. P., Beizer, J., Brandt, N., & Dombrowski, R., . . . Steinman, M. (2015, October 8). American Geriatrics Society 2015 updated Beers criteria for potentially inappropriate medication use in older adults. *Journal of the American Geriatrics Society, 63*(11), 2227–2246. Retrieved from http://onlinelibrary.wiley.com/doi/10.1111/jgs.13702/abstract. Accessed October 3, 2017.
9. Westra, B. L., Bliss, D. Z., Savik, K., Hou, Y., & Borchert, A. (2014). Effectiveness of wound, ostomy, and continence nurses on agency-level wound and incontinence outcomes in home care. *Home Healthcare Nurse*, 32(2), 119–127. DOI: 10.1097/NHH.0000000000000030

# Gastroesophageal Reflux Disease

## Definition[1,4,5]

Gastroesophageal reflux disease (GERD) is defined as the reflux of gastric contents into the esophagus.

## Causes[1,2,4,5]

- Incompetent lower esophageal sphincter (LES) muscle relaxation.

## Risk Factors[1,2,4,5]

- Family history of heartburn
- Advanced age
- Truncal obesity
- Hiatal hernia
- Tobacco smoking
- Alcohol
- Some foods
  - May include caffeinated beverages, spicy foods (limited evidence).
- Some medications
  - Includes nitrates, calcium channel blockers, antihistamines, antidepressants, anticholinergics, NSAIDs.
- Gastroparesis
- Scleroderma

## Signs & Symptoms[1,2,3,4,5]

- Heartburn
  - 30–60 min after eating and reclining.
- Sour regurgitation
- Dysphagia
  - May indicate development of esophageal stricture.
- Chronic cough
- Sore throat
- Atypical chest pain
- Worsening asthma
- Nausea or vomiting

## Tests[1,2,3,4,5]

- A trial round of a proton pump inhibitor (PPI)
  - Further workup recommended if no improvement noted after 2 months.
  - Positive response indicates 78% sensitivity and 54% specificity for GERD.

- Upper endoscopy (esophagogastroduodenoscopy)
  - Safe procedure, including in very frail elderly patients; should be done if reflux symptoms continue despite medication.
  - Determines severity of reflux disease and evaluates for complications such as esophageal cancer or Barrett's esophagus.
- Ambulatory pH monitoring, 24-hour
  - Not usually performed but is an option if upper endoscopy is negative and GERD symptoms are persistent despite PPI therapy. It will determine if symptoms are related to acid or not.
- Esophageal manometry
  - Not usually a benefit in older adults unless planning for antireflux surgery.

## Treatment & Management[1,2,3,4,5,6]

- **Nonpharmacological and nursing interventions:**
  - Encourage dietary changes
    - Avoid greasy or spicy foods, fats, caffeine, and/or alcoholic beverages.
    - Eat smaller, more frequent meals.
    - Avoid eating 3 hours before going to bed (if nocturnal symptoms present).
    - After eating, sit upright for about 3 hours and avoid reclining.
  - Encourage weight loss, if obese.
  - Avoid smoking and secondhand smoke.
  - Advise against wearing tight clothing.
- **Pharmacological and other interventions:**
  - Antacids (e.g., aluminum hydroxide/magnesium hydroxide/simethicone [Mylanta], calcium carbonate/magnesium hydroxide [Rolaids], calcium carbonate [Tums])
    - Example: Rolaids 2–4 chewable tabs PO PRN (max: 12 tabs/24 hrs).

    - Provides rapid relief of GERD symptoms; recommended with symptoms that occur less than once weekly.
    - Monitor for adverse effects: diarrhea, hypercalcemia, hypo-hypermagnesium, nephrolithiasis.
  - Proton-pump inhibitors (e.g., esomeprazole [Nexium], lansoprazole [Prevacid], omeprazole [Prilosec])
    - Example: omeprazole 20 mg PO QD-BID, 30 minutes before breakfast for 8 weeks *(some may need this longer)*.
      - Not to be given concomitantly with clopidogrel (Plavix).
    - Offers quick symptom relief and promotes healing in erosive esophagitis.
    - Preferred over H2 blockers in the short- and long-term treatment of GERD.
    - Adverse reactions include risk of osteoporosis, fracture, low magnesium, infectious gastroenteritis (*Clostridium difficilie*), pneumonia, and vitamin B12-deficiency with long-term use.
  - Histamine-2 receptor antagonists (e.g., famotidine [Pepcid AC], ranitidine [Zantac])
    - Example: ranitidine 150 mg PO QD or BID (may require decreased dose based off renal function).
    - Cimetidine (Tagamet) avoided in older adults given increased risk of delirium and drug interactions.
    - Provides heartburn relief for about 8–12 hours.
    - Can be used as an adjunct to proton-pump inhibitor (PPI) therapy if symptoms are still present.
    - Caution use in patients with delirium (or high risk of delirium). Adverse reactions include headache, constipation or diarrhea, dizziness, and xerostomia.
  - Gastroenterology consultation/referral
    - Refer when patients do not respond to the typical treatment.

- Can determine if surgery is the right option, especially if medications control symptoms but patient not willing to take long-term PPI therapy or if GERD symptoms continue despite PPI therapy. Surgery is unlikely to be beneficial if PPIs are ineffective.

Note: Beers listed items, as mentioned above, include proton-pump inhibitors (avoid use beyond 8 weeks) and H2-receptor antagonists.

## Differential Diagnosis[1,2,3]

- Peptic ulcer disease (PUD): Endoscopy would show an ulcer and patient typically will have nocturnal symptoms that awaken them at night. Compared to GERD, an upper endoscopy would show the severity or extent of tissue damage; about one-third will have erosion or ulcers in the esophagus. GERD does not typically cause nighttime symptoms or disrupt sleep. Heartburn as the main symptom indicates GERD, not PUD.
- Malignancy: Will have other symptoms such as anemia, worsening dysphagia, GI bleeding, and/or unintentional weight loss. May have abnormal blood work, such as anemia or elevated LFTs.

### CLINICAL PEARLS[1,2,3]

- Complications of GERD after the age of 65 years include Barrett's esophagus, esophageal adenocarcinoma, esophagitis, bleeding, and peptic stricture.
- The mainstay of treatment includes lifestyle changes (e.g., head of bed elevation, losing weight) and controlling symptoms with acid-suppressing therapy.

## References

1. Zuckerman, M. J., & Othman, M. O. (2017, February 7). Gastroesophageal Reflux Disease. Epocrates. Retrieved from https://online.epocrates.com/diseases/82/GERD-gastroesophageal-reflux-disease. Accessed December 9, 2017.
2. McQuaid, K. R. (2018). Gastrointestinal disorders. In *Current Medical Diagnosis & Treatment 2018*. New York, NY: McGraw-Hill. Retrieved from http://accessmedicine

.mhmedical.com/content.aspx?bookid=2192&sectionid=168013478. Accessed December 9, 2017.

3. Hall, K. E. (2014). Gastrointestinal and abdominal complaints. In *Current Diagnosis & Treatment: Geriatrics* (2nd ed.). New York, NY: McGraw-Hill. Retrieved from http://accessmedicine.mhmedical.com/content.aspx?bookid=953&sectionid=53375659. Accessed December 9, 2017.
4. Mayo Clinic. (2017, November 1). Gastroesophageal Reflux Disease (GERD). Retrieved from https://www.mayoclinic.org/diseases-conditions/gerd/symptoms-causes/syc-20361940. Accessed December 9, 2017.
5. National Institute of Diabetes and Digestive and Kidney Diseases (NIDDK). (2014, November 1). Definition & Facts for GER & GERD. U.S. Department of Health and Human Services, National Institute of Health. Retrieved from https://www.niddk.nih.gov/health-information/digestive-diseases/acid-reflux-ger-gerd-adults/definition-facts. Accessed December 9, 2017.
6. American Geriatrics Society 2015 Beers Criteria Update Expert Panel, Fick, D. M., Semla, T. P., Beizer, J., Brandt, N., & Dombrowski, R., . . . Steinman, M. (2015, October 8). American Geriatrics Society 2015 updated Beers criteria for potentially inappropriate medication use in older adults. *Journal of the American Geriatrics Society, 63*(11), 2227–2246. Retrieved from http://onlinelibrary.wiley.com/doi/10.1111/jgs.13702/abstract. Accessed October 8, 2017.

SECTION VI

# Genitourinary

## Benign Prostatic Hyperplasia

### Definition[2,3,4,5,6]

Benign prostatic hyperplasia (BPH) is a histologic condition characterized by benign proliferation of the cellular components within the prostate.

Note: BPH is the most common benign tumor in men; according to autopsy data, it affects about 90% of men ≥ age 80 years.

### Cause[2,5]

- Cause is unknown.

### Risk Factors[1,2,4,5,6,9]

*Poorly understood.*

- Age > 50 years
- Family history
- Race
    - Higher in African American and Caucasian men
- Physical inactivity
- Obesity
- Diabetes mellitus
- High fat and/or meat consumption

### Signs & Symptoms[1,2,3,4,5,6,9]

- Weak stream.
- Urinary frequency.
    - This can occur also at night; will void small amounts at a time.
- Urinary urgency.
- Incomplete bladder emptying.
- Straining to urinate.

- Postvoid dribbling (small amounts).
- Symmetrical, smooth, and firm enlarged prostate on digital rectal exam (DRE).
  - If induration or asymmetry is noted, further workup required (can indicate malignancy).
  - The size of the prostate on digital rectal examination does not correlate with symptoms.
- Bladder distention may be present.
  - Seen with significant urinary retention.
- Hematuria, dysuria, and pelvic pain are **not** common.
  - Further workup required, these are suggestive of underlying infection, stone, or malignancy.

## Tests[1,2,3,4,5,6,7,8,9,10]

- Perform a patient questionnaire (to guide management decisions); the American Urological Association symptom index (AUASI) to determine severity of symptoms (see Table 6-1).
  - Score of < 7 equals mild BPH.
  - Score of 8–19 equals moderate BPH.
  - Score of 20–35 equals severe BPH.
- Urinalysis.
  - Should be ordered in **all** men with lower urinary tract symptoms; used to check for microscopic hematuria.
  - This helps to exclude infection.
- Prostate specific antigen (PSA).
  - Screening for prostate cancer is not recommended by the U.S. Preventive Services Task Force (USPSTF).
  - The American Urological Association (AUA) does not recommend screening in men > age 70 years (unless in excellent health) or any man with limited life expectancy (less than 10 years).
- Postvoid residual.
  - Not usually required unless patient has failed empiric therapy, presence of urinary retention, or is on medications that impair detrusor contractility (e.g., anticholinergics).

- Urine flow rate.
  - Recommended in the AUA guideline.
- Cystoscopy.
  - Not routinely recommended.
  - Ordered when hematuria, pelvic pain, and risk factors for bladder cancer are present.
- Baseline creatinine, upper urinary tract imaging, or renal ultrasound should not be routinely ordered.

## Treatment & Management[2,3,4,5,6]

- **Nonpharmacologic and nursing interventions:**
  - Assess for underlying pain or discomfort, and hematuria.
    - Can be a sign of urinary tract infection (UTI).
  - Encourage lifestyle modifications.
    - Limit fluids before bedtime (to avoid nocturia and improve sleep).
    - Void prior going to bed.
    - Encourage fluids; however be mindful that overhydration can aggravate bladder distention.
    - Limit use of caffeinated beverages (e.g., coffee) to decrease urgency.
    - Consumption of moderate alcohol, vegetables, foods high in protein and low in fat, or meat can slow the progression of BPH.
    - Increase physical activity and weight loss.
  - Watchful waiting (conservative approach).
    - Recommended in those with no or mild symptoms (not likely to benefit from medical therapy).
    - These patients should be re-examined yearly.
- **Pharmacological and other interventions:**
  - Perform a medication review, given some drug effects can lead to lower urinary tract symptoms.
    - This includes anticholinergics (e.g., antihistamines), diuretics, and decongestants.

- Alpha blockers (e.g., alfuzosin [Uroxatral], doxazosin [Cardura], tamsulosin [Flomax]). Prazosin should **not** be used.
  - Example: tamsulosin 0.4–0.8 mg PO daily; takes 2–4 weeks to see effects.
  - Used as first-line agent for bothersome, moderate, or severe symptoms.
  - Improves urine flow and causes relaxation of the smooth muscle.
  - Ophthalmologists need to be aware if a patient is taking these medications prior to cataract surgery (risk of floppy iris syndrome, particularly with tamsulosin).
  - Monitor for adverse effects such as significant hypotension, dizziness, abnormal ejaculation (especially with higher dosages).
- 5-alpha-reductase inhibitors (e.g., finasteride [Proscar], dutasteride [Avodart]).
  - Example: dutasteride 0.5 mg PO daily.
  - Decreases prostate size, reduces risk of urinary retention, and likelihood of surgery; improvement in symptoms can take 6 months.
  - Can be used in combo with an alpha blocker.
  - Known to cause adverse sexual effects (e.g., decreased libido, erectile dysfunction).
    - There may be a risk of high-grade prostate cancer when used long term.
- Phosphodiesterase inhibitors (e.g., tadalafil [Cialis]).
  - Example: tadalafil 5 mg PO daily.
  - Improves BPH symptoms and treats erectile dysfunction.
  - If sildenafil [Viagra] is used in doses above 25 mg, avoid administration within 4 hours of an alpha blocker.
  - Can cause significant hypotension when combined with alpha blockers, except tamsulosin.
- Urinary antimuscarinics (e.g., tolterodine [Detrol], fesoterodine [Toviaz], solifenacin [Vesicare]).
  - Example: tolterodine extended release 4 mg PO daily.

        - Improves urinary urgency and frequency with minimal to moderate efficacy.
        - Commonly combined with an alpha blocker and ordered in those who do not have an elevated postvoid residual (above 250–300 mL).
        - Carries anticholinergic drugs effects (e.g., constipation, xerostomia, delirium).
    - Herbal therapy (e.g., saw palmetto).
        - The AUA does not recommend these therapies in the management of BPH.
- Urology and/or surgical referral
    - Referral recommended: When the above medications fail, distended bladder, urinary retention (acute or chronic), recurrent UTIs, gross hematuria, abnormal DRE findings, and for consideration of minimally invasive treatment or surgical intervention (e.g., transurethral resection of the prostate [TURP]).

Note: Beers listed items, as mentioned above, include urinary antimuscarinics and peripheral alpha blockers (doxazosin and terazosin).

## Differential Diagnosis[2,3,4]

- Bladder calculi (stones): Hematuria and pain are commonly associated with these (not as common in BPH).
- Urinary tract infection: Will have the irritative symptoms of BPH; may exhibit dysuria, hematuria, fever, and/or chills and can be identified by urinalysis and culture.
- Prostate cancer: May have abnormal findings on DRE, an elevated PSA, along with weight loss and/or night sweats. Other symptoms such as radiculopathy and/or back pain can imply metastases to the bone.
- Certain medications: Always consider this when patients present with BPH given diuretics, anticholinergics, and over-the-counter decongestants (e.g., pseudoephedrine [Sudafed]) mimic or worsen symptoms associated with BPH.

**Table 6-1** American Urological Association Symptom Index

| American Urological Association Symptom Index | | | | | | |
|---|---|---|---|---|---|---|
| ***Over the past month or so:*** | **Not at all** | **Less than 1 in 5 times** | **Less than one-half of the time** | **About one-half of the time** | **More than one-half of the time** | **Almost always** |
| How often have you had the sensation of not completely emptying your bladder after you finished urinating? | 0 | 1 | 2 | 3 | 4 | 5 |
| How often have you had to urinate again less than 2 hours after you finished urinating? | 0 | 1 | 2 | 3 | 4 | 5 |
| How often have you found that you stopped and started again when urinating? | 0 | 1 | 2 | 3 | 4 | 5 |
| How often have you found it difficult to postpone urination? | 0 | 1 | 2 | 3 | 4 | 5 |
| How often have you had a weak urinary stream? | 0 | 1 | 2 | 3 | 4 | 5 |
| How often have you had to push or strain to begin urination? | 0 | 1 | 2 | 3 | 4 | 5 |
| | None | 1 time | 2 times | 3 times | 4 times | 5 times |
| How many times do you typically get up to urinate from the time you go to bed at night until the time you get up in the morning? | 0 | 1 | 2 | 3 | 4 | 5 |
| | | | | | Total score: ______ | |

Reproduced from Barry MJ, et al. (1992). American Urological Association symptom index for benign prostatic hyperplasia. *Journal of Urology*, 148(5): 1555.

## CLINICAL PEARLS[4,5]

- American Urological Association (AUA) score index (Table 6-1).
- The impact of BPH symptoms should not be underestimated, given it can disrupt the patient's quality of life. Focus on the top bothersome symptoms to base treatment decisions, while keeping in mind that medication to target nocturia is not very effective.
- Not effectively treating the patient's BPH can disrupt his or her daily activities, sexual function, and sleep; it causes physical discomfort, leading to embarrassment.
- Some of the medications (e.g., alpha blockers) are on the Beers list and must be considered when prescribing these agents.

# References


1. Pearson, R., & Williams, P. M. (2014). Common questions about the diagnosis and management of benign prostatic hypertrophy. *American Family Physician, 90*(11), 769–774. Retrieved from https://www.aafp.org/afp/2014/1201/p769.html. Accessed December 30, 2017.
2. Meng, M. V., Walsh, T. J., & Chi, T. D. (2018). Urologic disorders. In *Current Medical Diagnosis & Treatment 2018*. New York, NY: McGraw-Hill. Retrived from http://accessmedicine.mhmedical.com/content.aspx?bookid=2192&sectionid=168019217. Accessed December 30, 2017.
3. Chao, S., & Chippendale, R. (2014). Benign prostatic hyperplasia and prostate cancer. In *Current Diagnosis & Treatment: Geriatrics* (2nd ed.). New York, NY: McGraw-Hill. Retrieved from http://accessmedicine.mhmedical.com/content.aspx?bookid=953&sectionid=53375664. Accessed December 30, 2017.
4. DuBeau, C. E. (2017). Benign prostate disorders. In *Hazzard's Geriatric Medicine and Gerontology* (7th ed.). New York, NY: McGraw-Hill. Retrieved from http://accessmedicine.mhmedical.com/content.aspx?bookid=1923&sectionid=144521381. Accessed December 30, 2017.
5. American Urological Association. (2010). Clinical Guideline: Management of Benign Prostatic Hyperplasia. Retrieved from https://auanet.org/guidelines/benign-prostatic-hyperplasia-(2010-reviewed-and-validity-confirmed-2014)#x2466. Accessed December 30, 2017.
6. Deters, L. A. (2017, December 18). Benign Prostatic Hyperplasia (BPH) (F. Talavera, F., & Kim, E. D., Eds.). Medscape. Retrieved from https://emedicine.medscape.com/article/437359-overview#a1. Accessed December 30, 2017.
7. Mcvary, K. T., Roehrborn, C. G., Avins, A. L., Barry, M. J., Bruskewitz, R. C., & Donnell, R. F., . . . Wei, J. T. (2011). Update on AUA guideline on the management of benign prostatic hyperplasia. *Journal of Urology, 185*(5), 1793–1803. doi:10.1016/j.juro.2011.01.074
8. Arma, A. V., & Wei, J. T. (2012, July 19). Benign prostatic hyperplasia and lower urinary tract symptoms. *New England Journal of Medicine, 367*, 248–257. doi:10.1056/NEJMcp1106637

9. Gulanick, M., & Myers, J. L. (2017). *Nursing Care Plans: Diagnoses, Interventions, & Outcomes*. St. Louis, MO: Elsevier.
10. American Urological Association. (2015). Early Detection of Prostate Cancer. Retrieved from http://www.auanet.org/guidelines/early-detection-of-prostate-cancer-(2013-reviewed-and-validity-confirmed-2015). Accessed February 17, 2018.
11. American Geriatrics Society 2015 Beers Criteria Update Expert Panel, Fick, D. M., Semla, T. P., Beizer, J., Brandt, N., & Dombrowski, R., . . .Steinman, M. (2015, October 8). American Geriatrics Society 2015 updated Beers criteria for potentially inappropriate medication use in older adults. *Journal of the American Geriatrics Society, 63*(11), 2227–2246. Retrieved from http://onlinelibrary.wiley.com/doi/10.1111/jgs.13702/abstract. Accessed October 8, 2017.
12. Therapeutic Research Center. (2015, December). PL Detail-Document, Potentially Harmful Drugs in the Elderly: Beers List. Pharmacist's Letter/Prescriber's Letter.

# Urinary Incontinence

## Definition[1,2,3,4,5,6]

Urinary incontinence (UI) is a syndrome defined as the involuntary loss of bladder control.

## Classification[1,2,3,4,5,6]

**Urge incontinence:** Leakage of urine due to inability to delay voiding following the sensation of a full bladder.

Note: This is the most common type of urinary incontinence in older adults.

**Stress incontinence:** Leakage of urine coincident with an increase in intraabdominal pressure; common in older women.
**Overflow incontinence (some experts prefer the term high postvoid residual):** Leakage of urine due to impaired urinary sphincter relaxation or bladder wall contraction; usually occurs in men due to obstruction of urinary flow.
**Functional incontinence:** Occurs in the presence of normal urine control, but inability to reach the toilet in time; common in nursing home patients or facilities.
**Mixed incontinence:** Leakage of urine due to mixed etiology (combination of stress and urgency incontinence seen in older women is most common). It is typical for older adults to have more than one type of incontinence.

## Causes[1,2,3,4,5,6]

| Type | Causes |
|---|---|
| Urge incontinence | Stroke, dementia, parkinsonism, multiple sclerosis, detrusor overactivity, tumors, stones, cystitis |
| Stress incontinence | Internal sphincter damage or pelvic floor weakness, prior vaginal childbirths, prior urinary tract surgery, genitourinary atrophy or prolapse, postprostatectomy |
| Overflow incontinence | Outlet obstruction (e.g., BPH, prostate cancer), bladder contractile dysfunction (e.g., diabetic neuropathy, spinal cord injury), certain medications (e.g., anticholinergics) |
| Functional incontinence | Impaired physical mobility (e.g., arthritis), cognitive or psychological impairment (e.g., severe depression, dementia), environmental barriers |

## Risk Factors[1,2,3,4,5,6]

*Risk factors of UI coincide with causes.*

- Advanced age *(not an inevitable condition of aging)*
  - About 50% of community-dwelling older adults and 50%–75% of those residing in institutions (e.g., nursing homes) have urinary incontinence.
- Female sex
- Morbid obesity
- Neurological disorders (e.g., dementia, stroke, Parkinson's disease)
- Impaired physical mobility (e.g., arthritis)
- History of genitourinary surgery
- Diabetes
- Decreased estrogen or atrophic vaginitis

- Medications (e.g., diuretics, anticholinergics, caffeine)
- Other causes: delirium, stool impaction, smoking, urinary tract infection, consumption of large amounts of water

## Signs & Symptoms[1,2,3,4,5,6]

| Type | Signs/Symptoms |
|---|---|
| Urge incontinence | The urgent need to urinate suddenly and inability to reach a restroom in time, frequent loss of urine (small to large volume), and nocturia. |
| Stress incontinence | Leakage of urine (usually small amount) when coughing, sneezing, laughing. |
| Overflow incontinence | Dribbling of urine and/or continual leakage, feeling of incomplete bladder emptying, high postvoid urinary volume, nocturia. |
| Functional incontinence | Loss of urine due to inability to reach a bathroom fast enough due to impaired cognitive, psychological, or physical function, may have altered cognition; large-volume leakage. |

## Tests[1,2,3,4]

- Urinalysis with culture
    - Ordered in the setting of new onset incontinence and if concerned for underlying urinary tract infection.
- Serum glucose, calcium, and creatinine levels
    - Reserved in adults with unexplained polyuria (check for hyperglycemia, hypercalcemia).
    - Renal function ordered in those with significant urinary retention (can cause renal impairment).
- Ultrasound bladder scanner or postvoid urinary catheterization
    - Used to assess urinary volume after voiding to identify urinary retention.
    - Under 50 mL is expected whereas over 200 mL suggests considerable bladder dysfunction (requiring further evaluation).

- Renal ultrasound, CT urogram
  - Not routinely ordered; evaluates the urinary systems structure and function.
  - Identifies cysts, tumors, blockages.
- Urodynamic studies
  - Determines the cause(s) of urinary retention, however not routinely ordered, especially in frail or demented older adults.
  - Consider in those considering surgery for UI.
- Cystoscopy
  - Looks for urinary tract structural abnormalities and can provide tissue sample.

## Treatment & Management[1,2,3,4,5,6,7,8,9,10,11]

- **Nonpharmacological and nursing interventions:**
  - Educate on pelvic muscle exercises (i.e., Kegel exercises).
    - This treats stress, urge, and mixed incontinence, including incontinence following prostatectomy.
  - Biofeedback.
  - Encourage urinating on a set schedule (about every 2–3 hours during the day).
    - This can be used in patients with impaired cognitive or physical function; used in urge and functional incontinence.
  - Bladder training.
    - Requires adequate cognitive and physical functioning; used in stress and urge incontinence.
  - Encourage lifestyle changes (e.g., increase physical activity, weight loss, stop smoking, drink less caffeine, take measures to prevent constipation, avoid extremes of fluid intake).
  - Ensure safe and effective passage to the bathroom; avoid clutter and keep light on at all times.
    - Treatment for functional incontinence.

- Unless indicated, avoid indwelling catheters. Alternatives include disposable or absorbent bed pads and undergarments (result in less morbidity than catheters). Many products aren't covered by Medicare.

- **Pharmacological and other interventions:**
  - Identify and treat the underlying issue(s), such as:
    - Reduce or discontinue the offending agent (e.g., diuretic).
    - Treat the delirium.
    - Treat underlying infection.
  - Urinary antimuscarinics (e.g., darifenacin [Enablex], fesoterodine [Toviaz], oxybutynin [Ditropan])
    - Example: oxybutynin 2.5–5.0 mg PO TID.
    - These medications increase bladder capacity and reduce bladder contractions; used to treat urge incontinence.
    - These are *only* recommended in older adults if no other alternatives are available.
    - Monitor for anticholinergic effects (e.g., dry mouth, confusion, constipation).
  - Beta-3 agonist (i.e., mirabegron [Myrbetriq])
    - Example: mirabegron 25–50 mg PO daily (dosage depends on renal/hepatic function).
    - This drug inhibits bladder contraction; treats urge incontinence.
    - Monitor for adverse effects such as hypertension, tachycardia, headache.
  - Vaginal estrogen (e.g., topical, vaginal ring [Estring])
    - Example: estrogen topical 0.5–1.0 g vaginal cream applied daily up to 2 weeks, followed by two to three times per week.
    - Useful in women with urge or stress incontinence.
    - This drug reduces inflammation from atrophic vaginitis and irritative voiding symptoms.
    - Not to be used in women with history of breast cancer.

- Alpha blockers (e.g., doxazosin [Cardura], terazosin [Hytrin], tamsulosin [Flomax])
    - Example: doxazosin 1–8 mg PO daily.
    - These agents relax muscle of urethra and prostatic capsule to improve urine flow; useful in men with symptoms associated with BPH.
    - Monitor for possible adverse effects, such as hypotension and dizziness.
- Wound, ostomy, and continence (WOC) nurse consultation/referral
  - Enhances the care for patients suffering from UI; research has shown agencies with WOC nurses have significantly better outcomes than those without WOC nurses.
- Physical therapist consultation/referral
  - They can provide women with a variety of methods to improve UI. They develop an exercise treatment program and use techniques such as biofeedback, electrical stimulation, and weighted vaginal cones.
- Urology consultation/referral
  - Recommended if postvoid residual is above 200 mL.
  - Recommended in men with pelvic pain, significant lower urinary tract symptoms, or history of pelvic radiation.
  - Surgical intervention may be necessary in the following: men with outflow obstruction and complete urinary retention, men with stress urinary incontinence and continual urinary leakage, women with significant pelvic prolapse or with stress UI who do not respond to treatment.
  - Other options: pessary (UI due to prolapsed bladder or uterus), injections of Botox for overactive bladder (not FDA approved), sacral nerve stimulators, and percutaneous tibial nerve stimulator for overactive bladder.

Note: Beers listed items, as mentioned above, include peripheral alpha blockers, estrogen (however low-dose intravaginal estrogen typically safe), and urinary antimuscarinics.

## Differential Diagnosis[1,2]

- Atrophic vaginitis or urethritis: Can present with dysuria, urgency, and frequency, contributing to UI; will result in thinning and drying of vagina and urethra. Symptoms are relieved with low-dose, topical estrogen.
- Acute urinary tract infection: Incontinence will come on quickly, and will have other symptoms, such as burning. Urinary culture would be positive.

### CLINICAL PEARLS[1,2,3,4,5]

- Be sure to discuss urinary incontinence with older adults, although it may be an embarrassing topic. Not addressing UI can lead to social isolation, depression, skin irritation and breakdown, skin infections, recurrent urinary tract infections, and predisposition to institutionalization.
- Indwelling catheters are often ordered for UI unnecessarily, placing the patient at risk for catheter-induced infection, and should therefore be avoided, unless indicated.
    - Indications for chronic indwelling catheter: care of terminally ill patients, skin wounds or pressure ulcers and urine would contribute to impaired healing, urinary retention that causes renal impairment or symptomatic infections, and/or urinary retention that fails medical management or unable to undergo surgical intervention.
    - If a catheter has been placed for urinary retention, try using an alpha blocker 48 hours prior to removing the catheter.

## References


1. Bass, J., & Knight, A. L. (2015). Kidney disease. In Burggraf, V., Kim, K. Y., & Knight, A. L. (Eds.) *Healthy Aging: Principles and Clinical Practice for Clinicians* (pp. 328–338). Philadelphia, PA: Lippincott Williams & Wilkins.
2. Vaughan, C. P., & Johnson, II, T. M. (2017). Incontinence. In *Hazzard's Geriatric Medicine and Gerontology* (7th ed.). New York, NY: McGraw-Hill. Retrieved from http://accessmedicine.mhmedical.com/content.aspx?bookid=1923&sectionid=144522371. Accessed January 4, 2018.
3. Kane, R. L., Ouslander, J. G., Resnick, B., & Malone, M. L. (Eds.). (2015). *Essentials of Clinical Geriatrics* (8th ed.). New York, NY: McGraw-Hill; Chapter 8: Incontinence. Retrieved from http://accessmedicine.mhmedical.com/content.aspx?bookid=678&sectionid=44833886. Accessed January 4, 2018.

4. Gammack, J. K. (2014). Urinary incontinence. In *Current Diagnosis & Treatment: Geriatrics* (2nd ed.). New York, NY: McGraw-Hill. Retrieved from http://accessmedicine.mhmedical.com/content.aspx?bookid=953&sectionid=53375663. Accessed January 4, 2018.
5. Hersh, L., & Salzman, B. (2013). Clinical management of urinary incontinence in women. *American Family Physician,* 87(9), 634–640. Retrieved from https://www.aafp.org/afp/2013/0501/p634.html. Accessed January 6, 2018.
6. National Institute of Aging. (2017, May 16). Urinary Incontinence in Older Adults. U.S. Department of Health and Human Services. Retrieved from https://www.nia.nih.gov/health/urinary-incontinence-older-adults. Accessed January 6, 2018.
7. Madhuvrata, P., Cody, J. D., Ellis, G., Herbison, G. P., & Hay-Smith, E. J. (2012, January 18). Which anticholinergic drug for overactive bladder symptoms in adults. *Cochrane Database of Systematic Reviews, 1,* CD005429. doi:10.1002/14651858.cd005429.pub2
8. Rogers, R. G. (2008, March 6). Clinical practice: Urinary stress incontinence in women. *New England Journal of Medicine,* 358(10), 1029–1036. doi:10.1056/NEJMcp0707023
9. American Geriatrics Society 2015 Beers Criteria Update Expert Panel, Fick, D. M., Semla, T. P., Beizer, J., Brandt, N., & Dombrowski, R., . . . Steinman, M. (2015, October 8). American Geriatrics Society 2015 updated Beers criteria for potentially inappropriate medication use in older adults. *Journal of the American Geriatrics Society,* 63(11), 2227–2246. Retrieved from http://onlinelibrary.wiley.com/doi/10.1111/jgs.13702/abstract. Accessed October 3, 2017.
10. Therapeutic Research Center. (2015, December). PL Detail-Document, Potentially Harmful Drugs in the Elderly: Beers List. Pharmacist's Letter/Prescriber's Letter.
11. Westra, B. L., Bliss, D. Z., Savik, K., Hou, Y., & Borchert, A. (2014). Effectiveness of wound, ostomy, and continence nurses on agency-level wound and incontinence outcomes in home care. *Home Healthcare Nurse,* 32(2), 119–127. doi: 10.1097/NHH.0000000000000030

# Urinary Tract Infection

## Definitions[2,4,6]

Urinary tract infection (UTI)* is defined as the presence of bacteriuria and pyuria, including signs and symptoms attributable to the genitourinary tract.

Note: There is currently *no clear definition* as to what defines symptomatic UTI in older adults.

* UTI can easily be confused with asymptomatic bacteruria (ASB), which has bacteriuria, with or without pyuria, however *not* accompanied with symptoms suggestive of a urinary tract infection (considered a colonization state).[1,2,4,6]

## Causes[1,2,4,6,7,9]

- Bacteria gaining entry into the urinary tract
  - Most common organisms include *Escherichia coli* (most common), *Proteus mirabilis* (more common in men), *Klebsiella pneumoniae.*

## Risk Factors[1,2,4,5,6,7,9]

- Advanced age
- History of UTI
- Presence of a urinary catheter
- Residing in a long-term care facility
- Structural or functional abnormalities (*prevents the removal of uropathogens*)
  - Benign prostatic hypertrophy, cystoceles
- Postmenopausal women, estrogen deficiency
- Sexual activity
- Diabetes mellitus
- Acquired neurologic disorders
  - Stroke, Alzheimer's disease, Parkinson's disease
- Functional disability

## Signs & Symptoms[1,2,3,4,5,6,7]

*Older adults often lack typical signs/symptoms of a UTI.*

- Nonspecific symptoms: lethargy, new or worsening confusion, odorous urine, decline in functional status

| Type | Signs/Symptoms |
|---|---|
| Acute uncomplicated UTI or cystitis | Dysuria, frequency, urgency, suprapubic pain, hematuria (with a structurally normal urinary tract). |
| Pyelonephritis | May include same symptoms as cystitis, including: fever*, nausea/emesis, chills, and flank pain. |

| Type | Signs/Symptoms |
|---|---|
| Catheter-associated UTI (i.e., suprapubic, indwelling urethral catheter, or catherization) | Will have no other identifiable etiology to explain new or worsening fever, chills, delirium, or malaise; flank pain, new hematuria, pelvic discomfort; costovertebral angle discomfort; OR if catheter removed in past 2 days, will demonstrate dysuria, urgency or frequency, or suprapubic pain. |

* Fever definition in long-term care facilities (per the Infectious Diseases Society of America [IDSA]): an oral temperature of ≥ 100°F, a temperature ≥ 2°F than the baseline, repeated temperature > 99°F (oral) or >99.5°F (rectal).

Note: Complicated UTI includes pyelonephritis, symptomatic UTI in patients with functional or anatomic abnormality of the urinary tract, urinary catheters, men with UTIs, and in patients with chronic kidney disease, diabetes, or immunodeficiency. It is unclear if all patients above the age of 65 with symptomatic UTI should be categorized as complicated.

## Labs[1,2,3,4,5,6,7,9]

- Urinary dipstick, urinalysis with culture and sensitivity
  - Should be ordered in symptomatic patients.
  - Bacteriuria (> 100,000 colonized forming units (CFU)/mL in a clean catch specimen or > 100 CFU/mL in a catheterized specimen) can indicate contamination of the specimen, UTI, or asymptomatic bacteriuria.
    - Squamous cells in high amounts suggest contamination.
  - Pyuria (≥ 10 white blood cells/$mm^3$ per high-power field) suggests genitourinary tract inflammation.
    - This will be seen in almost all patients residing in long-term care with bacteriuria and is NOT an indicator for antibiotics
    - The absence of pyuria and nitrate excludes underlying UTI.

Note: The presence of bacteriuria and pyuria does not confirm presence of UTI. Both of these will be present in almost all patients with an indwelling urinary catheter.

- CBC with differential, renal and hepatic function (blood urea nitrogen/creatinine [BUN/Cr], liver function test [LFT])
  - Evaluates for leukocytosis and the degree of renal and/or hepatic impairment for antibiotic prescribing.
    - A white blood count (WBC) of ≥ 14,000 should make the provider suspicious for underlying infection, with or without fever.
- Blood cultures
  - Not usually beneficial in most long-term care patients. The exception: presumed bacteremia.

## Treatment & Management[2,4,5,6,7,9,13,14]

- **Nonpharmacological and nursing interventions:**
  - Prevention of catheter-associated urinary tract infection(CAUTI).
    - Insert catheter using sterile technique, washing hands before and after catheter insertion, advise against routine bladder irrigations (unless catheter is obstructed), encourage adequate hydration and nutritional status, keep the collection bag below the bladder, maintain a closed drainage system, and remove the catheter (if appropriate).
    - Antibiotic-coated catheters are pricey and have not been shown to significantly prevent catheter-associated UTIs.
    - Alternatives to an indwelling urethral catheter include condom catheter, intermittent catheterization, suprapubic catheter (*carries lower risk of bacteriuria*), diapers, or pads.
  - Encourage ambulation.
    - Improving mobility in skilled nursing facilities reduces the risk of hospitalization from a UTI.

- Encourage fluids.
  - Encourage about 2–3 L/day (if no contraindications such as heart failure) to promote the removal of bacteria.
- Encourage regular toileting.
  - This can prevent infection. Encouraging patient to void about every 3 hours during the day enhances bacterial clearance.
- Teach the patient about importance of hygienic measures.
  - Cleaning the perineal area reduces the concentration of pathogens to go up in the urinary tract. This is also important following a bowel movement.
  - Change underwear daily; encourage loose fitting clothing and cotton fabric.

- **Pharmacological and other interventions:**
  - Choose antibiotic based on current bacterial susceptibility; empiric treatment can be based off prior cultures.
  - Prior to prescribing antibiotics, consider the following: the facility's resistance patterns, the facility's practice patterns and standards/protocol, patient's allergy profile and threshold for noncompliance, renal and hepatic impairment, cost and availability of the antibiotic, and drug-drug interactions.
  - Nitrofurantoin monohydrate/macrocrystals (Macrobid).
    - Administered at 100 mg PO BID for 5 days (avoid if CrCl < 30 mL/min).
    - Recommended for uncomplicated UTIs.
    - Compared to trimethoprim/sulfamethoxazole [Bactrim] and fluoroquinolones, has lower rate of resistance.
    - Carries potential for pulmonary toxicity (if used long term).
  - Trimethropim/sulfamethoxazole (TMP/SMX).
    - Administered at 160/800 mg PO BID for 3 days or up to 2 weeks, if UTI complicated.

- Known to increase serum creatinine and interact with warfarin (Coumadin) (increased risk of bleeding).
- Fosfomycin trometamol (Monurol).
  - Administered at 3 g PO × 1 dose.
  - Used for uncomplicated UTIs; is not FDA approved to treat complicated UTIs.
  - Known side effects include diarrhea, dizziness, vaginitis.
- Fluoroquinolone (e.g., ciprofloxacin [Cipro], levofloxacin [Levaquin]).
  - Example: ciprofloxacin 250 mg or 500 mg BID for 3 days or up to 2 weeks, if complicated.
  - Used as second-line treatment due to increased resistance rates.
  - Recommended treatment for pyelonephritis.
  - Side effects may include *Clostridium difficile* infection; tendon rupture rarely occurs.
- Amoxicillin/clavulanate (Augmentin).
  - Administed at 500/125 mg PO BID for 3–7 days.
  - Used as second-line treatment.
  - Side effects may include diarrhea and rash.
- Parental therapy (e.g., piperacillin/tazobactam [Zosyn], cefepime [Maxipime], meropenem [Merrem]).
  - Used in older adults who decline and are severely ill, despite oral antibiotics.

Note: The actual number of days recommended in older adults with a UTI is unknown; if there is delay in response to treatment, longer courses of up to 2 weeks is appropriate. Men with UTIs, catheter-associated UTIs, and pyelonephritis usually require 10–14 days of treatment.

- Suppressive antibiotics.
  - Consider in women with no urological abnormalities and more than three UTIs annually.
  - Rarely indicated; drug adverse reactions (e.g., *Clostridium difficilie* colitis, drug reactions) usually outweigh any benefit.

- Cranberry supplements.
  - Capsules containing 36–108 mg of cranberry proanthocyanidin may lower bacteriuria and pyuria in female patients residing in long-term care facilities.
  - The efficacy of cranberry products in the prevention of UTI is still uncertain.
  - Well tolerated and have minimal risks (juice supplement may increase glucose).
- Vaginal estrogens.
  - Example: vaginal cream with 0.5 mg estriol.
  - Efficacious in reducing UTI in postmenopausal women.
  - No evidence to suggest that oral estrogen reduce UTI recurrence.

- Urology consultation/referral
  - Patients with recurrent UTI.

Note: Beers listed items, as mentioned above, include estrogen (however acceptable to use low-dose intravaginal estrogen for lower urinary tract infections) and nitrofurantoin.

## Differential Diagnosis[2,8,9,10,11]

- Asymptomatic bacteriuria: Can be difficult to differentiate from a UTI. Prevalence is high in nursing home patients. Urine results positive; however will not have genitourinary symptoms.
- Interstitial cystitis: Symptoms come and go, and includes similar symptoms as a UTI (e.g., frequency, urgency, pelvic pain). Certain foods and emotional stress can worsen the symptoms. Urinalysis is usually normal. Treatment options do not include antibiotics. Compared to UTI, symptoms do not come and go, is caused by bacteria, and is not exacerbated by foods or emotional stress. Will have positive urine cultures and will respond to antibiotics.
- Prostatitis: This is an important diagnosis to consider in men because it can take several weeks to cure (i.e., up to 6 weeks).

It is associated with BPH. Acute bacterial prostatitis will present with tender prostate gland; chronic bacterial prostatitis is characterized by recurrent urinary tract infections, intermittent dysuria, and obstructive urinary symptoms. Men with UTI will require about 10–14 days of treatment and will lack the urinary obstruction symptoms, as seen with BPH.

## CLINICAL PEARLS[1,2,3,4,5,6,7,12]

- If patient has no clear indication for using a urinary catheter, remove as soon as possible to prevent infection and bacteremia.
  - Indications for a catheter: urinary incontinence (used for comfort in the terminally ill), urinary retention not responsive to medical therapy or surgery not an option, presence of skin wounds or pressure ulcers and urine would contribute to impaired healing, and urinary retention that causes renal impairment or symptomatic infections.
- If urinalysis reveals high amounts of squamous cells (> 20 cells/hpf) or multiple bacterial species, this likely represents contamination.
- Asymptomatic bacteriuria, which is easily confused with a UTI, is prevalent in older adults residing in long-term care facilities, ranging around 15%–50%. It usually resolves on its own, without the need for antibiotics.
- Treating asymptomatic bacteriuria with antibiotics does not improve mortality rates, genitourinary symptoms, or decrease the frequency of future infection. It can lead to antibiotic-resistant pathogens, *Clostridium difficile* colitis, and drug interactions.
- Screening for and treating asymptomatic bacteriuria is discouraged with the exception of prior to urologic procedures associated with mucosal bleeding to prevent bacteremia (e.g., transurethral prostatic resection).
- In patients with nonspecific symptoms (e.g., confusion, malodorous urine), encourage fluids for 48 hours and reduce or stop diuretics to see if symptoms fade, while considering other diagnosis. If symptoms are still present, then check urine for leukocyte esterase and nitrite; if positive, antibiotics may be indicated for symptomatic UTI.

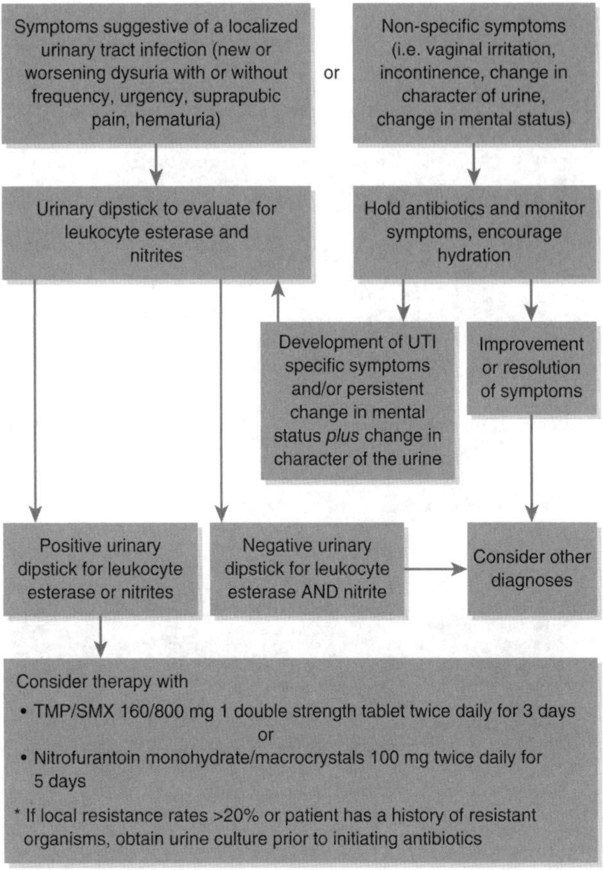


**Figure 6-1** Diagnostic Algorithm for UTI in Community-Dwelling Older Adults

Reproduced from Rowe T. A., Juthani-Mehta M. Diagnosis and Management of Urinary Tract Infection in Older Adults. *Infectious disease clinics of North America*; 2014;28(1):75-89. doi:10.1016/j.idc.2013.10.004. Figure 2.

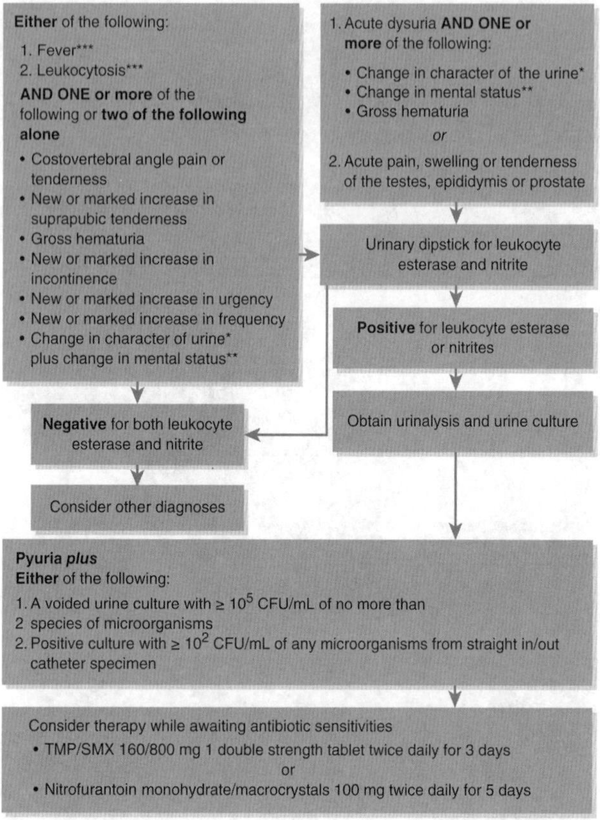
Either of the following:
1. Fever***
2. Leukocytosis***
AND ONE or more of the following or two of the following alone
• Costovertebral angle pain or tenderness
• New or marked increase in suprapubic tenderness
• Gross hematuria
• New or marked increase in incontinence
• New or marked increase in urgency
• New or marked increase in frequency
• Change in character of urine* plus change in mental status**
1. Acute dysuria AND ONE or more of the following:
• Change in character of the urine*
• Change in mental status**
• Gross hematuria
or
2. Acute pain, swelling or tenderness of the testes, epididymis or prostate
Urinary dipstick for leukocyte esterase and nitrite
Positive for leukocyte esterase or nitrites
Obtain urinalysis and urine culture
Negative for both leukocyte esterase and nitrite
Consider other diagnoses
Pyuria plus
Either of the following:
1. A voided urine culture with ≥ 10^5 CFU/mL of no more than 2 species of microorganisms
2. Positive culture with ≥ 10^2 CFU/mL of any microorganisms from straight in/out catheter specimen
Consider therapy while awaiting antibiotic sensitivities
• TMP/SMX 160/800 mg 1 double strength tablet twice daily for 3 days
or
• Nitrofurantoin monohydrate/macrocrystals 100 mg twice daily for 5 days

* Change in color or odor of urine

** Change in level of consciousness, periods of altered perception, disorganized speech, or lethargy

*** Fever: Single temperature ≥ 37.8°C (>100°F), or > 37.2°C (>99°F) on repeated occasions, or an increase of >1.1°C (>2°C) over baseline

**** Leukocytosis: >14,000 cells/mm or Left shift > 6% or 1,500 bands/mm

**Figure 6-2** Diagnostic Algorithm for UTI in Older Adults in Long-Term Care Facilities

Reproduced from Rowe T. A., Juthani-Mehta M. Diagnosis and Management of Urinary Tract Infection in Older Adults. *Infectious disease clinics of North America*; 2014;28(1):75-89. doi:10.1016/j.idc.2013.10.004. Figure 3.

## References

1. Nicolle, L. E., Bradley, S., Colgan, R., Rice, J. C., Schaeffer, A., & Hooton, T. M. (2005, March 1). Infectious Disease Society of America Guidelines for the Diagnosis and Treatment of Asymptomatic Bacteriuria in Adults. Retrieved from https://www.idsociety.org/uploadedFiles/IDSA/Guidelines-Patient_Care/PDF_Library/Asymptomatic%20Bacteriuria.pdf. Accessed December 23, 2017.
2. Genao, L., & Buhr, G. T. (2012). Urinary tract infections in older adults residing in long-term care facilities. *Annals of Long-Term Care: Clinical Care and Aging*, 20(4), 33–38.
3. High, K. P., Bradley, S. F., Gravenstein, S., Mehr, D. R., Quagliarello, V. J., Richards, C., & Yoshikawa, T. T.; Infectious Diseases Society of America. (2009). Clinical practice guideline for the evaluation of fever and infection in older adult patients of long-term care facilities: 2008 update by the Infectious Diseases Society of America. *Journal of the American Geriatrics Society*, 57(3), 375–394. doi:10.1111/j.1532-5415.2009.02175.x
4. Rowe, T., & Juthani-Mehta, M. (2017). Urinary tract infections. In *Hazzard's Geriatric Medicine and Gerontology* (7th ed.). New York, NY: McGraw-Hill. Retrieved from http://accessmedicine.mhmedical.com/content.aspx?bookid=1923&sectionid=144563864. Accessed December 23, 2017.
5. Mody, L., Riddell, J., IV, Kaye, K. S., & Chopra, T. (2014). Common infections. In *Current Diagnosis & Treatment: Geriatrics* (2nd ed.). New York, NY: McGraw-Hill. Retrieved from http://accessmedicine.mhmedical.com/content.aspx?bookid=953&sectionid=53375671. Accessed December 26, 2017.
6. Rowe, T. A., & Juthani-Mehta, M. (2014). Diagnosis and management of urinary tract infection in older adults. *Infectious Disease Clinics of North America,* 28(1), 75–89. doi:10.1016/j.idc.2013.10.004
7. Hooton, T. M., Bradley, S. F., Cardenas, D. D., Colgan, R., Geerlings, S. E., & Rice, J. C., . . . Nicolle, P. T. (2010). Diagnosis, prevention, and treatment of catheter-associated urinary tract infections in adults: 2009 international clinical practice guidelines from the Infectious Diseases Society of America. *Clinical Infectious Diseases,* 50(5), 625–663. Retrieved from https://doi.org/10.1086/650482. Accessed December 27, 2017.
8. Epocrates. (n.d.). Retrieved from https://www.epocrates.com (used for brand names and dosing instructions).
9. Gulanick, M., & Myers, J. L. (2017). *Nursing Care Plans: Diagnoses, Interventions, & Outcomes*. St. Louis, MO: Elsevier.
10. Lipsky, B. A. (1999, March). Prostatitis and urinary tract infection in men: What's new; what's true? *American Journal of Medicine, 106*(3), 327–334. doi: 10.1016/S0002-9343(99)00017-0
11. Turek, P. J. (2017, March 20). Prostatitis Clinical Presentation (Talavera, F., Lang, E. S., & Taylor, J. P., Eds.). Medscape. Retrieved from https://emedicine.medscape.com/article/785418-clinical. Accessed December 28, 2017.
12. Vaughan, C. P, & Johnson, II T. M. (2017). Incontinence. In *Hazzard's Geriatric Medicine and Gerontology* (7th ed.). New York, NY: McGraw-Hill. Retrieved from http://accessmedicine.mhmedical.com/content.aspx?bookid=1923&sectionid=144522371. Accessed January 4, 2018.
13. American Geriatrics Society 2015 Beers Criteria Update Expert Panel, Fick, D. M., Semla, T. P., Beizer, J., Brandt, N., & Dombrowski, R., . . . Steinman, M. (2015, October 8). American Geriatrics Society 2015 updated Beers criteria for potentially inappropriate medication use in older adults. *Journal of the American Geriatrics*

*Society,* 63(11), 2227–2246. Retrieved from http://onlinelibrary.wiley.com/doi/10.1111/jgs.13702/abstract. Accessed October 3, 2017.

14. Terrery, C. L., & Nicoteri, J. A. (2016). The 2015 American Geriatric Society Beers criteria: Implications for nurse practitioners. *Journal for Nurse Practitioners, 12*(3), 192–200. doi:10.1016/j.nurpra.2015.11.027.
15. Pasterneck, M. S. (2018, April 11). Approach to the adult with recurrent infections (E. R. Stiehm & A. M. Feldweg, Eds.). Retrieved from https://www.uptodate.com/contents/approach-to-the-adult-with-recurrent-infections?search=urinary tract infection referral to urology&source=search_result&selectedTitle=3~150&usage_type=default&display_rank=3. Accessed April 25, 2018.
16. DuBeau, C. E. Benign Prostate Disorders. In: Halter J. B., Ouslander J. G., Studenski S., High K. P., Asthana S., Supiano M. A., Ritchie C. eds. *Hazzard's Geriatric Medicine and Gerontology, 7e* New York, NY: McGraw-Hill; . http://accessmedicine.mhmedical.com/content.aspx?bookid=1923&sectionid=144521381. Accessed April 25, 2018.
17. Gupta, K., & Trautner, B. W. Urinary Tract Infections, Pyelonephritis, and Prostatitis. In: Jameson J., Fauci A. S., Kasper D. L., Hauser S. L., Longo D. L., Loscalzo J. eds. *Harrison's Principles of Internal Medicine, 20e* New York, NY: McGraw-Hill; . http://accessmedicine.mhmedical.com/content.aspx?bookid=2129&sectionid=186949849. Accessed April 25, 2018.

SECTION VII

# Rheumatology

## Gout

### Definition[1,4,5,6]

Gout is a form of arthritis that results from abnormal deposits of monosodium urate crystals in a joint space.

### Cause[1,4,5]

- Hyperuricemia

### Risk Factors[1,2,3,4,5,6]

- Age > 60 years
- Family history of gout
- Dietary factors (e.g., meat, seafood, alcohol, fructose)
- Metabolic syndrome
- Hypertension
- Obesity
- Some medications (e.g., loop and thiazide diuretics, cyclosporine)
- Chronic renal disease
- History of bypass surgery

### Signs & Symptoms[1,3,4,5,6]

- Intense and sudden joint pain.
  - Lasts between 1–2 weeks; can be disabling.
  - Pain may be episodic.
- Involvement of one or more joints (usually one joint at a time).
  - Most common joints affected: first metatarsophalangeal, metatarsal, ankle, or knee.
  - When gout is left untreated, it can affect many joints.
- Affected joint will be painful, erythematous, and swollen.
- Will not be able to tolerate light touch of socks or bed linen.

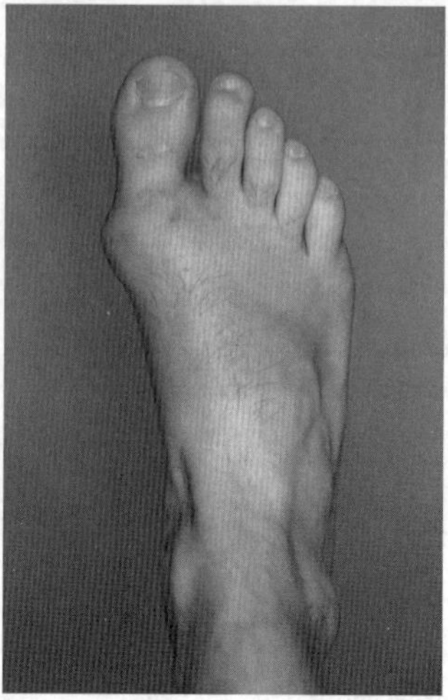

**Figure 7-1** Gout [See **Figure CP-1** at end of book for color version]


- Tophi (seen with untreated gout).
- Loss of mobility, chronic pain, and deformed joints.
    - Seen in chronic gout.

## Tests[1,4,5,6]

- Joint aspiration
    - Ordered when gout diagnosis is uncertain.
    - Confirms the diagnosis; monosodium urate crystals will be present.
    - Elevated leukocytes can cloud the picture and be confused with septic arthritis.
- Serum uric acid level
    - Levels above 6.8 mg/dL (405 μmol per L) is consistent with hyperuricemia.
- X-ray of affected joint
    - Asymmetric swelling within a joint will be noted.

## Treatment & Management[1,2,4,5,6,8]

- **Nonpharmacological and nursing interventions:**
  - Encourage lifestyle changes (e.g., limiting purine-rich foods and sweet sodas, avoiding heavy beer and wine consumption, encouraging fluids (*dehydration triggers gout*), avoiding crash diets and fasting, managing weight and being more active).
  - Encourage low-fat or nondairy products (may reduce gout flares) and vegetables.
  - Ice and elevate the affected joint.
- **Pharmacological and other interventions:**
  - Nonsteroidal anti-inflammatory drugs (NSAIDs) (e.g., ibuprofen [Motrin, Advil], naproxen [Naprosyn], Indocin ([ndomethacin])
    - Example: ibuprofen 600 mg PO q8 hours (for up to 10 days or 2 days after relief of symptoms).
    - Indocin often the go-to NSAID in gout, however more adverse effects than the others.
    - Used for an acute attack; used in addition with colchicine as first-line treatment.
    - There is no significant difference from one NSAID to another.
    - These carry a risk of gastrointestinal (GI) bleeding (use of proton pump inhibitor [PPI] decreases this risk), can exacerbate heart failure, and worsen renal function.
  - Colchicine (Colcrys)
    - Example: colchicine 1.2 mg initially for acute attack, followed by 0.6mg an hour later.
      - Caution use in renal impairment (creatinine clearance [CrCl] < 30 mL/min).
    - If used for gout prophylaxis, it is dosed at 0.6 mg PO daily or BID.
    - Used for an acute attack (given with an NSAID) and/or for gout prophylaxis.
    - May cause gastrointestinal side effects (e.g., diarrhea, nausea, cramping).

- Corticosteroids (available per os [by mouth, PO], intra-muscular [IM] or intra-articular [IA])
  - Example: prednisone 40 mg PO daily for 4 days.
  - Used for an acute attack; considered when NSAIDs and/or colchicine are contraindicated.
  - Can cause psychosis, worsen heart failure, increase glucose.
- Xanthine oxidase inhibitors (i.e., allopurinol [Zyloprim], febuxostat [Uloric])
  - Example: allopurinol 100 mg PO initially (max: 800 mg/day).
    - Caution use in renal impairment.
    - Single doses not to exceed 300 mg.
  - These drugs reduce uric acid levels; used as first-line treatment for prevention of recurrent gout.
  - Allopurinol side effects includes upset stomach or skin rash whereas febuxostat includes nausea and joint or muscle pain.
- Probenecid (Benemid, Probalan)
  - Dosed at 250 mg PO daily to BID (max of 2–3 g/daily)
    - Caution use in renal impairment (avoid use for CrCl < 30 ml/min).
  - Used to lower uric acid levels and prevent chronic gout (second-line treatment).
  - Carries multiple drug interactions and a risk of neph-rolithiasis (hydration should be encouraged).
- Uricase agents (e.g., pegloticase [Krystexxa])
  - Prescribed only by specialists.
  - Used in refractory chronic gout; are expensive.
  - Side effects may include gout flares, nausea/vomiting, infusion reaction.

- Rheumatology consultation/referral

Note: Beers listed items, as mentioned above, include probenecid, oral corticosteroids, colchicine, and NSAIDs.

## Differential Diagnosis[1,2,4,6]

- Pseudogout (also known as calcium pyrophosphate deposition disease): Can be diagnosed with joint fluid analysis of the crystals; is more likely to affect the knee or wrist. Both pseudogout and gout will respond to NSAIDs.
- Rheumatoid arthritis: Occurs symmetrically; hands affected more than feet.
- Septic arthritis: Arthrocentesis is required to differentiate this from gout. It is commonly associated with fever and leukocytosis.

### CLINICAL PEARLS[1,4,5,6,7]

- Gout comes on quickly; a patient can be asymptomatic, and within a few hours have excruciating pain in a joint.
- Look for hallmark symptoms of gout, such as erythema, pain, and swelling of a joint, especially the big toe.
- Gout attacks become unlikely when the serum uric acid level is under 6 mg/dl.
- Urate-lowering therapy should be initiated in older adults with a minimum of two gout attacks in a year, uric acid level above 12, history of nephrolithiasis, or if tophi present. When initiating these medications, there is a risk of precipitating a gout flare; they should be administered in combination with an NSAID, colchicine, or corticosteroid.

## References


1. Strano-Paul, L. (2014). Managing joint pain in older adults. In *Current Diagnosis & Treatment: Geriatrics* (2nd ed.). New York, NY: McGraw-Hill. Retrieved from http://accessmedicine.mhmedical.com/content.aspx?bookid=953&sectionid=53375690. Accessed January 17, 2018.
2. Baker, J. F., & Schumacher, H.R. (2010). Update on gout and hyperuricemia. *International Journal of Clinical Practice, 64*(3), 371–377.
3. Shah, A., & St. Clair, E. (2015). Rheumatoid arthritis. In Kasper, D., Fauci, A., Hauser, S., Longo, D., Jameson, J., & Loscalzo, J.*Harrison's Principles of Internal Medicine* (19th ed.). New York, NY: McGraw-Hill. Retrieved from http://accessmedicine.mhmedical.com/content.aspx?bookid=1130&sectionid=79750035. Accessed January 17, 2018.

4. Bankole, A. A., & Whitebrown, P. B. (2015). Arthritis, gout, and chronic pain. In Burggraf, V., Kim, K. Y., & Knight, A. L. (Eds.) *Healthy Aging: Principles and Clinical Practice for Clinicians* (pp. 297–300). Philadelphia, PA: Lippincott Williams & Wilkins.
5. Arthritis Foundation. (n.d.). Gout. Retrieved from http://www.arthritis.org/about-arthritis/types/gout/. Accessed January 19, 2018.
6. Hainer, B. L., Matheson, E., & Wilkes, R. T. (2014). Diagnosis, treatment, and prevention of gout. *American Family Physician, 90*(12), 831–836. Retrieved from https://www.aafp.org/afp/2014/1215/p831.html. Accessed January 19, 2018.
7. Goicoechea, M., Vinuesa, S. G., Verdalles, U., Ruiz-Caro, C., Ampuero, J., & Rincon, A., . . . Luno, J. (2010). Effect of allopurinol in chronic kidney disease progression and cardiovascular risk. *Clinical Journal of the American Society of Nephrology,* 5(8), 1388–1393. doi:10.2215/cjn.01580210
8. American Geriatrics Society 2015 Beers Criteria Update Expert Panel, Fick, D. M., Semla, T. P., Beizer, J., Brandt, N., & Dombrowski, R., . . . Steinman, M. (2015, October 8). American Geriatrics Society 2015 updated Beers criteria for potentially inappropriate medication use in older adults. *Journal of the American Geriatrics Society,* 63(11), 2227–2246. Retrieved from http://onlinelibrary.wiley.com/doi/10.1111/jgs.13702/abstract. Accessed October 8, 2017.

# Osteoarthritis

## Definition[1,2,3,5,6,7]

Osteoarthritis (OA), formerly known as degenerative joint disease, is a chronic arthropathy associated with hypertrophic bone changes, loss of cartilage, and other joint changes. It is an inevitable consequence of aging and referred to as age-related arthritis.

## Classification[2,3,5,6]

**Primary OA:** OA that occurs despite no prior injury to the joint (cause is unknown). If OA involves multiple joints, it is primary generalized OA; otherwise it is categorized based on site involvement (typically the hands, knee, spine, or hip).

**Secondary OA:** OA that occurs following injury or damage to a joint, such as trauma, infections, inflammatory arthropathies (e.g., chronic gout, rheumatoid arthritis), or a congenital abnormality.

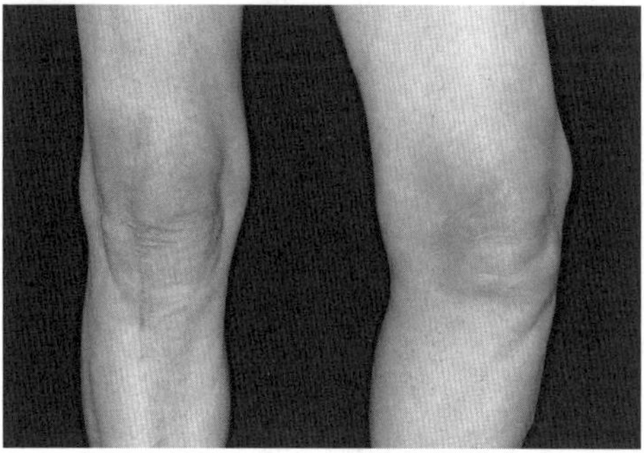

**Figure 7-2** Osteoarthritis [See **Figure CP-2** at end of book for color version]



## Causes[3,6]

- Exact cause is unknown

## Risk Factors[1,3,4,5,6]

- Advanced age
- Genetics
- Female sex
- Joint injuries (e.g., sport-related injuries)
- Obesity
- Certain occupations (e.g., agricultural workers, miners, heavy-labor related)
- Malalignment (e.g., varus or valgus deformity)
- Congenital hip dysplasia

## Signs & Symptoms[1,2,3,4,5,6,7]

- Joint pain.
  - Worse with activity and improves with rest.
  - Described as dull, sharp, or achy.
  - Joint line tenderness.
  - Morning stiffness that improves in about 30 minutes.

- Crepitus on range of motion.
- Limitation of function.
  - Such as knee or joint locking, difficulty climbing stairs.
- Restricted range of motion.
- Pain on range of motion.
- Hypertrophic changes at the distal *(Heberden nodes)* and proximal *(Bouchard nodes)* interphalangeal joints.
- Joint involvement is usually asymmetric.
- Joint effusion (knee).
  - Occurs intermittently, without warmth.

## Tests[1,2,4,5,6]

- Radiograph of the affected joint.
  - Confirms the diagnosis.
  - Findings may include joint space narrowing, bony remodeling, osteophytes, subchondral sclerosis or cysts.
- Serum lab testing not necessary.
  - Erythrocyte sedimentation rate (ESR) and C-reactive protein (CRP) usually normal.
  - Ordered if suspicious for other causes of arthritis (e.g., rheumatoid arthritis, gout, infectious arthritis).
- Joint fluid analysis.
  - Performed if suspicious for joint pain due to underlying gout or infection.
- Magnetic resonance imaging (MRI) or computed tomography (CT) are rarely required.
  - Used to investigate for other etiologies.

## Treatment & Management[1,2,3,4,5,7,8,9,10,11]

- **Nonpharmacological and nursing interventions:**
  - Encourage involvement in an exercise program.
    - Water-based exercise is beneficial in older adults with severe OA and limited physical activity.
    - Exercise programs are associated with reduced pain and improved performance in hip OA.

- Encourage weight loss (e.g., healthier eating practices and increased physical activity).
  - Especially helpful for knee and hip OA.
- Use of biomechanical devices (e.g., orthotics, braces).
  - Lateral wedge insoles are not effective for medial knee OA.
  - Knee braces improves stability and improve pain in some older adults with knee OA.
- Use of heat and/or cold therapy to reduce pain.
  - Should not be used for more than 20 minutes at a time.
- Encourage appropriate use of assistive devices.
  - A cane should be fitted to about the level of the hip and be used in the contralateral hand of the affected joint.
  - Walkers are reserved in individuals with severe disability and bilateral knee or hip OA.
- Acupuncture.
  - Recommended in older adults with hip or knee OA (reduces pain).
- Transcutaneous electrical nerve stimulation (TENS).
  - Offers pain relief in knee or hip OA and is well tolerated.

- **Pharmacological and other interventions:**
  - Topical agents
    - Capsaicin cream (SalonPas) 0.025%–0.075%, applied topically to affected joint 3–4 times daily PRN
      - Used to alleviate hand and knee OA pain.
      - May cause skin burning and/or erythema.
    - NSAID: Diclofenac sodium gel (Voltaren gel)
      - Used to alleviate hand and knee OA pain.
      - Not as effective as oral NSAIDs, however are well tolerated and not associated with acute renal failure.
  - Acetaminophen (Tylenol)
    - Example: acetaminophen 325–1,000 mg PO q6 hr PRN, not to exceed 3 g/day.
    - Effective as first-line treatment in mild to moderate knee or hip OA. Used in conjunction with a topical agent.

    - Monitor for hepatotoxicity, especially in patients with alcohol abuse or using known hepatotoxic agents.
- Oral NSAIDs (e.g., meloxicam [Mobic], naproxen, ibuprofen)
    - Example: ibuprofen 400–800 mg PO q6–8 hr PRN (max. 3,200 mg/day).
    - Effective in patients with moderate-severe related OA pains not controlled with acetaminophen. Added in conjunction to acetaminophen and a topical agent.
    - One NSAID is no more effective than another.
    - Monitor for bleeding or gastritis (reduced with proton pump inhibitor) and nephrotoxicity. Avoid in patients with glomerular filtrate rate < 30 cc/min. Caution use in patients with cardiovascular disease.

Note: A COX-2 inhibitor (e.g., celecoxib [Celebrex]) can be used as an alternative because the GI risk profile is lower; however, should also be used with caution in patients with cardiovascular risk factors.

- Serotonin and norepinephrine reuptake inhibitors (SNRIs, e.g., duloxetine [Cymbalta])
    - Example: duloxetine 30 mg PO daily (max: 60 mg/day).
    - May be modestly effective at reducing OA-related pains; improves function in knee OA.
    - Monitor for hyponatremia, xerostomia, impaired appetite, nausea, and constipation.
- Opioids
    - Tramadol (Ultram, Conzip) is a weak opioid that is effective at relieving hand, knee, or hip OA pain.
        - Start out at 25 mg daily, and slowly increase afterwards (max: 400 mg/day).
        - Lowers seizure threshold; however does not carry the side effects of respiratory depression like other opioids.
    - Stronger opioids (e.g., oxycodone [Oxaydo, Oxycontin, Roxicodone], hydrocodone [Hysingla ER, Zohydro

ER]), or morphine sulfate [Arymo ER, Kadian, MS Contin]).
  - Should be ordered starting with low doses.
  - Can be ordered if the above medications are ineffective, severe pain and/or debilitating OA, and in those not able to have joint replacement surgery.
  - Monitor for respiratory depression, sedation, confusion, and constipation. These increase the risk for falls; opioids should be used with caution and could be habit forming if used long term.
 - The above opioids can be added in conjunction to acetaminophen, a topical agent, and an NSAID.
- Joint injection with glucocorticoid (e.g., methylprednisolone [Medrol], triamcinolone acetonide [Zilretta])
  - Significantly reduces hip or knee OA pain.
  - Relief is temporary (4–8 weeks); injection is recommended for acute exacerbation of joint pain.
  - Can have four injections yearly.
  - Well tolerated; complications are rare.
- Hyaluronic acid injection (viscosupplementation)
  - Provides relief of symptoms for about 4 months; however pricier option.
  - Used by orthopedic surgeons in addition to steroid injection for ongoing knee OA pains.
  - Can be repeated in 6 months if effective.
- Nutritional supplements, glucosamine and chondroitin sulfate
  - These agents are controversial; several studies have shown they are no more efficacious than placebo.
  - Stop medication if no relief seen in 6 months.

- Pain specialist consultation/referral
  - This would be appropriate if opioids are considered. Be aware of your state regulations and guidelines; some states require referral when going above specific dosage levels.

- Orthopedic surgery consultation/referral
  - Surgery considered when pain is significant, there is a loss of function, and failed nonpharmacological and pharmacological options.
- Physical and/or occupational therapist consultation/referral
  - A physical therapist provides individualized exercise techniques, and can determine if assistive devices (e.g., cane or walker) are appropriate.
  - An occupational therapist recommends lifestyle modification changes to make daily tasks easier.

Note: Beers listed items, as mentioned above, include SNRIs, opioids, and NSAIDs (oral).

## Differential Diagnosis[1,3,4]

- Rheumatoid arthritis: Will typically have joint stiffness lasting more than an hour, pain improves with activity, ongoing joint swelling, joint involvement is symmetric, and involves the metacarpophalangeal (MCP) joints.
- Gout: Symptoms come on abruptly; affected joint is red, warm, and tender. It usually involves the $1^{st}$ metatarsophalangeal (MTP) joint and pseudogout affects the wrist or knees.

### CLINICAL PEARLS[1,2,3,4,5,6]

- Older adults often avoid activity as a result of their OA-related pains, which leads to physical disability. It is therefore critical to educate older adults with OA to avoid limiting their activity, treat their joint pain with medical therapy, and implement nonpharmacological interventions.
- OA symptoms come on gradually; affected joint is not typically red or warm. OA typically involves the hands, knees, hips, or spine.
- The joint stiffness will typically go away in under 30 minutes, pain worsens with activity, joint swelling is intermittent, joint involvement is usually asymmetric (starts from one joint at a time) and spares the MCP joints.
- The goal of OA is to reduce joint pain and stiffness, improve physical performance, and enhance quality of life.

## References


1. Sinusas, K. (2012, January 1). Osteoarthritis: Diagnosis and treatment. *American Family Physician,* 85(1), 49–56. Retrieved from http://www.aafp.org/afp/2012/0101/p49.html#afp20120101p49-c1. Accessed December 6, 2017.
2. Kontzias, A. (2017, February). Osteoarthritis (OA) – Musculoskeletal and Connective Tissue Disorders. Merck Manuals: Professional. Retrieved from http://www.merckmanuals.com/professional/musculoskeletal-and-connective-tissue-disorders/joint-disorders/osteoarthritis-oa. Accessed December 6, 2017.
3. Badlissi, F. (2017, March 23). Osteoarthritis. Epocrates. Retrieved from https://online.epocrates.com/diseases/192/Osteoarthritis. Accessed December 6, 2017.
4. Vina, E. R., & Kwoh, C. (2017). Osteoarthritis. In *Hazzard's Geriatric Medicine and Gerontology* (7th ed.). New York, NY: McGraw-Hill. Retrieved from http://accessmedicine.mhmedical.com/content.aspx?bookid=1923&sectionid=144562421. Accessed December 6, 2017.
5. Kwoh, C., & Hwang, Y. (2014). Osteoarthritis. In *Current Diagnosis & Treatment: Geriatrics* (2nd ed.). New York, NY: McGraw-Hill. Retrieved from http://accessmedicine.mhmedical.com/content.aspx?bookid=953&sectionid=53375650. Accessed December 6, 2017.
6. Cleveland Clinic. (2017, September 8). Osteoarthritis: What You Need to Know. Retrieved from https://my.clevelandclinic.org/health/articles/osteoarthritis-what-you-need-to-know. Accessed December 7, 2017.
7. Gulanick, M., & Myers, J. L. (2017). *Nursing Care Plans: Diagnoses, Interventions, & Outcomes*. St. Louis, MO: Elsevier.
8. American Geriatrics Society 2015 Beers Criteria Update Expert Panel, Fick, D. M., Semla, T. P., Beizer, J., Brandt, N., & Dombrowski, R., . . . Steinman, M. (2015, October 8). American Geriatrics Society 2015 updated Beers criteria for potentially inappropriate medication use in older adults. *Journal of the American Geriatrics Society,* 63(11), 2227–2246. Retrieved from http://onlinelibrary.wiley.com/doi/10.1111/jgs.13702/abstract. Accessed October 8, 2017.
9. Ebell, M. H. (2018). Osteoarthritis: Rapid evidence review. *American Family Physician,* 97(8), 523–526.
10. Dowell, D., Haegerich, T. M., & Chou, R. (2016, March 18). CDC guideline for prescribing opioids for chronic pain—United States, 2016. *Morbidity and Mortality Weekly Report Recommendations and Reports,* 65(1), 1–49. Retrieved from http://dx.doi.org/10.15585/mmwr.rr6501e1. Accessed December 6, 2017.
11. The American Academy of Pain Medicine. For the Primary Care Provider: When to Refer to a Pain specialist. (2016, December 1). www.painmed.org/files/when-to-refer-a-pain-specialist.pdf. Accessed April 25, 2018.


# Osteoporosis

## Definition[1,3,5,6]

Osteoporosis is defined as a skeletal disorder in which bone strength is compromised, with bone fragility, and increased risk of fractures. The bone becomes weak, then fractures occur with little to no trauma, sometimes just doing activities of daily living.

## Causes[1,5,6]

- Primary cause includes aging in both men and women.
- Secondary causes include bone loss associated with medications, disease states, and medical conditions.

## Risk Factors[1,2,3,5,6]

- Caucasian or Asian
- Age > 70 years men, > 65 women
- Inactivity/sedentary
- Family history of osteoporotic fracture
- Excessive alcohol intake
- Tobacco use
- Low calcium or vitamin D intake
- Small bone structure
- Some medications (e.g., glucocorticoids, chemotherapeutics, heparin, lithium, proton pump inhibitors, tacrolimus [Prograf], tamoxifen [Nolvadex])

## Signs & Symptoms[1,6]

- Osteoporosis is silent; there are no outward signs or symptoms.
- Can experience kyphosis and back and/or neck pain.
- Height loss.
- Fracture (even with minor injuries).

## Tests[1,2,3,4,5,6]

- Dual-energy X-ray absorptiometry (DEXA)
  - Used to measure bone mineral density; its painless and quick. Levels –2.5 or lower indicate osteoporosis (will likely need treatment).
  - Recommended screening for osteoporosis in all women ≥ 65 years of age.
  - Some organizations recommended screening in men > 70 years.
- Creatinine, calcium, parathyroid hormone (PTH), thyroid-stimulating hormone (TSH), and 25-hydroxy vitamin D level

  - Renal insufficiency or failure, vitamin D deficiency, primary hyperparathyroidism and hyperthyroidism are all common causes of secondary osteoporosis.[1,4,5,6]
  - Target vitamin D level should be at least 30 ng/mL.
- FRAX tool (www.sheffield.ac.uk/FRAX/)

## Treatment & Management[1,2,3,5,6,8]

- **Nonpharmacological and nursing interventions:**
  - Encourage good nutrition, calcium and vitamin D intake.
  - Take measures to prevent falls (e.g., remove hazards such as throw rugs, use walking aids if indicated, wearing appropriate footwear).
  - Consider hip protectors to decrease fracture risk.
  - Risk factor modification to maintain bone health: Encourage smoking cessation, limiting alcohol intake (*less than four drinks in 24 hours in men and less than two drinks in 24 hours in women*), limiting caffeinated beverages (*less than 2.5 cups of coffee in 24 hours*), and encourage activity including walking and resistance and/or weight bearing exercise.
  - Encourage sunlight exposure, for about 30 minutes per day most days of the week.
- **Pharmacological and other interventions:**
  - Calcium supplements.
    - 1,000 mg daily for men age 51–70 and 1,200 mg PO daily for women over age 50 and men over age 70.
  - Vitamin D supplementation.
    - Recommended to have 800–1,000 international units (IU) daily in older adults
  - Bisphosphonates (e.g., alendronate [Fosamax], ibandronate [Boniva]).
    - These have daily, weekly, and monthly preparations; if taken orally, should be taken only with water and avoid reclining for about 30 minutes (this reduces gastrointestinal adverse effects).

    - Recommended first-line treatment for osteoporosis; if unable to tolerate, alternatives include: teriparatide (Forteo) and denosumab (Prolia).
    - Consider discontinuing this therapy in women after 5 years without a history of vertebral fractures; optimal length of therapy is unknown.
    - May cause upper gastrointestinal events, osteonecrosis of the jaw *(rare)*, bleeding events.
  - Selective estrogen-receptor modulators (e.g., raloxifene [Evista], bazedoxifene [Viviant]).
    - Example: raloxifene 60 mg by mouth daily.
    - Recommended in women who do not tolerate bisphosphonate therapy and no history of venous thromboembolism.
    - Has shown to reduce vertebral fractures.
  - Calcitonin is administered daily by nasal spray or injection, approved for the treatment of postmenopausal osteoporosis, also has some pain relief benefit in vertebral fractures.
    - There have been reports of increased cancer rates with this drug.
  - Estrogen, without or without progesterone, reduces the risk of osteoporotic fractures in women; however is associated with risks (e.g., stroke, breast cancer).
- Physical therapy consultation/referral (to assist in fall prevention)
- Rheumatology consultation/referral (helpful in determining secondary causes of osteoporosis)

Note: Beers listed items, as mentioned above, include estrogens with or without progestins.

## Differential Diagnosis[7]

- Trauma as cause of fracture.
- Osteomyelitis: Can have bone pain (at site of infection), along with signs/symptoms of infection, such as low-grade fever and/or malaise.

- Multiple myeloma: Will have bone pain, along with anemia, hypercalcemia, and renal failure (creatinine above 2 mg/dL).
- Metastatic bone malignancy: DEXA can be normal, will have bone pain (also in atypical locations), may have a known history of cancer; diagnosed confirmed with bone biopsy.

## CLINICAL PEARLS[1,6]

- Pay attention to the shape of an older person's neck and shoulders; a slight roll forward in position could be a clue to vertebral compression fractures.
- A small weight (anything more than an empty hand) lifted over the head several times a day, can help strengthen bone.
- The most serious consequence of osteoporosis is sustaining a fracture. Osteoporotic fractures lead to chronic pain, nursing home placement, and mortality. It is therefore very important to take measure in preventing falls and encourage risk factor modification (e.g., limit alcohol and caffeine intake, exercise).

## References

1. Malik, R. A. (2014). Osteoporosis and hip fractures. In *Current Diagnosis & Treatment: Geriatrics* (2nd ed.). New York, NY: McGraw-Hill. Retrieved from http://accessmedicine.mhmedical.com/content.aspx?bookid=953&sectionid=53375651. Accessed January 9, 2018.
2. American College of Obstetricians and Gynecologists (ACOG). (2013. August 15). ACOG releases practice bulletin on osteoporosis. *American Family Physician, 88*(4), 269–275. Retrieved from https://www.aafp.org/afp/2013/0815/p269.html. Accessed January 11, 2018.
3. Lim, S. Y., & Bolster, M. B. (2015). Current approaches to osteoporosis treatment. *Current Opinion in Rheumatology, 27*(3), 216–224. doi:10.1097/bor.0000000000000169
4. Baliram, R., Sun, L., Cao, J., Li, J., Latif, R., & Huber, A. K., . . . Davies, T. F. (2012). Hyperthyroid-associated osteoporosis is exacerbated by the loss of TSH signaling. *Journal of Clinical Investigation, 122*(10), 3737–3741. doi:10.1172/jci63948
5. Jeremiah, M. P., Unwin, B. K., Greenawald, M. H., & Casiano, V. E. (2015). Diagnosis and management of osteoporosis. *American Family Physician, 92*(4), 261–268. Retrieved from https://www.aafp.org/afp/2015/0815/p261.html. Accessed January 11, 2018.
6. Udell, J. (2017, March). Osteoporosis. American College of Rheumatology. Retrieved from https://www.rheumatology.org/I-Am-A/Patient-Caregiver/Diseases-Conditions/Osteoporosis. Accessed January 11, 2018.

7. Sakhaee, K., & Cabo Chan, Jr., A. V. (2017, November 13). Osteoporosis. Epocrates. Retrieved from https://online.epocrates.com/diseases/85/Osteoporosis (used for diagnoses – multiple myeloma and metastatic bone). Accessed January 11, 2018.
8. American Geriatrics Society 2015 Beers Criteria Update Expert Panel, Fick, D. M., Semla, T. P., Beizer, J., Brandt, N., & Dombrowski, R., . . . Steinman, M. (2015, October 8). American Geriatrics Society 2015 updated Beers criteria for potentially inappropriate medication use in older adults. *Journal of the American Geriatrics Society, 63*(11), 2227–2246. Retrieved from http://onlinelibrary.wiley.com/doi/10.1111/jgs.13702/abstract. Accessed October 8, 2017.

# Rheumatoid Arthritis

## Definition[1,2,4,5]

Rheumatoid arthritis (RA) is a chronic, systemic, inflammatory disease; classified as an autoimmune disease where the immune system attacks body tissues, such as the lining of the joints (synovium), eventually leading to bone erosion and joint deformities. RA will go through periods of remission and prolonged exacerbation of the disease.

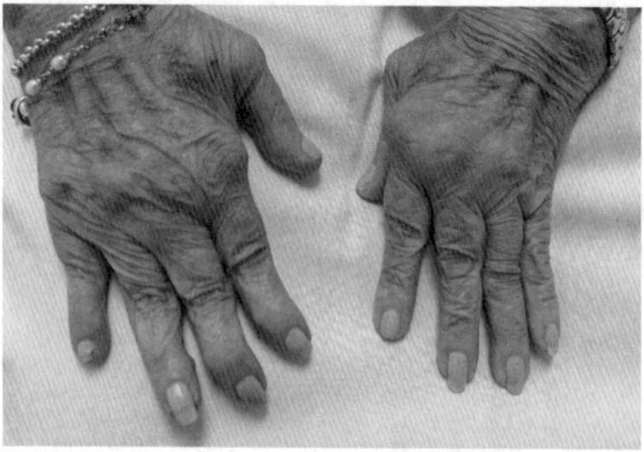

**Figure 7-3** Rheumatoid Arthritis [See **Figure CP-3** at end of book for color version]

## Causes[1,4,5]

- Cause of RA is unknown.

## Risk Factors[1,3,4,5]

- Age 25–55
    - Plateaus until age 75 and then disease rate decreases.
- Female sex
- Family history of RA
- Cigarette smoking

## Signs & Symptoms[1,2,4,5]

- Symmetric arthritis of the hands and feet (small joints).
    - May be monoarticular, oligoarticular, or polyarticular (usually $\geq$ 3 joints)
- Joint pain and swelling (lasting 6 weeks or longer).
    - The wrists and metacarpophalangeal and proximal interphalangeal joints are most frequently involved.
    - Larger joints (e.g., knees, shoulders) remain asymptomatic for several years following disease onset.
- Early morning joint stiffness.
    - Lasts more than 60 minutes and improves with physical activity.
- Flexor tendon tenosynovitis (hallmark of RA).
    - It can lead to decreased range of motion, trigger finger development, and reduced grip strength.
- Complaint of feeling systemically ill (e.g., low-grade fever, chills, decreased appetite, weight loss).
- Joint deformities are seen as the disease progresses.
- Cachexia in severe cases.
- Extraarticular manifestations: fatigue, lung involvement (e.g., pulmonary nodules, pleural effusions), pericarditis, ischemic heart disease, peripheral neuropathy, rheumatoid nodules, anemia, osteoporosis.

## Tests[1,2,4,5]

*RA diagnosis is established clinically; the following tests provide prognostic information more-so than diagnostic confirmation.*

- Rheumatoid factor (RF) or RA antibody
    - It lacks diagnostic specificity and is elevated in other chronic inflammatory diseases. It is found in about 80% of adults with RA.
    - A positive antibody titer will not always be present in those with RA.
- Anticyclic citrullinated peptides (anti-CCP) antibodies in serum
    - Has greater specificity for RA diagnosis than a positive RA. It is found in 60%–70% of adults with RA.
    - It carries the most value at predicting prognosis.
- Radiographs of the affected joints
    - Show joint space narrowing, osteopenia, and erosions.
- Acute phase reactants (e.g., CRP and ESR)
    - These are nonspecific inflammatory markers and are usually abnormal in RA.
- Hemoglobin and hematocrit
    - Patients with RA can develop iron deficiency anemia.
- Hepatic and renal function tests
    - The possibility of treatment adverse effects should be monitored.

## Treatment & Management[3,4,5,6,7,8]

- **Nonpharmacological and nursing interventions:**
    - Encourage daily exercise to promote weight loss, increase mobility, and reduce cardiovascular risk.
        - Exercise program should aim for low-impact aerobics (a physical therapist can assist with this).
    - Encourage sleep, about 8–10 hours and periods of rest during the daytime.
        - Sleep improves the immune system and reduces inflammation. Fatigue is associated with increased joint pains.

- Apply hot or cold packs on affected joints.
  - Alternating hot and cold can reduce local inflammatory process in painful, inflamed joints.
- Inform patients and family members of resources, such as the Arthritis Foundation.
- Encourage patient to continue with their medication treatment for RA (e.g., disease-modifying antirheumatic drugs [DMARDs] and/or biological response modifier therapy).
  - May take weeks to months for full therapeutic effect.
  - Educate patients that **nonopioid analgesics PRN can relieve inflammatory pain more effectively than opioids.**
- Wear splints as necessary.
  - Splints allow the inflamed joints to rest and reduces muscle spasms.

- **Pharmacological and other interventions:**
  - Disease-modifying antirheumatic drugs (DMARDs) (e.g., hydroxychloroquine [Plaquenil], methotrexate [Rheumatrex], gold salts [Ridaura, Solganal], sulfasalazine [Azulfidine])
    - Example: methotrexate 7.5–25 mg PO/IM/subcutaneous (SC) once weekly.
    - Methotrexate is the preferred DMARD agent for most RA patients.
    - DMARDs significantly reduce inflammation in RA, prevent joint damage, and enable a person to continue with activities of daily living.
    - DMARDs are associated with severe adverse events, especially in elderly patients with multiple comorbidities.
  - NSAIDs (e.g., ibuprofen [Motrin, Advil], naproxen [Naprosyn])
    - Example: ibuprofen 400–800 mg PO q4–6 hours PRN.
    - Relieves mild to moderate pain and used in adjunct to DMARDs.

    - These carry a risk of gastrointestinal bleeding (use of PPI decreases this risk), can exacerbate heart failure, and worsen renal function. Cox-2 selective NSAIDs are associated with lower risk of adverse effects.
  - Corticosteroids (e.g., prednisone [Deltasone], methyl-prednisolone [Medrol])
    - Example: prednisone 5–10 mg PO daily.
    - Used short term during exacerbations.
    - May be used for 1–2 weeks to allow DMARD therapy to take effect.
    - Can worsen heart failure, increase glucose, and cause or worsen delirium.
  - Biological response modifiers (e.g., etanercept [Enbrel], adalimumab [Humira])
    - Example: adalimumab 40 mg SC q2 weeks.
    - Reserved in those who have not responded or unable to tolerate DMARDs.
    - These are not to be used in those with serious infections because they interfere with the body's ability to fight infection.
- Physical and occupational therapy consultation/referral
  - To maintain and improve physical strength and determine what equipment works best for the individual.
- Rheumatology consultation/referral
  - They are aware of the latest treatment regimen(s).
  - Older adults in complete remission need to be seen once or twice yearly, whereas those with frequent exacerbations and persistent activity require closer monitoring.
  - Can help decide if surgical intervention is the right option (e.g., due to limitation in daily function or mobility due to joint damage).

Note: Beers listed items, as mentioned above, include oral corticosteroids and NSAIDs.

## Differential Diagnosis[2,6]

- Gout: May be polyarticular (especially recurrent gout) and can involve the hands; RA is however more likely to involve the hands. Radiographs can distinguish between the two diagnoses.
- Osteoarthritis: More likely to involve the distal interphalangeal joints; morning stiffness usually goes away after 30 minutes.

### CLINICAL PEARLS[1,3,4,5,9]

- Patients more likely to develop extraarticular manifestations have a history of smoking, early onset physical disability, and positive testing for serum RF.
- The most common cause of death in patients with RA is cardiovascular disease. Coronary artery disease and carotid atherosclerosis is higher compared to the general population, despite managing risk factors (e.g., diabetes, smoking, hypertension). Systolic and diastolic heart failure is also more likely to occur in patients with RA.
- The goal of RA is to relieve pain and inflammation, reduce joint damage, and improve physical function.
- The use of folic acid (5 mg weekly) has been recommended to reduce hematologic, GI, and hepatic adverse events in those receiving methotrexate. Folic acid is not generally given on the day of methotrexate.

## References

1. Shah, A., & St. Clair, E. (2015). Rheumatoid arthritis. In Kasper, D., Fauci, A., Hauser, S., Longo, D., Jameson, J., & Loscalzo, J.*Harrison's Principles of Internal Medicine* (19th ed.). New York, NY: McGraw-Hill. Retrieved from http://accessmedicine.mhmedical.com/content.aspx?bookid=1130&sectionid=79750035. Accessed January 17, 2018.
2. Strano-Paul, L. (2014). Managing joint pain in older adults. In *Current Diagnosis & Treatment: Geriatrics* (2nd ed.). New York, NY: McGraw-Hill. Retrieved from http://accessmedicine.mhmedical.com/content.aspx?bookid=953&sectionid=53375690. Accessed January 17, 2018.
3. Carey, S. A. (2015). Women with rheumatoid arthritis: The unspoken risk factor. *Journal for Nurse Practitioners, 11*(8), 829–846. doi:10.1016/j.nurpra.2015.05.009
4. Gulanick, M., & Myers, J. L. (2017). *Nursing Care Plans: Diagnoses, Interventions, & Outcomes*. St. Louis, MO: Elsevier.
5. Arthritis Foundation. (n.d.). Rheumatoid Arthritis. Retrieved from http://www.arthritis.org/about-arthritis/types/rheumatoid-arthritis/. Accessed January 25, 2018.

6. Yazici, Y. (2017, November 13). Rheumatoid Arthritis. Epocrates. Retrieved from https://online.epocrates.com/diseases/10511/Rheumatoid-arthritis/Key-Highlights. Accessed January 25, 2018.
7. American Geriatrics Society 2015 Beers Criteria Update Expert Panel, Fick, D. M., Semla, T. P., Beizer, J., Brandt, N., & Dombrowski, R., . . . Steinman, M. (2015, October 8). American Geriatrics Society 2015 updated Beers criteria for potentially inappropriate medication use in older adults. *Journal of the American Geriatrics Society, 63*(11), 2227–2246. Retrieved from http://onlinelibrary.wiley.com/doi/10.1111/jgs.13702/abstract. Accessed October 8, 2017.
8. Singh, J. A., Saag, K. G., Bridges, S. L., Akl, E. A., Bannuru, R. R., & Sullivan, M. C., . . . Mcalindon, T. (2015). 2015 American College of Rheumatology guideline for the treatment of rheumatoid arthritis. *Arthritis & Rheumatology, 68*(1), 1–26. doi:10.1002/art.39480
9. Shea, B., Swinden, M. V., Ghogomu, E. T., Ortiz, Z., Katchamart, W., & Rader, T., . . . Tugwell, P. (2014). Folic acid and folinic acid for reducing side effects in patients receiving methotrexate for rheumatoid arthritis. *Journal of Rheumatology, 41*(6), 1049–1060. doi:10.3899/jrheum.130738

# Spinal Stenosis

## Definition[1,5,6,7]

Spinal stenosis is defined as compression of the contents of the spinal canal, caused by narrowing of the canal (most commonly in the lower back and neck).

## Causes[1,2,5,7]

- Degenerative changes as a person ages
- Osteoarthritis
- Herniated disks
- Tumors
- Thickened ligaments
- Spinal injuries (e.g., motor vehicle accident)

## Risk Factors[1,2,5,6,7]

- Age > 65 years
- Congenital shortened pedicles
  - Symptoms are more severe and show up in the fifth decade or sooner.
- Degenerative arthritis appearing after the fifth decade of life

## Signs & Symptoms[1,2,4,5,6,7,10]

- Symptoms not seen until they are moderate to severe.
- Numbness, weakness, or tingling in a hand, arm, foot, or leg.
- Back pain (*lumbar spine stenosis*); neck pain (*cervical spine stenosis*).
  - Leg numbness, weakness, and/or paresthesia may accompany back pain (includes one or both legs).
- Reduction in the ability to walk (*lumbar spine stenosis*).
- Insidious onset of radiating buttock and leg pain.
  - Worse when standing or walking (downhill especially) and improves when sitting or leaning forward (e.g., placing weight on a cart): classic for lumbar spine stenosis.
- Wide-based gait.

Note: Neurological deficits are uncommon; straight leg test is usually negative; diminished ankle or knee reflex may be present, however is nonspecific.

## Tests[1,2,5,6,7]

- Plain X-rays
  - Are not necessary; sometimes ordered to ensure no spinal instability or deformity.
- Noncontrast MRI
  - Most useful diagnostic tool for identifying spinal stenosis.
  - Best for soft tissue and disc evaluation.
- CT myelogram
  - Reserved for individuals who cannot tolerate MRI scans (e.g., pacemaker)
- Plain CT
  - Little role in evaluating spinal stenosis.
  - Best for seeing bone structures, narrowing, facets, osteophytes.
  - Will show a flattening of the spinal canal.

## Treatment & Management[1,3,4,5,6,7,11,12]

- **Nonpharmacological and nursing interventions**:
  - Therapeutic exercise.
    - Works best with lumbar flexion.
    - Walking is less tolerated.
  - Abdominal core strengthening in combination with weight loss.
  - Lumbar corsets for posture training and maintenance.
  - Application of hot or cold packs to relieve symptoms.
  - Encourage massage, acupuncture, or spinal manipulation.
  - Use of assistive devices (e.g., cane or walker) to relieve pain.
- **Pharmacological interventions:**
  - Acetaminophen (Tylenol)
    - Used to ease the discomfort of spinal stenosis (used short term).
    - Strength of evidence is low for acute or subacute low back pain.
    - Carries potential adverse effects: hepatotoxicity (with overdose), thrombocytopenia, agranulocytosis.
  - NSAIDs (e.g., ibuprofen [Motrin, Advil], naproxen [Naprosyn])
    - Recommended for short-term use.
    - These carry a risk of gastrointestinal bleeding (use of PPI decreases this risk), can exacerbate heart failure and worsen renal function. Cox-2 selective NSAIDs are associated with lower risk of adverse effects.
  - Skeletal muscle relaxants (e.g., cyclobenzaprine [Flexeril], metaxalone [Skelaxin])
    - Moderate-quality evidence in the management of acute or subacute low back pain.
    - May cause sedation, drowsiness, dizziness.

- Antidepressant, duloxetine (Cymbalta)
  - Moderate-quality evidence shows this drug improves pain intensity and function in lower back pain.
  - May cause drowsiness, dizziness, dry mouth, constipation. Avoid use if CrCl <30 mL/min.
- Gabapentin (Gralise, Neurontin) or pregabalin (Lyrica)
  - Used to treat neuropathic pain.
  - The use of these to treat chronic lower back pain is limited due to central nervous system (CNS) adverse effects; they may require reduced dosage based off renal function.
- Opioids (e.g., tramadol [Ultram, ConZip], oxycodone [Oxycontin, Roxicodone], hydrocodone [Norco])
  - Consider tramadol as second-line therapy when nonpharmacological therapy and NSAIDs have failed.
  - Stronger opioids offer a short-term improvement in pain scores and function.
  - Recommended for short-term pain relief.
  - Use with caution if used long term (habit forming); may cause somnolence, constipation (short term).
- Steroid injections
  - Will reduce inflammation and relieve some pain.

- Pain specialist consultation/referral.
  - This would be appropriate if opioids are considered. Be aware of your state regulations and guidelines; some states require referral when going above specific dosage levels.
- Physical therapy consultation/referral.
  - Improve mobility, gait, strength and endurance.
- Surgical intervention is reserved in individuals who have failed conservative treatment or progressive neurologic deficits.

Note: Beers listed items, as mentioned above, include opioids, gabapentin, pregabalin, duloxetine, skeletal muscle relaxants, and NSAIDs.

## Differential Diagnosis[4,7,10]

- Hip osteoarthritis: Hip pain will worsen with internal rotation (diagnosed by ordering plain X-ray of the hip).
- Claudication due to vascular insufficiency (PVD): Leg pain is described as crampy, begins distally and travels proximally. Symptoms will not improve with lumbar flexion, whereas it would with lumbar spinal stenosis. Patients will experience difficulty walking uphill whereas flexing forward would relieve symptoms in lumbar spinal stenosis.
- Disk herniation: This causes unilateral radiculopathy rather than neurogenic claudication. Straight leg test would be positive and is more commonly seen in individuals under age 60 years. MRI can be ordered to differentiate this from spinal stenosis.

### CLINICAL PEARLS[7]

- Neurogenic claudication (seen with lumbar spinal stenosis) is worse with walking down hill; it's not enough to ask if pain present with walking, the direction of the walking matters.
- Spinal stenosis is more common in the lumbar spine and sometimes, the cervical spine. Lumbar spinal stenosis is managed based on severity of symptoms and it rarely progresses to paralysis whereas cervical stenosis can lead to paralysis and is more likely to require surgery.
- A neurological exam is not helpful, as there are too many variables; spinal stenosis does not have a single pathognomonic physical finding.

## References

1. Czervionke, L. F., & Fenton, D. S. (2011). *Imaging Painful Spine Disorders*. London, UK: Elsevier Health Sciences.
2. Tay, B. B., Freedman, B. A., Rhee, J. M., Boden, S. D., Skinner, H. B. (2014). Disorders, diseases, and injuries of the spine (Chapter 4). In Skinner, H. B., & McMahon, P. J. (Eds.) *Current Diagnosis & Treatment in Orthopedics* (5th ed.). New York, NY: McGraw-Hill; 2014. Retrieved from http://accessmedicine.mhmedical.com/content.aspx?bookid=675&sectionid=45451710. Accessed January 20, 2018.
3. American Geriatrics Society 2015 Beers Criteria Update Expert Panel, Fick, D. M., Semla, T. P., Beizer, J., Brandt, N., & Dombrowski, R., . . . Steinman, M. (2015, October 8). American Geriatrics Society 2015 updated Beers criteria for potentially inappropriate medication use in older adults. *Journal of the American Geriatrics Society, 63*(11), 2227–2246. Retrieved from http://onlinelibrary.wiley.com/doi/10.1111/jgs.13702/abstract. Accessed October 8, 2017.

4. Browne, K. L., Diersing, D., & Hilliard, T. (2017). Musculoskeletal assessment and management of patients participating in a walking program. *Journal for Nurse Practitioners, 13*(1), 26–33. doi:10.1016/j.nurpra.2016.08.033
5. Mayo Clinic. (2017, August 4). Spinal Stenosis. Retrieved from https://www.mayoclinic.org/diseases-conditions/spinal-stenosis/symptoms-causes/syc-20352961. Accessed January 20, 2018.
6. Parks, E. (Ed.) (2017). *Practical Office Orthopedics*; Low back pain. New York, NY: McGraw-Hill. Retrieved from http://accessmedicine.mhmedical.com/content.aspx?bookid=2230&sectionid=172778778. Accessed January 23, 2018.
7. Stern, S. C., Cifu, A. S., & Altkorn, D. (Eds.) (2014). *Symptom to Diagnosis: An Evidence-Based Guide* (3rd ed.); Back pain. New York, NY: McGraw-Hill. Retrieved from http://accessmedicine.mhmedical.com/content.aspx?bookid=1088&sectionid=61697331. Accessed January 23, 2018.
8. Qaseem, A., Wilt, T. J., Mclean, R. M., & Forciea, M. A.; Clinical Guidelines Committee of the American College of Physicians. (2017, April 4). Noninvasive treatments for acute, subacute, and chronic low back pain: A clinical practice guideline from the American College of Physicians. *Annals of Internal Medicine, 166*(7), 514–530. doi:10.7326/m16-2367
9. Shanthanna, H., Gilron, I., Rajarathinam, M., Alamri, R., Kamath, S., Thabane, L., & Bhandari, M. (2017). Benefits and safety of gabapentinoids in chronic low back pain: A systematic review and meta-analysis of randomized controlled trials. *PLoS Medicine, 14*(8), e1002369. doi:10.1371/journal.pmed.1002369
10. Pearson, A. M. (2017, January 9). Spinal Stenosis. Epocrates. Retrieved from https://online.epocrates.com/diseases/19111/Spinal-stenosis/Key-Highlights. Accessed January 24, 2018.
11. Dowell, D., Haegerich, T. M., & Chou, R. (2016, March 18). CDC guideline for prescribing opioids for chronic pain—United States, 2016. *Morbidity and Mortality Weekly Report Recommendations and Reports, 65*(1), 1–49. Retrieved from http://dx.doi.org/10.15585/mmwr.rr6501e1.
12. The American Academy of Pain Medicine. For the Primary Care Provider: When to Refer to a Pain specialist. (2016, December 1). www.painmed.org/files/when-to-refer-a-pain-specialist.pdf. Accessed April 25, 2018.

SECTION VIII

# Dermatology

## Candidiasis/Intertrigo

### Definition[1,2,3,4,5,6]

Candidiasis (see Figure 8-1) is the formation of *Candida* in the warm, moist environment of the skin folds on the body. Intertrigo is an inflammatory condition of the skin folds that is aggravated by heat, moisture, friction, and lack of air circulation. Intertrigo can be worsened if colonized by infection such as bacterial, viral, or fungal sources.

### Causes

- *Candida albicans* is the primary cause

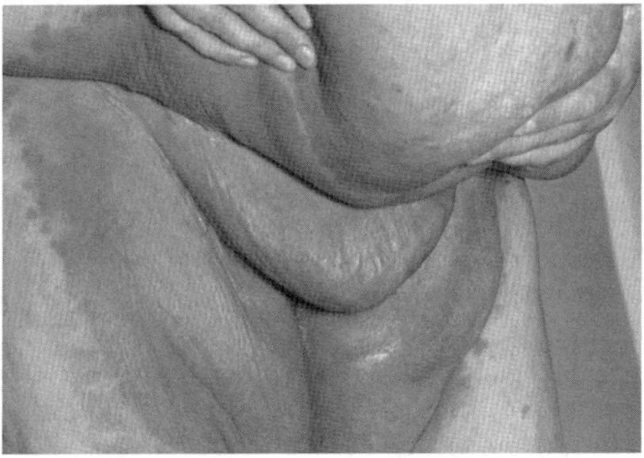

**Figure 8-1** Candidiasis [See **Figure CP-4** at end of book for color version]
© Mediscan/Alamy Stock Photo.

### Risk Factors[1,2,3,4,5,6]

- Obesity
- Tight clothing
- Incontinence
- Increased skin friction

- Diabetes
- Hyperhidrosis
- Use of topical and systemic steroids
- Frequent use of antibiotics
- Human immunodeficiency virus (HIV) infection
- Chemotherapy
- Immunosuppressive medications

## Signs & Symptoms[1,2,3,4,5,6]

Candidal intertrigo exhibits as:

- Erythematous, macerated (softening and breaking down of skin resulting from prolonged exposure to moisture) plaques and erosions that have mild scaling and satellite papules or pustules.
- The pustules are easily ruptured.
- Sudden onset of itching, burning, pain, and stinging in the skin folds.
- Typical locations affected: inguinal folds, axillae, scrotum, intergluteal folds, inframammary folds, web spaces of toes and fingers, abdominal folds, and the corners of the mouth in the elderly.

## Tests[1,2,3,4,5,6]

- Potassium hydroxide (KOH) examination or culture of skin scrapings
  - Confirms the diagnosis.
- Skin culture
  - Pustules can be cultured if bacterial infection is suspected.
- Skin biopsy
  - If treatment measures do not improve areas affected, a skin biopsy of the site should be done to confirm diagnosis.

## Treatment & Management[1,2,3,4,5,6,9,10]

- **Nonpharmacologic and nursing interventions:**
  - Take steps to eliminate heat and friction.
    - Keep skin folds cool and dry.
    - Always dry skin folds well after bathing.

    - The use of cotton and linen clothing is recommended.
    - Avoid constrictive clothing.
  - Emphasize weight control, glycemic control in diabetes, along with good hygiene in the prevention of candida skin infections.
- **Pharmacologic and other interventions:**
  - Topical antifungal medications (e.g., clotrimazole [Mycelex], econazole [Ecoza], ciclopirox [Luprox], miconazole [Zeasorb, Micatin], nystatin [Nystop, Nyamc])
    - Can be applied after bathing; applied in between skin folds BID until the area has resolved (usually 2–4 weeks).
    - Used as first-line therapy for candidal intertrigo.
    - May cause skin irritation or erythema.
  - Low-potency topical steroids (e.g., desonide [Verdeso, Tridesilon, Desowen], triamcinolone acetonide)
    - These are used in conjunction with antifungal therapy to reduce pruritus, pain, and burning.
    - May cause skin atrophy, burning, and/or dryness.
  - Drying solution (e.g., aluminum acetate topical [Domeboro])
    - Domeboro should be applied for 15 minutes 3 times per day, followed by topical application of antifungal cream.
    - Recommended if weeping is present.
    - May cause skin irritation.
  - Systemic antifungals
    - Fluconazole 50–100 mg daily or 150 mg weekly and itraconazole 200 mg twice daily may be used for 2–6 weeks or until signs and symptoms are clear.
    - Oral ketoconazole should not be used due to high risk of liver injury.
    - These are recommended only if topical antifungals have failed.
    - For prolonged use of oral antifungals, liver enzymes should be monitored.
  - Treatment for angular cheilitis (candidiasis in oral commissures):

    - Zinc oxide paste or petrolatum should be applied twice daily (well tolerated).
  - Oral fluconazole plus topical antifungal
    - 1–2 doses of oral fluconazole 150 mg plus miconazole cream BID for 7 days.
    - This combination is used to treat vulvovaginal candidiasis.
    - For recurrent infections, weekly doses of fluconazole 150 mg can be given for 6–12 months.

## Differential Diagnosis[4,7,8,9]

- Bacterial intertrigo: Manifests as areas of skin erythema, edema, and warmth. Fever may be present. Bacterial skin infections are almost always unilateral, and the lower extremities are the most common sites of involvement. Bacterial skin infections are in deeper dermis and subcutaneous fat. Purulent drainage may be present. Symptoms usually present suddenly.
- Seborrheic dermatitis: Characterized by erythema and scales, with some pruritus. The margins are usually less sharply demarcated. The distribution is characteristic: lateral sides of the nose and the nasolabial folds, eyebrows and glabella, and scalp.
- Inverse psoriasis: This is often mistaken for candida intertrigo because presentation is similar. KOH preparation can help determine if area is candida or not.
- Herpes simplex: Small blisters are often present with clear drainage. Not usually seen in large skin folds. Often seen around mouth and in perineal area.

### CLINICAL PEARLS

- Be careful in using steroid creams in skin folds. Applying steroid creams in skin folds make the steroid more potent and can cause atrophy of the skin if used long term.
- Monitor liver enzymes q2 weeks with the use of prolonged oral antifungal medications.
- Keeping skin cool, dry, and friction free will help prevent reoccurrences.

## References


1. Hidalgo, J. A. (2017, December 1). Candidiasis. Medscape. Retrieved from http://emedicine.medscape.com/article/213853-overview. Accessed January 19, 2018.
2. Linton, C. P. (2011, July–August). Describing the shape of individual skin lesions. *Journal of the Dermatology Nurses' Association*, 3(4), 230–231.
3. Linton, C. P. (2012, January–February). Intertrigo: Describing the distribution of the skin lesions. *Journal of the Dermatology Nurses' Association*, 4(1), 62–63.
4. Lyons, F., & Ousley, L. (2015). *Dermatology for the Advanced Practice Nurse*. New York, NY: Springer Publishing Company.
5. Paras, V. (2017, April 28). Intertrigo. Medscape. Retrieved from http://emedicine.medscape.com/article/1087691-overview. Accessed January 19, 2018.
6. Parker, E. R. (2017, July 14). Candidal Intertrigo. UpToDate. Retrieved from http://uptodate.com/contents/candida-intertrigo. Accessed January 19, 2018.
7. Raff, A. B., & Kroshinsky, D. (2016). Cellulitis: A review. *JAMA*, *316*(3), 325–337.
8. Spelman, D. (2017, Sept 6). Cellulitis and Skin Abscess: Clinical Manifestations and Diagnosis. UpToDate. Retrieved from http://www.uptodate.com/contents/cellulitis-and-skin-abcess-clinical-manifestations-and-diagnosis?source=see_link. Accessed January 19, 2018.
9. Weston, W. L., & Howe, W. (2014, March 5). Overview of Dermatitis. UpToDate. Retrieved from http://uptodate.com/contents/overview-of-dermatitis. Accessed January 19, 2018.
10. Epocrates. (n.d.). Retrieved from https://www.epocrates.com (used for adverse effects).


# Cellulitis/Erysipelas

## Definition[1,2,4,5,6,8]

Cellulitis (see Figure 8-2) has inflammation involving the subcutaneous tissue that is caused most frequently by *Streptococcus pyogenes or Staphylococcus aureus* and usually follows some apparent wound. Erysipelas (see Figure 8-3) is a bacterial skin infection involving the upper dermis and extends into the superficial lymphatics. The area is very tender with extreme erythema.

## Causes[1,2,4,5,6,8]

| Cellulitis | Erysipelas |
|---|---|
| • Beta-hemolytic streptococci (groups A, B, C, G, and F)<br>• Streptococcus or streptococcus pyogenes<br>• *S. aureus* (including methicillin-resistant *S. aureus* [MRSA]) | • Beta-hemolytic streptococci |

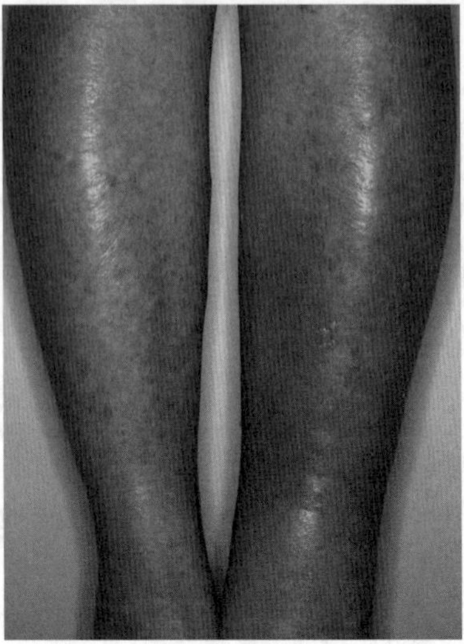

**Figure 8-2** Cellulitis [See **Figure CP-5** at end of book for color version]


## Risk Factors[1,2,4,5,6]

| Cellulitis | Erysipelas |
| --- | --- |
| • Skin barrier disruption due to trauma or existing infection (tinea or bacterial)<br>• Skin inflammation<br>• Edema due to impaired lymphatic drainage<br>• Obesity<br>• Immunosuppression (HIV, diabetes) | • Lymphatic obstruction or edema (lymphedema is an immense risk factor)<br>• Saphenous vein grafting to lower extremities<br>• Status post mastectomy<br>• HIV<br>• Arterial insufficiency<br>• Paretic limbs<br>• Nephrotic syndrome<br>• Venous insufficiency, stasis ulcerations, inflammatory dermatoses, dermatophyte infection, insect bites, and surgical incisions |

## Signs & Symptoms[1,2,4,5,6,8]

| Cellulitis | Erysipelas |
|---|---|
| • Erythema, warmth, and tenderness.<br>• Malaise and chills.<br>• Affected skin may become pitted from edema and have nodular components with vesicles.<br>• Local lymph nodes may be tender and enlarged. | • Local redness, heat, and swelling, and a classic raised border.<br>• The lymph nodes are commonly involved, and streaking is present.<br>• Malaise, high fever, headaches, nausea/vomiting, and joint pains. |

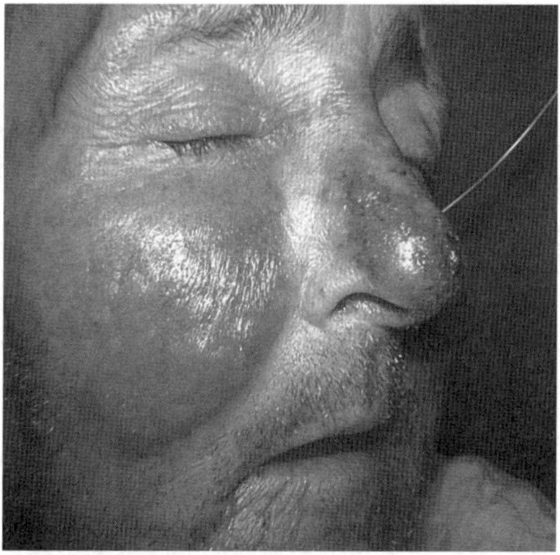

**Figure 8-3** Erysipelas [See **Figure CP-6** at end of book for color version]
Courtesy of Dr. Thomas F. Sellers, Emory University/CDC.

## Tests[1,2,4,5,6]

- Uncomplicated cellulitis usually does not warrant a workup.
- Complete blood count (CBC), basic metabolic panel (BMP), erythrocyte sedimentation rate (ESR), C-reactive protein (CRP), and blood cultures.

  - Recommended if fever and chills are present with cellulitis.
  - Recommended labs with erysipelas.
- Culture and sensitivity.
  - If drainage is present.

## Treatment & Management[2,3,7,8,9]

- **Nonpharmacologic and nursing interventions:**
  - Warm compresses to site
  - Dressing to cover any skin openings
- **Pharmacological and other interventions:**
  - Treatment of MRSA includes clindamycin (Cleocin), sulfamethoxazole/trimethoprim (Bactrim DS, Sulfatrim), tetracycline, and linezolid (Zyvox). Duration of treatment should be for 10 days.
    - Sulfamethoxazole/trimethoprim can worsen renal function; adjust dose based on renal function. Linezolid interacts with several medications. All of the above antibiotics carry the potential for *Clostridium difficile*-associated diarrhea.
  - Penicillin (PCN) and cephalosporin agents are dosed for 10 days. If allergic to PCN, then consider clarithromycin 500 mg BID for 10 days.
  - Erysipelas may require intravenous (IV) antibiotics (if severe).
  - An underlying cause for lower extremity cellulitis is often tinea pedis. Treatment with an antifungal cream prevents recurrent cellulitis.
  - OTC acetaminophen (Tylenol), ibuprofen (Motrin, Advil) can be used for pain.
    - Nonsteroidal anti-inflammatory drugs (NSAIDs) may cause gastrointestinal (GI) bleeding, abdominal pain, fluid retention, and worsening in renal function.

Note: Beers listed item, as mentioned above, include NSAIDs.

## Differential Diagnosis[1,2,4,5,6,8]

- Erythema migrans: Early sign of Lyme's disease; has a bull's eye appearance with large circular erythematous macular patch and central clearing.
- Herpes zoster: Begins with area of erythema, but then papules and vesicles appear. Rash usually follows a dermatome and is unilateral.
- Acute gout: Consists of severe pain, warmth, erythema, and swelling around a joint.
- Drug reaction: Presents with an erythematous maculopapular rash that involves the trunk and extremities. It is usually accompanied by pruritus.
- Deep vein thrombosis: Usually involves the extremities; area will be firm and with some erythema. Venous ultrasound can confirm diagnosis.
- Vasculitis: Appears with macular and papular lesions that are nonblanchable. Diagnosis is confirmed by skin biopsy.

### CLINICAL PEARLS

- Patients should decrease physical activity and elevate extremity, if affected.
- Educate family and staff that patients who are immunocompromised, are diabetics, have cancer, or have chronic lymphedema are at higher risk and should bathe with antibacterial soaps.

## References


1. Baddour, L. M. (2016, November 2). Cellulitis and Skin Abscesses: Clinical Manifestations and Diagnosis. UpToDate. Retrieved from http://www.uptodate.com/contents/cellulitis-and-skin-abcesses-clinical-manisfestations-and-diagnosis. Accessed January 21, 2018.
2. Herchline, T. E. (2017, June 5). Cellulitis. Medscape. Retrieved from http://emedicine.medscape.com/article/214222-overview#a0156. Accessed January 21, 2018.
3. Lessing, J. N., & McGee, S. (2016). Therapy for cellulitis. *JAMA, 316(19)*, 2046–2047.
4. Linder, K. A., & Preeti, N. M. (2017). Cellulitis. *JAMA, 317(20)*, 2142.
5. Moran, G. J., & Talan, D. A. (2017). Cellulitis. Commonly misdiagnosed or just misunderstood? *JAMA, 317(3)*, 760–761.
6. Raff, A. B., & Kroshinsky, D. (2016). Cellulitis: A review. *JAMA, 316(3)*, 325–337.
7. Epocrates. (n.d.). Retrieved from https://www.epocrates.com (used for adverse effects).

8. Lyons, F., & Ousley, L. E. (2015). *Dermatology for the Advanced Practice Nurse*. New York, NY: Springer Publishing Company.
9. American Geriatrics Society 2015 Beers Criteria Update Expert Panel, Fick, D. M., Semla, T. P., Beizer, J., Brandt, N., & Dombrowski, R., . . . Steinman, M. (2015, October 8). American Geriatrics Society 2015 updated Beers criteria for potentially inappropriate medication use in older adults. *Journal of the American Geriatrics Society,* 63(11), 2227–2246. Retrieved from http://onlinelibrary.wiley.com/doi/10.1111/jgs.13702/abstract. Accessed October 3, 2017.

# Contact Dermatitis

## Definition

Contact dermatitis (CD) (see Figure 8-4) refers to any type of dermatitis that arises from direct skin exposure to a substance.

## Types[1,2,3,6,7,8]

**Allergic contact dermatitis (ACD):** An allergen induces an immune response.
**Irritant contact dermatitis (ICD):** The dermatitis is actually caused by direct contact of the irritant on the skin.

## Causes[1,2,3,4,5,6,7,8]

| ACD | ICD |
|---|---|
| • Contact with a specific substance that elicits a delayed (type IV) hypersensitivity reaction. Anyone with normal cell-mediated immunity can develop ACD.<br>• Due to allergens found in home or in the workplace (e.g., metals, glues, plastics, rubber, fragrances, topical antibiotics, preservatives, and chemicals used in hair care and cosmetic products). | • Results from exposure to substances that cause physical, mechanical, or chemical irritation of the skin. The irritant disrupts the normal epidermal skin barrier and secondary inflammation develops.<br>• Exposures encountered daily (e.g., soapy water, cleansers, rubbing alcohol). |

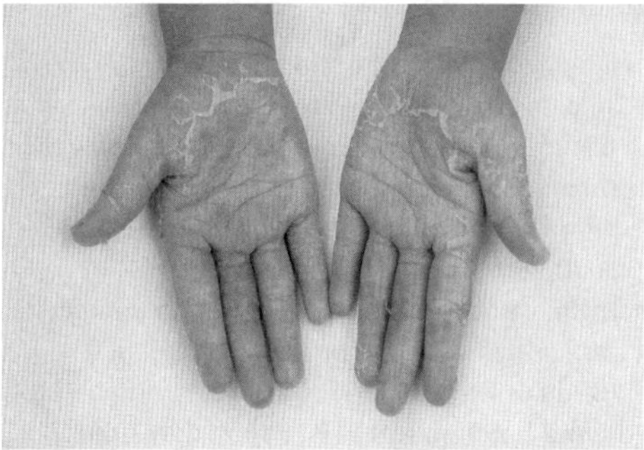

**Figure 8-4** Contact Dermatitis [See **Figure CP-7** at end of book for color version]



## Risk Factors[2,3,6,7]

- People with atopic dermatitis and fair skin tone are at higher risk for having ICD.
- Elderly exposed to harsh soaps or lotions with fragrances may exhibit signs of CD.

## Signs & Symptoms[2,3,5,6,7,8]

| ACD | ICD |
|---|---|
| • Sharp, demarcated, pruritic, eczematous eruption localized to the area of skin that comes in contact with the allergen.<br>• The affected area may have vesicles and weeping.<br>• Chronic ACD sites may have lichenified or scaled plaques.<br><br>*The initial site of dermatitis often provides the best clue regarding the potential cause of ACD.* | • Macular erythema, hyperkeratosis, and/or fissuring.<br>• Epidermis may appear dry or scalded; chapped skin, dryness.<br>• Pruritus that is mild to severe.<br>• Pain (common when erosions or fissures are present).<br>• Hands are the most common area; eyelids are often more affected due to thin skin.<br>• Severe cases: edema, serous oozing, and tenderness. |

## Tests[3,5,6,8]

- Potassium hydroxide preparation (KOH) and/or fungal culture to exclude tinea, especially if areas affected are on hands or feet.
- Patch testing to identify external chemicals causing the reaction.
- Repeat open application test (ROAT) to determine whether a reaction is significant in people who have a weak positive (1+) reaction to a chemical.
- Dimethylgloxime test to determine whether a metallic object contains enough nickel to provoke a reaction.
- For individuals who have widespread dermatitis, a CBC, CMP, and thyroid function test (TFT) should be done.
- Skin biopsy can help to exclude other disorders such as tinea, psoriasis, and cutaneous lymphoma.

## Treatment & Management[3,4,5,6,7,9]

- **Nonpharmacologic and nursing interventions:**
  - Use mild cleansing agents (e.g., Aquanil, Cetaphil cleanser).
  - Recommending ceramide creams or bland emollients after washing hands is useful.
  - Avoid any known irritants.
    - Gloves can be recommended to prevent ICD (hands are usually exposed to irritants at home and/or in the workplace). Gloves should be changed as soon as they become wet or damp to prevent maceration.
- **Pharmacological and other interventions:**
  - Topical soaks with cool tap water; aluminum acetate topical (Burow's solution, 1:40 dilution), saline (1 tsp/pint), or oatmeal baths can be soothing for ICD and ACD.
  - Emollients (e.g., white petrolatum [Eucerin]) may be beneficial in chronic cases of ICD and ACD.
  - Large vesicles should not be opened (this can introduce bacteria). Cover vesicles with dressings soaked in aluminum acetate topical (Burow's solution).
  - Cool compresses with saline or aluminum acetate solution are helpful for acute vesicular dermatitis (e.g., poison ivy).

- Oral antihistamines are beneficial for itching (however carry anticholinergic effects such as sedation).
- Topical corticosteroids are the mainstay of treatment, with the strength of the topical corticosteroid appropriate to the body site. For severe allergic contact dermatitis of the hands, 3-week courses of class I topical corticosteroids are required (e.g., clobetasol propionate [Clobex), fluocinonide [Lidex]), while class 6 or class 7 topical corticosteroids (e.g., triamcinolone acetonide, hydrocortisone) typically are used for allergic contact dermatitis of intertriginous areas or the face.
- Systemic corticosteroids are used for acute severe allergic contact dermatitis, such as from poison ivy. Most adults require an initial dose of 40–60 mg (prednisone [Deltasone]). The oral corticosteroid is tapered over a 2-week period (shorter courses often allow poison ivy dermatitis to relapse).
  - Alternative: Long-acting intramuscular (IM) triamcinolone acetonide (Kenalog) 40–60 mg may be used in place of oral prednisone.

Note: Beers listed items, as mentioned above, include oral antihistamines and oral corticosteroids.

## Differential Diagnosis[2,3,4,5,6,7,8]

- Allergic contact dermatitis: Differentiating between ACD and ICD is difficult. A positive patch test to allergen is diagnostic of ACD.
- Atopic dermatitis: This type of skin condition usually affects the flexural areas of the body (antecubital fossa of arms and popliteal fossa of legs). However, individuals who have atopic dermatitis are at higher risk for the development of ICD.
- Psoriasis: Psoriatic plaques are usually prominent at distant sites (elbows, knees); nail changes are clues to diagnosis of psoriasis.
- Hand/foot eczema: Dyshidrotic hand/foot eczema is characterized by vesicles and bullae on palms and soles of feet.
- Fungal infection: KOH examination can determine diagnosis. Fungal infections often have fine scales present.

**CLINICAL PEARLS**

- It is sometimes very difficult to differentiate between ACD and ICD. A thorough history of exposures and habits is often needed to determine etiology and diagnosis.
- Be careful in using clobetasol (Clobex) cream and potent steroid creams on elderly skin. Instead of twice-daily applications, consider daily application.
- Use very mild soap and nonfragrant lotions in elderly population to prevent potential ACD/ICD.
- Often the geriatric population can be poor historians. Dependence on family and nursing staff may be needed to obtain a comprehensive history of exposures.
- Wash new sheets, blankets, and clothing before use and use a mild detergent.

- Scabies: Scabies in interdigital spaces can simulate an irritant dermatitis. Pruritus is very prominent and severe. Skin scraping, adhesive tape test, or dermoscopy can provide a correct diagnosis.

## References

1. Fityan, A., & Ardern-Jones, M. R. (2013, February). Rashes in the elderly. *General Medicine, 41*.
2. Goldner, R., & Tuchinda, P. (2015, June 25). Irritant Contact Dermatitis in Adults. UpToDate. Retrieved from http://www.uptodate.com/contents/Irritant-contact-dermatitis-in-adults. Accessed January 25, 2018.
3. Helm, T. D. (2017, June 5). Allergic Contact Dermatitis. Medscape. Retrieved from http://emedicine.medscape.com/article/1049216-overview#a1. Accessed January 25, 2018.
4. Linton, C. P. (2011, July–August). Describing the shape of individual skin lesions. *Journal of the Dermatology Nurses' Association*, 3(4), 230–231.
5. Lyons, F., & Ousley, L. (2015). *Dermatology for the Advanced Practice Nurse*. New York, NY: Springer Publishing Company.
6. Savina, A. (2017, July 26). Irritant Contact Dermatitis. Medscape. Retrieved from http://emedicine.medscape.com/article/1049353-overview@a1. Accessed January 25, 2018.
7. Weston, W. L., & Howe, W. (2014, March 5). Overview of Dermatitis. UpToDate. Retrieved from http://uptodate.com/contents/overview-of-dermatitis. Accessed January 25, 2018.
8. Yiannias, J. (2017, December 11). Clinical Features and Diagnosis of Allergic Contact Dermatitis. UpToDate. Retrieved from http://www.uptodate.com/contents/clinical-features-and-diagnosis-of-allergic-contact-dermatitis. Accessed January 25, 2018.

9. American Geriatrics Society 2015 Beers Criteria Update Expert Panel, Fick, D. M., Semla, T. P., Beizer, J., Brandt, N., & Dombrowski, R., . . . Steinman, M. (2015, October 8). American Geriatrics Society 2015 updated Beers criteria for potentially inappropriate medication use in older adults. *Journal of the American Geriatrics Society, 63*(11), 2227–2246. Retrieved from http://onlinelibrary.wiley.com/doi/10.1111/jgs.13702/abstract. Accessed October 3, 2017.

# Pressure Injury

## Definition[2,4,5,6,12]

Although the terms *decubitus ulcer*, *pressure sore*, and *pressure ulcer* have often been used for the same diagnosis, the National Pressure Ulcer Advisory Panel (NPUAP) currently considers pressure injury the best term to use, given that open ulceration does not always occur. It is characterized as localized areas of damage to the skin, underlying tissue, or both, and is typically over a bony prominence (e.g., sacrum, calcaneus, ischium).

## Cause[2,4,5,6]

- Pressure, in combination with shear and/or friction

Note: The superficial skin is less susceptible to pressure-induced damage than deeper tissues, and thus, the external appearance may underestimate the extent of damage. Pressure-induced skin and soft tissue injuries can serve as a reservoir for resistant organisms such as methicillin-resistant *Staphylococcus aureus*, vancomycin-resistant enterococci, and multiply-resistant gram-negative bacilli, and colonized or infected ulcers pose a potential risk to patients in crowded facilities (e.g., nursing homes, facilities).

## Risk Factors[1,2,4,5,6,12]

- Advanced age (skin is less elastic and will have thinning of the epidermis)
- Immobility
- Poorly fitted cast
- Poorly fitted medical equipment or devices
- Neurologically impaired, heavily sedated, restrained, dementia, or patients recovering from trauma
- Contractures
- Inability to perceive pain

- Paralysis and insensibility
- Smoking
- Obesity
- Poor nutrition
- Diabetes and thyroid disease
- Poor circulation.

## Signs & Symptoms[2,3,4,5,6,12]

National Pressure Ulcer Advisory Panel (NPUAP) system consists of four main stages of ulceration, but is not intended to imply that all pressure ulcers follow a standard progression from stage I to stage IV, or that healing pressure ulcers follows a standard

### Stages of Ulceration

**Deep tissue injury:** A purplish area of intact skin or blister caused by damage of underlying soft tissue. Dark skin is more difficult to evaluate.

**Stage I:** Undamaged skin with signs of approaching ulceration; at first, the area will appear as blanchable erythema that indicates reactive hyperemia, which can resolve within 24 hours if pressure is relieved. The area can also have warmth and induration. The first signs of tissue destruction are present if the area is non-blanchable and the skin may have a white appearance from ischemia.

**Stage II:** A partial-thickness wound that involves the epidermis and dermis. There is ulceration with a pink wound bed.

**Stage III:** A full-thickness wound which extends into subcutaneous tissue. The fascia of skin is not involved. Tunneling to surrounding tissue may be present.

**Stage IV:** A full-thickness wound with extension into muscle, bone, tendon, or joint capsule. Sloughing may be present. Bone infection (osteomyelitis), pathologic fractures or dislocations may be present. Tunneling of surrounding skin is common.

**Unstageable:** A full-thickness wound in which the basement of the wound is covered by eschar/slough and the full extent of the wound cannot be determined. The eschar/slough must be removed to determine the stage and depth of wound.

regression from stage IV to stage I to a healed wound. The system is designed to describe the degree of tissue damage observed at a specific time of examination and is meant to facilitate communication among the various disciplines involved in the study and care of patients with these lesions.

The categories specified in the NPUAP staging system are shown in Figure 8-5.

## Tests[2,4,5,6,7,12,15]

- CBC with differential, ESR
  - Checks for anemia (weakens the body's ability for gas exchange) and leukocytosis (implies inflammation or infection).
  - Be concerned of possible osteomyelitis if ESR is above 120 mm/hr and white blood cell (WBC) count above 15,000/μL.
- Serum albumin, prealbumin, and protein
  - Used to determine nutritional status (inadequate intake of protein negatively impacts wound healing).
  - Albumin level under 2.5 g/dL is a grave sign; implies significant protein depletion.
- Stool test to evaluate for *Clostridium difficilie*
  - If concerned over this being the cause of fecal incontinence.
- Blood cultures
  - If concerned over underlying bacteremia.
- X-rays, bone scan, magnetic resonance imaging (MRI), bone biopsy
  - Plain films are usually ordered first to determine the presence of osteomyelitis; a positive bone scan strongly suggests osteomyelitis. This can further be investigated by ordering an MRI or bone biopsy (gold standard for diagnosing osteomyelitis).
- Tissue biopsy
  - Recommended in wounds that do not heal despite treatment. It also helps to check for the presence of an underlying malignancy.

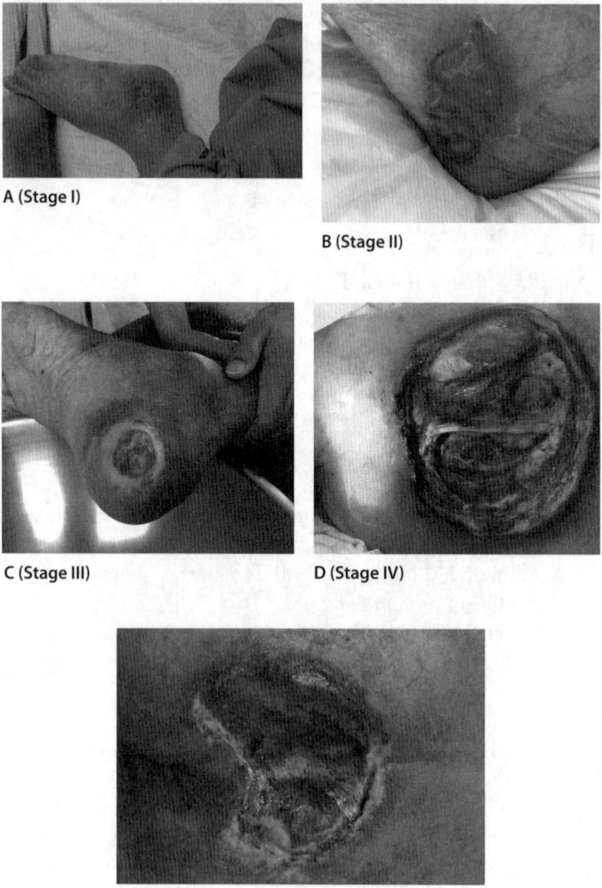


**Figure 8-5** The Four Stages of Ulceration [See **Figure CP-8A-8E** at end of book for color version]

## Treatment & Management[2,4,5,6,8,9,10,11,12,16,17,18]

- **Nonpharmacologic and nursing interventions:**
  - Use tools (e.g., Braden scale) to predict pressure ulcer risk.
    - In long-term care, assessment is recommended when the patient first arrives, then weekly for the first month, then quarterly and/or if their condition changes.
  - Reduction of pressure (especially in those with open wounds).
    - Patients should be repositioned a minimum of every 2 hours.
  - If intake is poor and patient has insufficient calories or proteins, consider nutritional supplementation (protein goal of at least 1.5 g/kg/day).
    - Increased dietary protein promotes wound healing.
  - Encourage smoking cessation (smoking is known to impair wound healing).
  - Implement thorough wound care.
    - Keep the wound free of urine and fecal matter by frequently inspecting the site and cleansing.
    - Monitor for necrotic tissue, eschar, and slough (may need wound debridement).
    - Cleanse the wound to rid of inflammatory contaminates.
      - Toxic agents such as hydrogen peroxide, acetic acid, hypochlorite, and povidone-iodine (Betadine) should be used with caution; evidence supports limiting its use.
      - If an agent is safe to drink, such as water, then this can be used to cleanse a wound.
      - Water, normal saline, and preparations (e.g., 2 tsp of salt/1 L of boiled water) are options to clean wounds.
    - Avoid excessive moisture given this prolongs wound healing (harms healthy cellular growth).

- Appropriate use of wound dressings.
  - Dressings that absorb (e.g., foams, alginates) are used to avoid maceration and decrease wound fluid build-up.
  - Transparent films, hydrocolloids, and hydrogels are used on desiccated wounds or wounds with low levels of exudate.
  - Use of classic wet-to-dry dressings is not supported in the literature; it is a nonselective wound debridement.
- Offer psychosocial support.
  - This is often overlooked and should be emphasized; these patients can feel like they have no control over their lives and feel stigmatized, resulting in isolation, depression, and impaired quality of life.
- Adjunctive therapy for wound healing: negative pressure wound therapy, hyperbaric oxygen therapy, ultrasound, electrical stimulation, and support surfaces (e.g., foam mattress, low air-loss systems).

- **Pharmacologic and other interventions**:
  - Pain control
    - Consider this especially prior to dressing changes and debridement.
    - Nonopioid agents (e.g., acetaminophen, NSAIDs, COX-2 inhibitors).
    - Opioids (e.g., oxycodone, ultram) are reserved in severe forms of acute pain.
  - Vitamin C and zinc supplementation
    - Often used to promote healing (effectiveness has not been conclusively confirmed).
  - Muscle relaxants (e.g., baclofen [Lioresal], diazepam [Valium], dantrolene [Dantrium])
    - Relief of spasticity is crucial in the treatment and prevention of pressure ulceration.
    - Some have anticholinergic adverse effects; can cause sedation.

- Empiric antibiotics (e.g., topical silver sulfadiazine [Silvadene], topical mafenide [Sulfamylon])
  - Silver sulfadiazine is commonly used and carries few complications; if wounds do not respond to this, then mafenide is used (penetrates eschar more effectively).
  - Goal is to cover aerobic gram-positive and gram-negative organisms and anaerobes.

Note: A 14-day course of topical antibiotics can be used for nonhealing, clean pressure ulcers. Antiseptics can be used for wounds not expected to heal and/or are colonized. Systemic antibiotics are reserved in the presence of sepsis, advancing cellulitis, or osteomyelitis.

- Physical, occupation, and speech therapy consultation/referral
  - Including rehabilitation therapist is key to a successful wound care program.
  - Physical therapist can provide the following services (but not limited to): wound debridement, edema management, mobility, and modalities (e.g., electrical stimulation).
  - Occupational therapist can also provide wound debridement, along with wheelchair management, and toileting programs.
  - Speech therapy can address nutrition, cognitive deficits, and chewing impairment.
- Wound specialist consultation/referral
  - Consider in patients with chronic, nonhealing wounds.
- Dietitian consultation/referral
  - To assist in optimizing nutrition.
- Pain specialist consultation/referral
  - This would be appropriate if opioids are considered. Be aware of your state regulations and guidelines; some states require referral when going above specific dosage levels.
- Surgical referral
  - Stage III and IV pressure ulcers usually require surgical intervention.

- Of note, colostomy procedure has high complication rate in older adults and its benefit is questionable.

Note: Beers listed items, as mentioned above, include skeletal muscle relaxants, NSAIDs, COX-2 inhibitors, and opioids.

## Differential Diagnosis[2,4,5,6,8,13,14,15]

- Cellulitis: Erythema, swelling, and tenderness on skin that is usually not on a pressure point area (e.g., lower extremities).
- Diabetic lower extremity ulcers: Will have a history of diabetes (supported by HbA1c); diabetic neuropathy will lead to diminished perception of pain; therefore, ulcers will be noted on the foot, due to pressure from shoes. These patients are at greater risk of peripheral artery disease, which can be screened by ordering an ankle-brachial index.
- Vascular ulcerations: From arterial and venous insufficiency. Usually found on lower extremities. The medial and lateral malleoli are common sites in venous stasis ulcers. Skin staining is also common. Arterial ulcers are usually found on feet, heels, or toes; the base will be pale.

### CLINICAL PEARLS

- Educate patients and support staff about methods of prevention for pressure ulcerations.
- Educate staff on signs of pressure ulcerations so early treatment can be initiated.
- Offer nutritional supplements to promote protein intake and adequate nutrition (especially important in patients with stage 3 and 4 pressure injuries).
- Wound care should be divided into operative and nonoperative methods:
  - Stage 1 and 2 pressure injuries are nonoperative and the use of conservative methods are recommended.
  - Stage 3 and 4 pressure injuries use surgical interventions.
  - Approximately 70%–90% pressure injuries heal by second intention.
- Debridement should be considered when conservative management fails and/or in the presence of necrotic tissue, eschar, and slough.

## References

1. Barratt, N. (2014, January–February). Nutrition and wound healing: Implications for practice. *Journal of the Dermatology Nurses' Association, 6(1)*, 27–32.
2. Berlowitz, D. (2017, April 17). Clinical Staging and Management of Pressure-Induced Skin and Soft Tissue Injury. UpToDate. Retrieved from http://www.uptodate.com/contents/clinical-staging-and-management-of-pressure-induced-skin-and-soft-tissue-injury. Accessed January 4, 2018.
3. Black, J., Baharestani, M. M., Cuddigan, J., Dorner, B., Edsberg, L., & Langemo, D., . . . Ratcliff, C. (2007, May). National Pressure Ulcer Advisory Panel's updated pressure ulcer staging system. *Advances in Skin & Wound Care: The Journal for Prevention and Healing, 20(5)*, 269–274.
4. Cheung, C. (2010, January). Older adults and ulcers: Chronic wounds in the geriatric population. *Advances in Skin & Wound Care: The Journal for Prevention and Healing, 23(1)*, 39–44.
5. Kirman, C. N. (2017, March 15). Pressure Ulcers and Wound Care. Medscapte. Retrieved from http://emedicine.medscape.com/article/190115-overview#a1. Accessed January 4, 2018.
6. Lyons, F., & Ousley, L. (2015). *Dermatology for the Advanced Practice Nurse*. New York, NY: Springer Publishing Company,.
7. Livesley, N., & Chow, A. (2002). Infected pressure ulcers in elderly individuals. *Clinical Infectious Diseases,* 35(11), 1390–1396. doi:10.1086/344059
8. Gorecki, C., Brown, J. M., Nelson, E. A., Briggs, M., Schoonhoven, L., & Dealey, C., . . . Nixon, J. (2009, May 21). Impact of pressure ulcers on quality of life in older patients: A systematic review. *Journal of the American Geriatrics Society,* 57(7), 1175–1183. Retrieved from http://onlinelibrary.wiley.com/doi/10.1111/j.1532-5415.2009.02307.x/abstract. Accessed January 4, 2018.
9. National Pressure Ulcer Advisory Panel, European Pressure Ulcer Advisory Panel. (2009). Pressure ulcer treatment recommendations. Prevention and Treatment of Pressure Ulcers: Clinical Practice Guideline. Washington, DC: National Pressure Ulcer Advisory Panel.
10. Langer, G., & Fink, A. (2014, June 12). Nutritional interventions for preventing and treating pressure ulcers. *Cochrane Database of Systematic Reviews, 6, CD003216.* Retrieved from http://onlinelibrary.wiley.com/doi/10.1002/14651858.CD003216/abstract. Accessed January 27, 2018.
11. Mercer, D. M. (2015). Pressure ulcers. In Burggraf, V., Kim, K. Y., & Knight, A. L. (Eds.) *Healthy Aging: Principles and Clinical Practice for Clinicians* (pp. 383–406). Philadelphia, PA: Lippincott Williams & Wilkins.
12. Gulanick, M., & Myers, J. L. (2017). *Nursing Care Plans: Diagnoses, Interventions, & Outcomes*. St. Louis, MO: Elsevier.
13. Berlowitz, D. R. (2017, November 18). Pressure ulcers. Epocrates. Retrieved from https://online.epocrates.com/diseases/37811/Pressure-ulcer/Key-Highlights (used for diagnoses only). Accessed January 5, 2018.
14. Chen, S., Hsiao, P., Huang, J., Lin, K., Hsu, W., & Lee, Y., . . . Shin, S. (2015). Abnormally low or high ankle-brachial index is associated with proliferative diabetic retinopathy in type 2 diabetic mellitus patients. *PLoS One, 10*(7), e0134718. doi:10.1371/journal.pone.0134718

15. Richlen, B., & Richlen, D. (2015). The role of rehab in wound care. *Wound Care Advisor, 4*(2), 18. Retrieved from https://woundcareadvisor.com/role-of-rehab-in-wound-care/. Accessed January 6, 2018.
16. American Geriatrics Society 2015 Beers Criteria Update Expert Panel, Fick, D. M., Semla, T. P., Beizer, J., Brandt, N., & Dombrowski, R., . . . Steinman, M. (2015, October 8). American Geriatrics Society 2015 updated Beers criteria for potentially inappropriate medication use in older adults. *Journal of the American Geriatrics Society, 63*(11), 2227–2246. Retrieved from http://onlinelibrary.wiley.com/doi/10.1111/jgs.13702/abstract. Accessed October 3, 2017.
17. Dowell, D., Haegerich, T. M., & Chou, R. CDC Guideline for Prescribing Opioids for Chronic Pain — United States, 2016. MMWR Recomm Rep 2016;65(No. RR-1):1–49. DOI: http://dx.doi.org/10.15585/mmwr.rr6501e1.
18. The American Academy of Pain Medicine. For the Primary Care Provider: When to Refer to a Pain specialist. (2016, December 1). www.painmed.org/files/when-to-refer-a-pain-specialist.pdf. Accessed April 25, 2018.

# Seborrheic Keratosis

## Definition[1,2,3,4,5]

Seborrheic keratoses (SK) (see Figure 8-6) are common epidermal tumors consisting of a benign proliferation of immature keratinocytes.

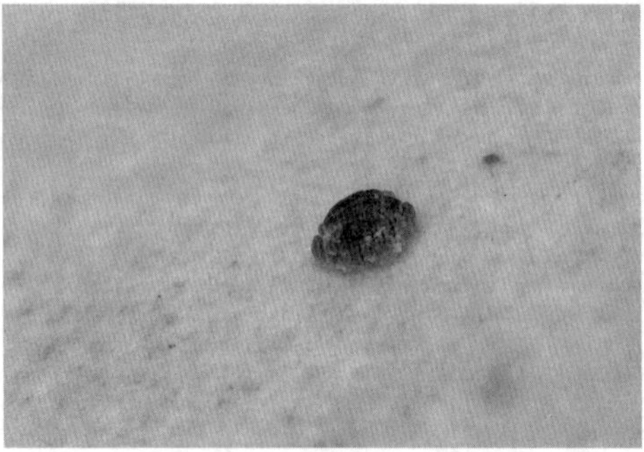

**Figure 8-6** Seborrheic Keratosis [See **Figure CP-9** at end of book for color version]



## Cause[1,2,3,4,5]

- Thought to result from a clonal expansion of a mutated epidermal keratinocyte.

## Risk Factors[1,2,3,4,5]

- Increased age (over age 50)
- Caucasian ancestry
- Sun exposure

## Signs & Symptoms[1,2,3,4,5]

- One or more light brown, flat lesions that have a velvety to finely verrucous surface that arise on normal skin.
- Lesions start as less than 1 cm, but the lesions can grow to several cm or more. Later, the lesions become thicker and have an appearance of being stuck or pasted on the skin surface; they may be pigmented and usually do not resolve.
- Lesions may be itchy (seborrheic keratoses can easily catch on clothing and become irritated; can be a site for the development of an infection).

## Tests

- No laboratory tests are required; they are easily diagnosed clinically.
- Skin biopsy (only recommended if the diagnosis is ambiguous).

## Treatment & Management[1,2,3,4,5,6,8]

- **Nonpharmacological and nursing interventions:**
  - Educate the patients and their families that SKs are benign lesions and do not become malignant. SKs grow larger with time, which is an expected finding (not dangerous).
  - Monitor for inflamed lesions or lesions suspicious for cancer.
- **Pharmacological and other interventions:**

  *No treatment is indicated unless the lesions become irritated or appear to be changing.*
  - Mineral oil can soften seborrheic keratosis lesions so that they may be peeled off manually.
  - Topical diclofenac 3% (Solaraze) can be used twice per day for 3 months; it is an NSAID that is effective at

clearing up actinic keratoses. Patient satisfaction with this agent is high; may cause skin itching, redness, drying, or localized edema.
    - Ammonium lactate and alpha hydroxy acids can be used to decrease the size or height of seborrheic keratosis lesions.
    - Superficial lesions can be treated by carefully applying trichloroacetic acid or topical treatment with tazarotene cream 0.1% applied twice daily for 16 weeks.
- Dermatologist referral
    - For surgical treatment with cryotherapy, electrodessication, electrodessication and cuttettage, curettage alone, shave biopsy or excision using a scalpel, or laser or dermabrasion surgery.

## Differential Diagnosis[1,2,3,4,5,6]

- Skin cancer (basal cell carcinoma, squamous cell carcinoma, and malignant melanoma): These can be mistaken for SK lesions and should be biopsied.
- Atypical nevi: Look for signs of irregular borders or color variations, but are not typically scaled. SKs are usually larger, thicker, and scaled versus a nevi.
- Acrochordon: Skin tags that hang on skin. Not scaled.
- Verruca vulgaris: These appear similar to SKs but are more flesh colored and typically occur on feet and hands, whereas SKs are typically found on the trunk.

### CLINICAL PEARLS[7]

- Seborrheic keratoses are benign and do not become malignant; they are easily mistaken for being a basal cell carcinoma or malignant melanoma (a biopsy will determine the difference). Skin cancers can however arise within a seborrheic keratosis, and be easily overlooked. It is therefore recommended in patients with multiple seborrheic keratoses to have routine skin examinations.
- Sudden onset of seborrheic keratoses on the abdomen can indicate an underlying internal cancer (Leser-Trélat sign) and should be investigated.

## References


1. Balin, A. K. (2017, September 12). Seborrheic Keratosis Treatment & Management. Medscape. Retrieved from http://emedicine.medscape.com/article/1059477-treatment#d7. Accessed January 11, 2018.
2. Chung, G. Y., Morrell, T. J., & Kerstetter, J. (2015, November–December). Seborrheic keratosis. *Journal of the Dermatology Nurses' Association*, 7(6), 359–361.
3. Goldstein, B. G., & Goldstein, A. O. (2017, July 26). Overview of Benign Lesions of the Skin. UpToDate. Retrieved from http://www.uptodate.com/contents/overview-of-benign-lesions-of-the-skin. Accessed January 11, 2018.
4. Lyons, F., & Ousley, L. (2015). *Dermatology for the Advanced Practice Nurse*. New York, NY: Springer Publishing Company.
5. Panther, D. J., & Jacob, S. E. (2015, March–April). Brown spot on the back. *Journal of the Dermatology Nurses' Association*, 7(2), 109–110.
6. Wolff, K., Johnson, R., Saavedra, A. P., & Roh, E. K. (Eds.) (2017, March 15). *Fitzpatrick's Color Atlas and Synopsis of Clinical Dermatology* (8th ed.); Benign neoplasms and hyperplasias. New York, NY: McGraw-Hill. Retrieved from http://accessmedicine.mhmedical.com/content.aspx?bookid=2043&sectionid=154898019. Accessed January 11, 2018.
7. Schwartz, R.A. (2017, June 2). Sign of Leser-Trélat. Medscape. Retrieved from http://emedicine.medscape.com/article/1097299-overview. Accessed January 11, 2018.
8. Nelson, C. (2011, June 15). Diclofenac gel in the treatment of actinic keratoses. *Therapeutics and Clinical Risk Management,* 7, 207–211. doi:10.2147/tcrm.s12498


# Herpes Zoster

## Definition[1,2,3,5,6,7,8,11]

Herpes zoster (shingles) (see Figure 8-7) is an infection that results from reactivation of latent varicella-zoster virus (VZV) infection within the sensory ganglia.

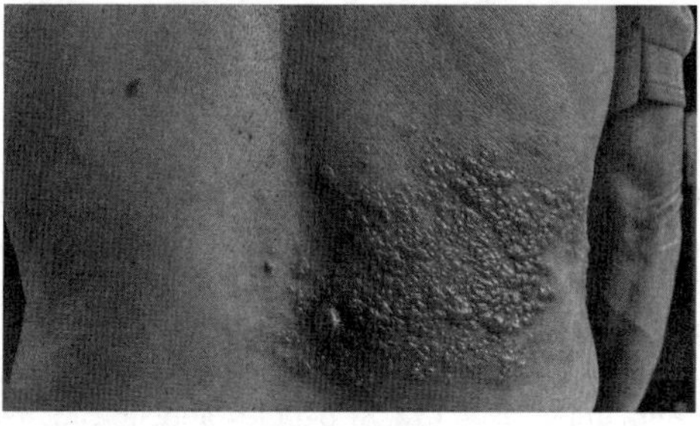

**Figure 8-7** Herpes Zoster [See **Figure CP-10** at end of book for color version]

Note: Primary infection with VZV results in varicella (chickenpox), characterized by vesicular lesions in different stages of development on the face, trunk, and extremities.

## Cause[1,2,3,5,6,7,8,11]

- Reactivation of latent VZV

## Risk Factors[1,2,3,5,6,7,8,11,12,13]

- Age: the most important risk factor for the development of herpes zoster

Note: Almost 100% of adults above 50 years of age are infected with VZV and one-third (33%) of Americans will develop shingles in their lifetime. This risk increases to one in two in those ≥ 85 years.

- Physical trauma
- Underlying malignancy
- HIV
- Immunosuppressed patients
- Transplant patients
- Autoimmune disease

## Signs & Symptoms[1,2,3,5,6,7,8,11]

- Painful, unilateral vesicular eruption, which usually occurs in a restricted dermatomal distribution.
- Systemic response of fever, anorexia, and body aches (mild-severe).
- Prodromal sensory phenomena along one or more skin dermatomes that last 1–10 days with associated pain, pruritus, and paresthesia.
- Painful grouped herpetiform vesicles on an erythematous base confined to the cutaneous surface innervated by a sensory nerve.
- Typically, the condition affects a single dermatome, most commonly a thoracic dermatome, on one side of the body.
- Regional lymphadenopathy.
- Erythematous macules and papules appear, progressing to vesicles within 1 day (this occurs after the prodromal period).

- The vesicles eventually cloud, rupture, crust, and involute.
- Postherpetic neuralgia (PHN) along the confined area of the dermatome.
  - PHN may last weeks to years after zoster resolution and can be very painful.
  - Symptoms include pain, burning, and tingling.

## Tests[1,2,3,5,6,7,8,11]

- Polymerase chain reaction (PCR)
  - Offers consistent fast and sensitive validation of VZV from clinical specimens obtained from skin lesions and body fluids such as cerebrospinal fluid (CSF) and bronchial lavage.
- Direct fluorescent antibody (DFA)
  - Prompt diagnosis of VZV infection can be done by DFA on skin scrapings of active non-crusted vesicular lesions.
- Viral culture
  - During the vesicular stage, a swab of the lesion or sterile body fluid (CSF) can be done and incubated for 1-2 weeks.
- Serologic testing with ELISA (enzyme-linked immunosorbent assay)
  - When IgG antibodies are present this confirms the history and protection of the Varicella infection.
- Tzanck smear of vesicular fluid (lower sensitivity and specificity than DFA or PCR)

## Treatment & Management[1,4,5,6,7,8,10,11,12,13,14,15,16]

- **Nonpharmacological and nursing interventions**:
  - Wet to dry dressings with sterile saline applied to skin for 30–60 minutes for four to six times per day can help with pruritus.
- **Pharmacological interventions:**
  - Herpes zoster subunit vaccine (Shingrix).

    - Used for the prevention of herpes zoster in adults above 50 years old (not indicated for prevention of primary varicella infection)
    - Preferred over Zoster vaccine live (Zostavax) for preventing shingles and related complications.
    - May cause injection site pain, myalgia, fatigue, and upset stomach.
  - Corticosteroids (e.g., prednisone [Deltasone]).
    - Although its use is controversial in herpes zoster, it helps to reduce inflammation and help with pain. Possibly helps to reduce PHN.
    - Corticosteroids increase the risk of secondary bacterial infections.
  - Pain medication: Narcotic and nonnarcotic pain medications can be used for pain control.
    - NSAIDs with or without acetaminophen can be used.
    - Weak opioids such as codeine or tramadol (Ultram) can be used; if pain is severe and disturbs sleep, consider stronger opioids (e.g., oxycodone or morphine).
    - Gabapentin (Neurontin) in low doses help control PHN.
  - Antiviral agents (e.g., valacyclovir [Valtrex], acyclovir [Zovirax], famciclovir [Famvir]).
    - Example: valacyclovir 1,000 mg PO three times daily for 7 days.
    - The sooner these are started, the less chance of PHN.
    - Adverse events are not common (may include gastrointestinal disturbance or headache).
- Pain specialist consultation/referral
  - This would be appropriate if opioids are considered. Be aware of your state regulations and guidelines; some states require referral when going above specific dosage levels.

Note: Beers listed items, as mentioned above, include NSAIDs, gabapentin, opioids, and oral corticosteroids.

## Differential Diagnosis[3,5,6,7,8,10,11]

- Herpes simplex: Pain and tingling is localized and does not follow a dermatome.
- Contact dermatitis: May cross midline of the body.

### CLINICAL PEARLS

- Educate patients about the progression of herpes zoster and what to expect in regards to pain and potential for postherpetic neuralgia. Patients should be treated aggressively with antivirals, steroids, and gabapentin for prevention of PHN.
- During the acute phase, people who are elderly, immunocompromised, pregnant women (such as family members or staff), and people with no history of chickenpox should avoid contact with infected persons.
- Treatment should be initiated within 72 hours to speed recovery of shingles and prevent PHN.
- Keep nails trimmed if patients are scratching lesions to prevent potential secondary bacterial infections.

## References


1. Albrecht, M. A. (2016, July 21). Treatment of Herpes Zoster in the Immunocompetent Host. UpToDate. Retrieved from http://www.uptodate.com/contents/treatment-of-herpes-zoster-in-the-immunocompetent-host. Accessed January 19, 2018.
2. Albrecht, M. A. (2016, October 25). Epidemiology and Pathogenesis of Varicella-Zoster Virus Infection: Herpes Zoster. UpToDate. Retrieved from http://www.uptodate.com/contents/epidemiology-and-pathogeneis-of-varicella-zoster-virus-infection-herpes-zoster. Accessed January 19, 2018.
3. Albrecht, M. A. (2017, May 31). Diagnosis of Varicella-Zoster Virus Infection. UpToDate. Retrieved from http://www.uptodate.com/contents/diagnosis-of-varicella-zoster-virus-infection. Accessed January 19, 2018.
4. Cernik, C., Gallina, K., & Brodell, R. (2008, June 9). The treatment of herpes simplex infections: An evidence-based review. *Archives of Internal Medicine, 168(11)*, 1137–1144.
5. Dworkin, R. H., Johnson, R. W., Breuer, J., & Gnann, J. W., Levin, M. J., Backonja, M., . . . Whitley, R. J. (2007, January 1). Recommendations for the management of herpes zoster. *Clinical infectious Diseases*, *44*(Supp 1), S1–26.
6. Folusakin, O. A. (2017, March 9). Herpes Simplex. Medscape. Retrieved from http://emedicine.medscape.com/article/218580-overview. Accessed January 19, 2018.
7. Janniger, C. K. (2017, October 24). Herpes Zoster. Medscape. Retrieved from http://emedicine.medscape.com/article/1132465-overview. Accessed January 19, 2018.
8. Lyons, F., & Ousley, L. (2015). *Dermatology for the Advanced Practice Nurse*. New York, NY: Springer Publishing Company.
9. Nassaji, M., Ghorbani, R., Taheri, R., Azizzadeh, M., & Zolfaghari, S. (2017, March–April). Herpes zoster: Dermographic and clinical severity of acute pain. *Journal of the Dermatology Nurses' Association*, 9(2), 80–84.

10. Perez, C., & Jacob, S. E. (2017, January–February). Herpes zoster: Localized vesicular lesion. *Journal of the Dermatology Nurses' Association*, 9(1), 39–40.
11. Wilson, D. D. (2014, May 12). Herpes zoster. *The Nurse Practitioner*, 39(5), 15–16.
12. SHINGRIX. (n.d.). Be one of the first to get information about SHINGRIX. Retrieved from https://www.shingrix.com/. Accessed January 19, 2018.
13. GlaxoSmithKlein. (2017, October 25). CDC's Advisory Committee on Immunization Practices recommends Shingrix as the preferred vaccine for the prevention of shingles for adults aged 50 and up. Retrieved from https://www.gsk.com/en-gb/media/press-releases/cdc-s-advisory-committee-on-immunization-practices-recommends-shingrix-as-the-preferred-vaccine-for-the-prevention-of-shingles-for-adults-aged-50-and-up/. Accessed January 19, 2018.
14. American Geriatrics Society 2015 Beers Criteria Update Expert Panel, Fick, D. M., Semla, T. P., Beizer, J., Brandt, N., & Dombrowski, R., . . . Steinman, M. (2015, October 8). American Geriatrics Society 2015 updated Beers criteria for potentially inappropriate medication use in older adults. *Journal of the American Geriatrics Society*, 63(11), 2227–2246. Retrieved from http://onlinelibrary.wiley.com/doi/10.1111/jgs.13702/abstract. Accessed October 3, 2017.
15. Dowell, D., Haegerich, T. M., & Chou R. CDC Guideline for Prescribing Opioids for Chronic Pain — United States, 2016. MMWR Rcomm Rep 2016;65(No. RR-1): 1–49. DOI: http://dx.doi.org/10.15585/mmwr.rr6501e1.
16. The American Academy of Pain Medicine. For the Primary Care Provider: When to Refer to a Pain specialist. (2016, December 01). Retrieved from www.painmed.org/files/when-to-refer-a-pain-specialist.pdf. Accessed April 25, 2018.

# Bullous Pemphigoid

## Definition[1,6,9]

Bullous pemphigoid (BP) (see Figure 8-8) is a chronic, inflammatory, subepidermal, blistering disease. It is an autoimmune

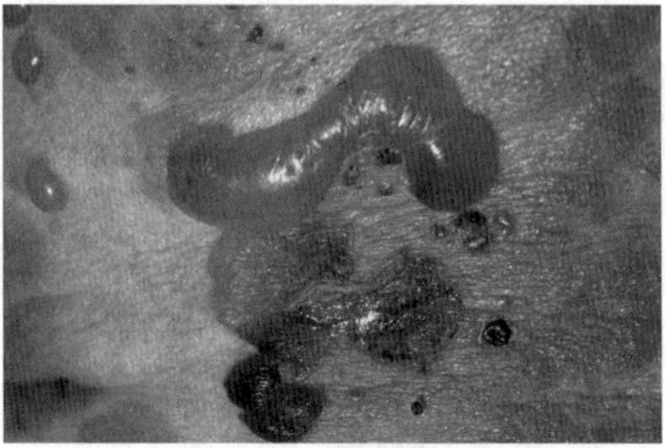

**Figure 8-8** Bullous Pemphigoid [See **Figure CP-11** at end of book for color version]

blistering disease that most commonly affects older adults. If not treated, it may persist for months to years, with episodes of remission and exacerbations. For those whom are incapacitated, this disease may be fatal.

## Types

- Generalized bullous form: The most common form of pemphigoid. Taut bullae can be present on any skin surface. Oral or ocular involvement is rare. The bullae may appear as erythematous or flesh colored on skin surfaces. These bullae will normally heal without scarring.
- Vesicular form: This is a rare form of pemphigoid. This form presents as multiple small, tense, pruritic, erythematous based blisters on skin surface.
- Vegetative form: Extremely rare. This form occurs in the skin folds of the skin such as the axillae, neck, groin, and inframammary areas.
- Generalized erythroderma form: This type of pemphigoid will often be confused with psoriasis, atopic dermatitis, or other skin conditions that present as scaled erythroderma.
- Urticarial form: Initially will present with pruritic lesions that convert to bullae eruptions.
- Nodular form: Very rare. Appears similar to prurigo nodules with blisters or nodules on normal skin surface.
- Acral form: Occurs in childhood.

## Causes[1,2,6,7,9]

- The etiology of BP is not well understood.
    - Blister formation occurs as a result of a breakdown in the immune system. The body's immune system will usually produce antibodies to fight infection or foreign substances. With BP, the body forms an antibody to that area of skins fiber that connects the epidermis to the dermis. Inflammation develops that produces the blisters and pruritus.

- Medications (may lead to a small percentage of cases).
    - Medications that can cause BP reactions are penicillin, etanercept (Enbrel), sulfasalazine (Azulfidine), and furosemide (Lasix).
- Light and radiation.
    - Light and radiation such as ultraviolet light that is routinely used to treat skin conditions or cancer can trigger BP reaction.

## Risk Factors[1,2,5,6,9]

- Age 50–70, with average age of 65
- Neurologic disorders
    - Dementia, Parkinson's disease, multiple sclerosis, bipolar disorders
- Patients with multiple comorbidities
    - Hypertension, diabetes, thromboembolism, heart disease
- High-dose steroids and immunosuppressants

## Signs & Symptoms[2,3,4,6,7,9]

- Tense, fluid-filled bullae on the skin (classic finding).
    - A prodromal phase may last from weeks to months preceding the development of cutaneous bullae.
- The primary feature of BP is the appearance of large bullae that do not rupture easily when touched.
- The fluid inside the blisters is usually clear to blood tinged.
- The surrounding skin around the blisters may appear normal, reddish, or darker than usual.
- Some people with BP develop eczema or hive-like rash rather than bullae.
- Most commonly, the bullae will appear on the lower abdomen, groin, upper thighs, and arms. The affected areas of skin can be very pruritic. The mucosa of the mouth and mucous membranes of the eyes may also be affected (this is called mucous membrane pemphigoid).

## Tests[6, 9]

- Histopathologic analysis: A skin biopsy is done from the edge of the blister.
- Direct immunofluorescence (DIF) studies are done on normal skin near infected site.
- Indirect immunofluorescence (IDIF) is done on patient's serum if the DIF is positive.
- Peripheral blood eosinophilia is common in patients with BP. Increased serum IgE levels are also common.

## Treatment & Management[1,2,6,8,10,11]

- **Nonpharmacologic and nursing interventions:**
  - Daily rupturing of tense blisters and bullae is helpful for reducing lateral extension of new bullae formation.
    - Patients and caregivers should cleanse areas with alcohol prior to rupturing the blisters/bullae with a sterile needle. The overlying epithelial layer can act as a natural wound dressing, so it should be left in place. Open erosions should be covered with a nonstick dressing to reduce pain and friction.
  - Patients and caregivers should be educated on signs and symptoms of infection at sites so that prompt treatment can be administered.
  - Active blister sites should be covered with bandage to prevent infection.
- **Pharmacologic and other interventions:**
  - Corticosteroids, topical
    - Example: clobetasol (Clobex) 0.5% cream applied topically BID, up to 2 weeks.
      - Order after disease is under control.
    - These are ordered as first-line therapy.
    - Common reactions may include skin atrophy, dryness, erythema.
  - Anti-inflammatory agents (e.g., corticosteroids, tetracycline [Aureomycin], dapsone [Aczone]) and

immunosuppressants (e.g., azathioprine [Imuran], methotrexate [Trexall], mycophenolate mofetil, cyclophosphamide).
  - Example: azathioprine 0.5–2.5 mg/kg per day ongoing until clear.
    - Monitor CBC, CMP q 2 weeks for the first 3 months and every 2–3 months thereafter.
- Antihistamines (e.g., loratadine [Claritin], diphenhydramine [Benadryl], doxepin [Silenor])
  - These provide relief from intense itching.
  - Monitor for side effects of these anticholinergic drugs (e.g., drowsiness, dry mouth).
- Systemic steroid therapy
  - Example: prednisone starting at 0.75 mg/kg to 1.25 mg/kg per day for up to 21 days.
    - Dose depends on severity of disease and patient's comorbidities.
    - Once itch and new blisters have resolved for at least 14 days and most of existing blisters have healed, start tapering the steroid slowly over several months.
  - Steroids increase the risk of osteoporosis (long-term use), hyperglycemia, and delirium.

- Dermatology consultation/referral
  - This is recommended as soon as possible if BP is suspected.

Note: Beers listed items, as mentioned above, include oral corticosteroids and oral antihistamines.

## Differential Diagnosis[2,3,4,6,7,9]

- Urticaria: When compared to BP, does not form blisters; urticarial lesions are dermal in nature and nodular.
- Eczematous dermatitis: If blisters are present, they are fragile. BP bullea are tense and do not rupture easy.
- Dermatitis herpetiformis: Blisters easily rupture and often have a small cluster formation of blisters, not bullae.

**CLINICAL PEARLS**[2]

- BP is an autoimmune bullous skin disease with treatment goals focused on decreasing blister formation and healing of blisters or erosions with minimal required medications to control symptoms.
- Be careful in using clobetasol (Clobex) cream and potent steroid creams on elderly skin. Instead of twice-daily applications, consider daily application.
- Using oral steroids and autoimmune drugs in geriatric population may increase risk of peptic ulcers, GI bleeds, agranulocytosis, and diabetes.

## References


1. Bastuji-Garin, S., Joly, P., Lemordant, P., Sparsa, A., Bedane, C., & Delaporte, E., . . . Richard, M. A.; French Study Group for Bullous Diseases. (2011, March). Risk factors for bullous pemphigoid in the elderly: A prospective case-control study. *Journal of Investigative Dermatology*, *131*(3), 637–643.
2. Chan, L. S. (2017, July 11). Bullous Pemphigoid. Medscape. Retrieved from http://emedicine.medscape.com/article/1062391-treatment#d7. Accessed January 29, 2018.
3. Christiaan, V. B., Jorrit, B. T., & Hendri, H. P. (2013). Bullous pemphigoid as pruritus in the elderly: A common presentation. *JAMA*, *149*(8), 950–953.
4. Fityan, A., & Ardern-Jones, M.R. (2013, February). Rashes in the elderly. *General Medicine*, *41*.
5. Langan, S. M., Groves, R. W., & West, J. (2011, March). The relationship between neurological disease and bullous pemphigoid: A population-based case-control study. *Journal of Investigative Dermatology*, *131*(3), 631–636.
6. Leiferman, K. M., Zone, J. J., & Ofori, A. O. (2017, November). Clinical Features and Diagnosis of Bullous Pemphigoid and Mucous Membrane Pemphigoid. UpToDate. Retrieved from http://www.uptodate.com/contents/clinical-features-and-diagnosis- of -bullous-pemphigoid-and-mucous-membrane-pemphigoid. Accessed January 29, 2018.
7. Mayo Clinic. (2017, August 04). Bullous Pemphigoid. Retrieved from http://www.mayoclinic.org/diseases-conditions/bullous-pemphigoid/symptoms-causes/syc-20350414. Accessed January 29, 2018.
8. Murrell, D. F., & Ramirez-Quizon, M. (2017, June 30). Management and Prognosis of Bullous Pemphigoid. UpToDate. Retrieved from http://www.uptodate.com/contents/management-and-prognosis-of-bullous-pemphigoid. Accessed January 29, 2018.
9. Schmidt, E., della Torre, R., & Borradori, L. (2011, July). Clinical features and practical diagnosis of bullous pemphigoid. *Dermatology Clinics*, 29(3), 427–438, viii–ix.
10. Epocrates. (n.d.). Retrieved from https://www.epocrates.com (used for adverse effects).

11. American Geriatrics Society 2015 Beers Criteria Update Expert Panel, Fick, D. M., Semla, T. P., Beizer, J., Brandt, N., & Dombrowski, R., . . . Steinman, M. (2015, October 8). American Geriatrics Society 2015 updated Beers criteria for potentially inappropriate medication use in older adults. *Journal of the American Geriatrics Society, 63*(11), 2227–2246. Retrieved from http://onlinelibrary.wiley.com/doi/10.1111/jgs.13702/abstract. Accessed October 8, 2017.

# Actinic Keratosis

## Defintion[1,4]

Actinic keratosis (AK) (see Figure 8-9) is a precancerous growth caused from repeated exposure to the sun or tanning bed.

## Cause[1]

- Ultraviolet radiation

## Risk Factors[1,3,4]

*Risk factors of AK coincide with causes, in addition to*:

- Age > 40 years
- Male gender
- Fair skin
- Light-colored or red hair
- Green or gray eyes

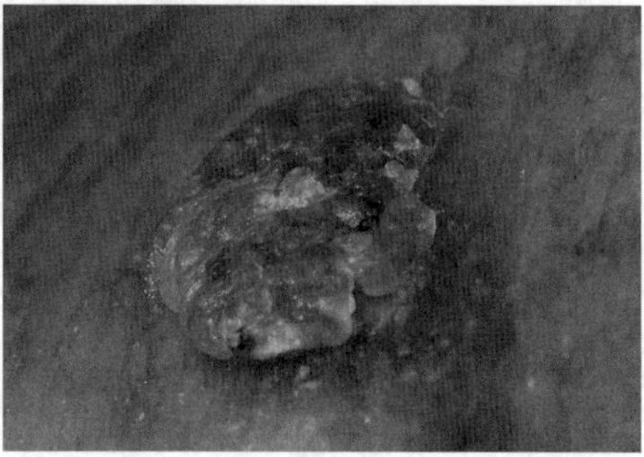

**Figure 8-9** Actinic Keratosis [See **Figure CP-12** at end of book for color version]

## Clinical Appearance[3,4]

- Erythematous, scaled plaques
- Macules or papules
- Hyperkeratotic surface
- Location of lesions: sun-exposed areas

## Tests[2,4]

- Usually none, if in doubt: skin biopsy

## Treatment & Management[1,2,3,4,5]

- **Nonpharmacological and nursing interventions:**
  - Encourage skin protection.
    - Avoid sunburns, encourage use of shade, wear appropriate clothing that covers the skin, use of sunscreen with SPF $\geq$ 15.
  - Encourage patients to inspect their skin for suspicious lesions, at least once every 30 days.
  - Education regarding avoid scratching lesions.
    - Can lead to secondary infections.
- **Pharmacological and other interventions:**
  - Imiquimod 5% gel (Aldara, Zyclara)
    - Example: Apply topically twice per week at night x 4 months.
  - Diclofenac sodium gel (Voltaren, Solaraze)
    - Not as effective as imiquimod; it does however decrease inflammation.
  - 5-fluorouracil (5-FU)
    - Example: 5% cream, apply BID for a month.
  - Cryotherapy
    - The AK is removed by freezing with liquid nitrogen.
  - Laser therapy
  - Dermabrasion
  - Chemical peels
  - Curettage
    - The surgeon removes damaged cells.

  - Photodynamic therapy
    - A solution is placed to the skin that makes it sensitive to light; the presence of light afterwards removes damaged cells.

## Differential Diagnosis[3,4]

- Squamous cell carcinoma (SCC): Has the potential to metastasize; lesions are usually larger and redder. AK carries potential to progress to SCC and appearance is similar to SCC. Biopsy rules out SCC.
- Seborrheic keratosis: Will often be tan to brown in color and be waxy, nonscaled benign lesions. AK has a different appearance; they are typically erythematous with scaling.

### CLINICAL PEARLS[3,4]

- Monitor patients a minimum of yearly with confirmed actinic keratosis, considering they can progress over to squamous cell carcinoma.

## References


1. Skin Cancer Foundation. (n.d.). Skin Cancer Information: What Is Skin Cancer? Retrieved from http://www.skincancer.org/skin-cancer-information. Accessed November 7, 2017.
2. Mayo Clinic. (2017, August 11). Actinic Keratosis. Retrieved from https://www.mayoclinic.org/diseases-conditions/actinic-keratosis/diagnosis-treatment/drc-20354975. Accessed November 7, 2017.
3. Berman, B., & Amini, S. (2016, October 18). Actinic Keratosis. Epocrates. Retrieved from https://online.epocrates.com/diseases/61635/Actinic-keratosis/Differential-Diagnosis. Accessed November 7, 2017.
4. Lyons, F., & Ousley, L. (2015). *Dermatology for the Advanced Practice Nurse*. New York, NY: Springer Publishing Company.
5. Spencer, J. M. (2017, July 14). Actinic Keratosis Treatment & Management (James, W. D., Ed.). Medscape. Retrieved from https://emedicine.medscape.com/article/1099775-treatment. Accessed November 10, 2017.
6. (2014, January–February). Actinic keratosis: A review of therapeutic options. *Journal of the Dermatology Nurses' Association*, 6(1), 15–16.
7. Berlin, J. M. (2014, January–February). Actinic keratosis: A review of therapeutic options. *Journal of the Dermatology Nurses' Association*, 6(1), 11–14.
8. Habif, T. P. (Ed.) (2010). *Clinical Dermatology: A Color Guide to Diagnosis and Therapy*. (5th ed.). Edinburgh, Scotland: Mosby.

9. James, W. D., Berger, T. G., & Elston, D. M. (2006). *Andrews' Diseases of the Skin: Clinical Dermatology*. (10th ed.). Philadelphia, PA: Saunders/Elsevier.
10. Nolen, M. E., Beebe, V. R., & King, J. M. (2011, Sept.Oct). Nonmelanoma skin cancer: Part 1. *Journal of the Dermatology Nurses' Association*. 3(5), 260–281.
11. Shulstad, R. M., & Proper, S. (2010, January–February). Squamous cell carcinoma: A review of etiology, pathogenesis, treatment, and varients. *Journal of the Dermatology Nurses' Association,* 2(1), 12–16.
12. Spencer, J. M. (2017, July 14). Actinic Keratosis. Medscape. Retrieved from http://emedicine.medscape.com/article/1099775-overview. Accessed November 10, 2017.

# Basal Cell Carcinoma

## Definition[1,2,4]

Basal cell carcinoma (BCC) (see Figure 8-10) is a common skin cancer seen on skin exposed areas; rarely metastasizes.

## Cause[2,3,4]

- Ultraviolet radiation

## Risk Factors[1,2,4]

*Risk factors of BCC coincide with causes, in addition to:*

- Fair skin
- Light-colored or red hair
- Green or blue eyes
- Transplant patients
- Radiation exposure

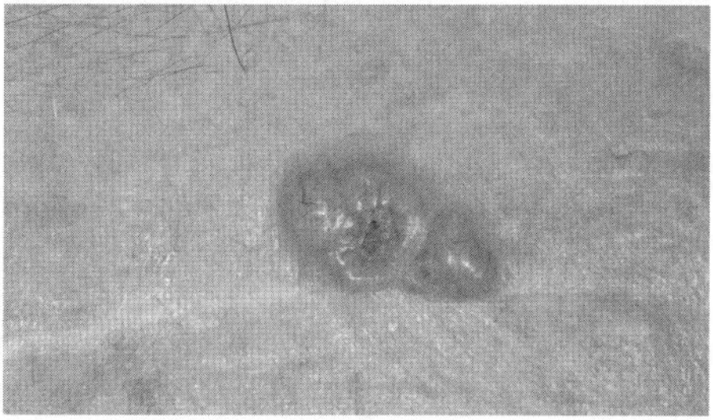

**Figure 8-10** Basal Cell Carcinoma [See **Figure CP-13** at end of book for color version]

## Clinical Appearance[2]

- Waxy papules with central ulceration and raised borders.
- Bleeds easily.
- Pink pearled appearance with telangiectasia present.
- Location of lesions: sun-exposed areas.

## Test[1,2,4]

- Skin biopsy

## Treatment & Management[2,4]

- **Nonpharmacological and nursing interventions:**
  - Encourage skin protection.
    - Avoid sunburns, encourage use of shade, wear appropriate clothing that covers the skin, use of sunscreen with SPF $\geq$ 15.
  - Encourage patients to inspect their skin for suspicious lesions, at least once every 30 days.
- **Pharmacological and other interventions:**
  - 5-fluorouracil 5% cream
    - Similar efficacy as imiquimod.
  - Interferon-alfa 2b protein product
  - Imiquimod 5% cream
  - Tazorac cream
  - Surgical excision and radiation

## Differential Diagnosis[1,2]

- Squamous cell carcinoma: Has more of a scaled appearance and larger patch. BCC appears more raised and often has a pearly hue with umbilicated center.
- Psoriasis or eczema: Will often be present on other parts of the body, on non-sun exposed skin and more widespread. Eczema often flares in flexure areas of body or will be an overall generalized dryness on skin. BCC is solitary and tends to be on sun-exposed skin.

**CLINICAL PEARLS**

- Educate patients about risk factors, the importance of self-skin examinations and yearly clinical skin examinations.
- Patients need to be educated on sun exposure and importance of wearing protective clothing and sunscreen.
- Patients should always follow up with clinician after receiving treatment for skin cancer to assure clearance.

## References

1. Schwartz, R. A. (2017, September 22). Basal Cell Carcinoma. Epocrates. Retrieved from https://online.epocrates.com/diseases/269/Basal-cell-carcinoma. Accessed November 7, 2017.
2. Skin Cancer Foundation. (n.d.). Skin Cancer Information. What Is Skin Cancer? Retrieved from http://www.skincancer.org/skin-cancer-information. Accessed November 7, 2017.
3. Centers for Disease Control and Prevention. (2017, January 24). Indoor Tanning Is Not Safe. Retrieved from https://www.cdc.gov/cancer/skin/basic_info/indoor_tanning.htm. Accessed November 7, 2017.
4. Lyons, F. & Ousley, L. (2015). *Dermatology for the Advanced Practice Nurse*. New York, NY. Springer Publishing Company.
5. Badar, R. S. (2017, Feb 27). Basal Cell Carcinoma. Medscape. Retrieved from http://emedicine.medscape.com/article/276624-overview
6. Morrell, T.J., Chung, G.Y., & Calame, A. (2015, September–October). Nodular basal cell carcinoma. *Journal of the Dermatology Nurses' Association,* 7(5), 293–295.

# Squamous Cell Carcinoma

## Definition[1,2,3]

Squamous cell carcinoma (SCC) (see Figure 8-11) is the second most common skin cancer that composes the skins top layer (epidermis).

## Cause[1,2,3]

- Ultraviolet radiation

## Risk Factors[1,2,3]

*Risk factors of SCC coincide with causes, in addition to:*

- Fair skin
- Light-colored hair

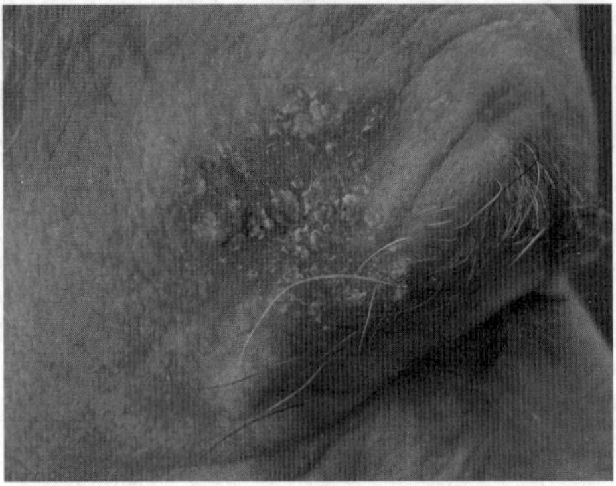

**Figure 8-11** Squamous Cell Carcinoma [See **Figure CP-14** at end of book for color version]



- Green or blue eyes
- Advanced age
- Male sex
- Immunosuppression
- Prior skin cancer

## Clinical Appearance

- Raised, firm, thick-scaled, pink or flesh-colored papule or plaque
- Location of lesions: sun-exposed areas

## Tests[1,3]

- Skin biopsy
- Computed tomography (CT), MRI, or positron emission tomography (PET) scan
  - If concern of metastases

## Treatment & Management[2,3]

- **Nonpharmacological and nursing interventions:**
  - Encourage skin protection.

        - Avoid sunburns, encourage use of shade, wear appropriate clothing that covers the skin, use of sunscreen with SPF $\geq$ 15.
    - Encourage patients to inspect their skin for suspicious lesions, at least once every 30 days.
- **Pharmacological and other interventions:**
    - Imiquimod gel
    - Mohs micrographic surgery
    - Excisional surgery
    - Curettage and electrodesiccation
    - Cryotherapy
    - Radiation
    - Photodynamic therapy
    - Laser therapy

## Differential Diagnosis[3]

- Actinic keratosis: Appearance is very similar to SCC; AK not as large as SCC. Biopsy rules out SCC. SCC will often be a larger, more scaled patch of erythema.
- Seborrheic keratosis: Will often be tan to brown in color and be a waxy, non-scaled benign lesion. SCC appearance is not typically tan to back; biopsy confirms SCC.

### CLINICAL PEARL[1,3]

- The skin should be inspected at a minimum of every 6 months with confirmed squamous cell carcinoma.

## References

1. Skin Cancer Foundation. (n.d.). Skin Cancer Information: What Is Skin Cancer? Retrieved from http://www.skincancer.org/skin-cancer-information. Accessed November 7, 2017.
2. Soltani, K., & Nwaneshidu, A. I. (2016, November 29). Squamous Cell Carcinoma of the Skin. Epocrates. Retrieved from https://online.epocrates.com/diseases/270/Squamous-cell-carcinoma-of-the-skin. Accessed November 7, 2017.
3. Lyons, F., & Ousley, L. (2015). *Dermatology for the Advanced Practice Nurse*. New York, NY: Springer Publishing Company.

4. Shulstad, R. M. (2009, March–April). Treatment of recurrent and inoperable squamous cell carcinomas with Imiquimod 5% cream: A case series. *Journal of the Dermatology Nurses' Association, 1*(2), 148.
5. Talib, N. (2017, October 11). Cutaneous Squamous Cell Carcinoma. Medscape. Retrieved from https://emedicine.medscape.com/article/1965430-overview. Accessed November 7, 2017.

# Malignant Melanoma

## Definition[1,2,4]

Malignant melanoma (MM) (see Figure 8-12) is the most dangerous form of skin cancer that arises from melanocytes.

## Cause[1,3,4]

- Ultraviolet radiation

## Risk Factors[1,2,3,4]

*Risk factors of BCC coincide with causes, in addition to:*

- Dysplastic nevi
- Fair skin
- Light-colored hair and eyes
- Personal or family history of melanoma
- History of sunburns
- Immunosuppression

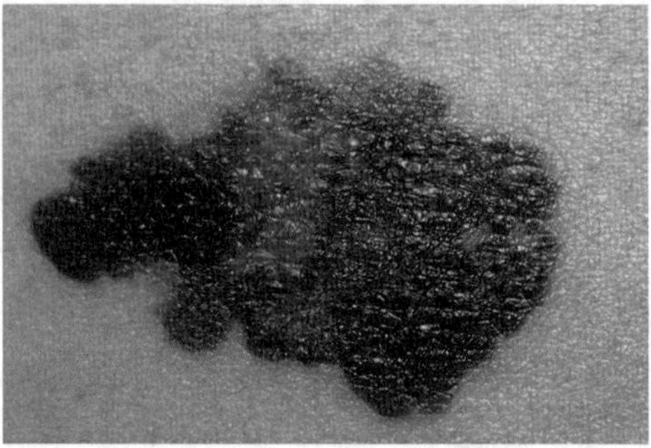

**Figure 8-12** Malignant Melanoma [See **Figure CP-15** at end of book for color version]

## Clinical Appearance

- Irregular, pigmented papule or plaque
- Fast growing
- Location of lesions: anywhere on the skin

## Tests[1]

- Dermatoscopy
  - Helps determine if a lesion should be biopsied.[1]
- Skin biopsy

## Treatment & Management[1,3,5]

- **Nonpharmacological and nursing interventions:**
  - Avoid excessive sun exposure.
  - Sunscreen.
  - Annual skin checks.
- **Pharmacological and other interventions:**
  - There are no pharmacological interventions; surgical removal is the treatment of choice.
  - Wide surgical excision based on TNM (tumor, node, metastases) classification system.
  - Chemotherapy.
- Palliative care referral
  - To improve quality of life and provide relief of symptoms; as patient declines consider transition to hospice services.

## Differential Diagnosis

- Atypical nevi, blue nevi, halo nevi, pigmented actinic keratosis, and pigmented BCC, benign melanocytic lesions, solar lentigos: Do not significantly change in size. MM will however change in color, size, and will have irregular borders. If MM is suspected, biopsy of lesion is recommended to confirm a diagnosis, especially if there is a family history of MM, or history of sun exposure.

## CLINICAL PEARLS[3,4]

- When obtaining medical history from patient, ask about history of skin cancers and malignant melanoma. This is often missed when obtaining medical history from patients. It is important to know if patient has a history of malignant melanoma due to risk of metastasis.
- If patient is unable to give history, ask family members about skin cancer history. Also ask patient's children if they have had MM. There is a 10% chance of MM if family history of MM is present.

## References


1. Skin Cancer Foundation. (n.d.). Skin Cancer Information: What Is Skin Cancer? Retrieved from http://www.skincancer.org/skin-cancer-information. Accessed November 7, 2017.
2. Menzies, A. M., Saw, R. P., & Fernandez-Penas, P. (2016, December 13). Melanoma. Epocrates. Retrieved from https://online.epocrates.com/diseases/268/Malignant-melanoma. Accessed November 7, 2017.
3. Tan, W. W. (2017, August 14). Malignant Melanoma. Medscape. Retrieved from https://emedicine.medscape.com/article/280245-overview. Accessed November 7, 2017.
4. Lyons, F., & Ousley, L. (2015). *Dermatology for the Advanced Practice Nurse*. New York, NY: Springer Publishing Company.
5. What Are Palliative Care and Hospice Care? (2017, May 17). https://www.nia.nih.gov/health/what-are-palliative-care-and-hospice-care#palliative-vs-hospice. Accessed May 8, 2018.


# Stasis Dermatitis

## Definition[1,2,3,4,5]

Stasis dermatitis (see Figure 8-13), or stasis eczema, is a common inflammatory dermatosis of the lower extremities.

## Cause[1,2,3,4,5]

- Direct consequence of venous insufficiency

## Risk Factors[1,2,3,4,5]

- Venous insufficiency
- Varicose veins
- Obesity

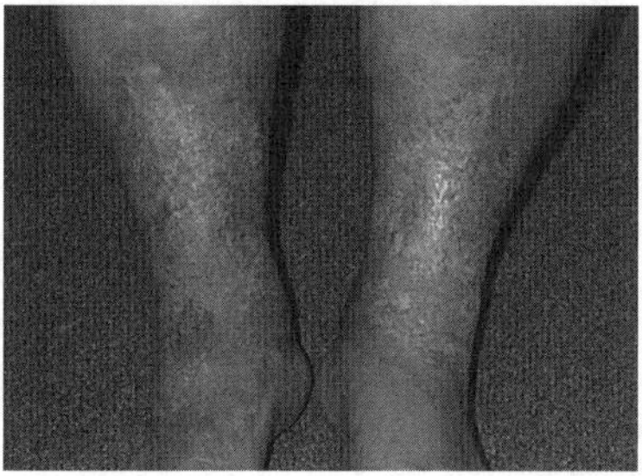

**Figure 8-13** Stasis Dermatitis [See **Figure CP-156** at end of book for color version]



- Lymphedema
- Advanced age
- Family history of venous disease
- Ligament hernias, flat feet
- Prolonged standing
- Smoking
- Sedentary lifestyle
- History of deep vein thrombosis (DVT)
- Presence of arteriovenous (AV) shunt

## Signs & Symptoms[1,2,3,4,5]

- Erythematous, scaling, and eczematous patches affecting the lower extremity.
- The medial ankle is most frequently and severely involved, due to limited blood supply as compared to the rest of the lower leg. In advanced cases of stasis dermatitis, the inflammation may encircle the ankle/foot and extend to just below the knee; this is sometimes referred to as stocking erythroderma.
- A solitary, small patch of stasis dermatitis may mimic basal cell carcinoma or squamous cell carcinoma.
- Secondary infection can cause typical honey-colored crusting due to bacteria or can produce pustules due to cutaneous candidiasis.

- Involved skin may exhibit changes seen in other eczematous conditions. Severe, acute inflammation may result in exudative, weeping patches and plaques.
- In long-standing lesions, lichenification and hyperpigmentation may occur as a consequence of chronic scratching and rubbing. In addition, patients with chronic stasis dermatitis can show changes, such as skin induration, that may progress to lipodermatosclerosis (with the classic inverted champagne bottle appearance).
- Violaceous plaques and nodules appear on legs and dorsal part of the feet.

## Test

- Arterial and venous Doppler studies to evaluate circulation

## Treatment & Management[1,2,3,4,5]

- **Nonpharmacological and nursing interventions:**
  - Compression stockings
  - Weight control
  - Exercise
  - Leg elevation
- **Pharmacological interventions**:
  - Midpotency corticosteroids (e.g., triamcinolone [Kenalog] 0.1% ointment)
    - Reduce the inflammation and itching in acute flares.
    - High-potency topical corticosteroids in stasis dermatitis should be avoided because of thinning of the skin, which can increase the risk of systemic absorption.
    - Steroid-induced cutaneous atrophy can predispose the patient to ulceration.
  - Aspirin 81 mg each day to promote circulation.
  - Infection is a particular concern in stasis dermatitis, since topical corticosteroids make the patient more susceptible to infection. Open excoriations and erosions should be treated with a topical antibiotic.
- Dermatology consultation/referral (improve diagnostic accuracy)

## Differential Diagnosis[1,2,3,4,5,6]

- Cellulitis: Characterized as unilateral extremity erythema, edema, warmth, and tenderness; requires antibiotic therapy.
- Psoriasis: Thick-scaled plaques with or without swelling of lower extremities.
- Eczema: Generalized dry skin all over. Appears as erythematous and mild-scaled patches.
- Tinea infections: Diagnosed by skin scrapings and biopsy. Erythematous, mild-scaled, powdery patches.
- Contact dermatitis: Erythematous papules with pruritus.

### CLINICAL PEARLS

- Be careful in using clobetasol (Clobex) cream and potent steroid creams on elderly skin. Instead of twice-daily applications, consider daily application.
- Stasis dermatitis is commonly misdiagnosed as cellulitis, leading to overtreatment and potential adverse effects of antibiotic therapy. It is important to remember the characteristics of cellulitis (i.e., unilateral extremity erythema, edema, warmth, and tenderness) and treatment is different than stasis dermatitis (cellulitis requires antibiotics).

## References

1. Alguire, P. C. (2017, November 15). Overview and Management of Lower Extremity Chronic Venous Disease. UpToDate. Retrieved from http://www.uptodate.com/contents/overview-and-management-of-lower-extremity-chronic-venous-disease. January 11, 2018.
2. Flugman, S. L. (2017, April 17). Stasis Dermatitis. Medscape. Retrieved from http://emedicine.medscape.com/article/1084813-overview. Accessed January 11, 2018.
3. Fransway, A. F. (2016, December 8). Stasis Dermatitis. UpToDate. Retrieved from http://www.uptodate.com/contnets/stasis-dermatitis. Accessed January 11, 2018.
4. Lyons, F., & Ousley, L. (2015). *Dermatology for the Advanced Practice Nurse*. New York, NY: Springer Publishing Company.
5. Weston, W. L., & Howe, W. (2014, March 5). Overview of Dermatitis. UpToDate. Retrieved from http://uptodate.com/contents/overview-of-dermatitis. Accessed January 11, 2018.
6. Brett, A. S. (2016, November 17). Misdiagnosis of cellulitis. *New England Journal of Medicine Journal Watch*. Retrieved from https://www.jwatch.org/na42798/2016/11/17/misdiagnosis-cellulitis. Accessed January 11, 2018.

SECTION IX

# Endocrinology

## Diabetes – Type 2

### Definition

Type 2 diabetes is a condition in which the body resists the effects of insulin, a hormone that regulates movements of glucose into cells, or the pancreas does not produce enough insulin to maintain normal glucose levels.

### Causes[10,11]

- Genetics
- Environmental factors (usually lifestyle related)

### Risk Factors[2,9,11]

- Aging *(insulin production decreases, insulin resistance increases)*
- Family history of diabetes (i.e., parents or siblings with diabetes)
- Overweight and obesity
- Smoking
- Physical inactivity
- Race/ethnicity (e.g., blacks, Hispanic-Americans, Native Americans, Asian-Americans, and Pacific Islanders)
- Previously identified impaired fasting glucose (IFG) or impaired glucose tolerance (IGT)
- Hypertension (≥ 140/90 mm Hg in adults)
- High-density lipoprotein (HDL) cholesterol ≤ 35 mg/dL (0.90 mmol/l) and/or a triglyceride level ≥ 250 mg/dL (2.82 mmol/l)

### Signs & Symptoms[3,10,11]

- Often asymptomatic or subtle symptoms in older adults and may be mistaken for a different chronic disease.
- Classic symptoms include polyuria, polydipsia, nocturia, and weight loss.

## Tests[1,3,4]

- HbA1c (or A1C), 2-hour plasma glucose (2-h PG) value following 75-g oral glucose tolerance test, or fasting plasma glucose (FPG)
  - Consider HbA1c in older adults to avoid fasting.
  - Criteria for diagnosis:
    - A1C ≥ 6.5% (48 mmol/mol)
    - 2-h PG ≥ 200 mg/dL (11.1 mmol/L)
    - FPG ≥ 126 mg/dL (7.0 mmol/L)
    - Random plasma glucose ≥ 200 mg/dL (11.1 mmol/L)
      - In individuals with symptoms of hyperglycemia or hyperglycemic crisis
  - Per the American Diabetes Association (ADA), recommendation is for routine screening for all individuals > 45 years old
  - In asymptomatic adults age 40–70 years old who are overweight or obese or with sustained blood pressure > 135/80 mm Hg
    - If initial screening normal, consider repeating every 3 years

## Treatment & Management[1,3,5,6,7,8,10,11,12]

- **Nonpharmacological and nursing interventions:**
  - Encourage lifestyle changes.
    - Nutrition (plant-based diet, calorie restriction, maintain optimal weight). Medical nutrition therapy is a covered benefit through Medicare for patients with diabetes.
    - Physical activity (consider barriers including safety and risk of hypoglycemia).
    - Sleep, behavioral support, and smoking cessation.
  - Hypoglycemia prevention through education of signs and symptoms is essential.
- **Pharmacological and other interventions:**
  - Metformin (Glucophage, Riomet, Fortamet, Glumetza)
    - Example: metformin 500 mg PO daily, initial dose (max of 2 g/day).

  - Preferred first-line agent (in combination with lifestyle therapy).
  - Avoid use in patients with an eGFR under 30 mL/minute; starting this drug with an eGFR between 30–45 mL/minute is not recommended.
  - Discontinue medication prior to iodinated contrast imaging procedures if eGFR is between 30–60 mL/minute, in patients with liver disease, alcoholism, or heart failure. Re-evaluate renal function 48 hours after the procedure.
  - Carries an unlikely risk for hypoglycemia; has gastrointestinal adverse effects (e.g., diarrhea, nausea, upset stomach).
- Sulfonylureas (e.g., glyburide [DiaBeta], glipizide [Glucotrol], glimepiride [Amaryl])
  - Example: glimepiride 1–2 mg PO daily (max 8 mg/day).
  - Risk of hypoglycemia, especially with glyburide. Glimepiride carries a lower risk and may be the preferred sulfonylurea in older adults.
- Thiazolidinediones (e.g., pioglitazone [Actos], rosiglitazone [Avandia])
  - Example: pioglitazone 15 mg PO once daily (max: 45 mg/day).
  - Carries a high risk of hypoglycemia.
  - May cause weight gain and worsen fluid retention (use with caution in older adults with heart failure, edema, or hepatic failure); carries an increased risk of fracture and bladder cancer.
- Glucagon-like peptide (GLP)-1 agonists (e.g., exenatide [Byetta], liraglutide [Victoza], dulaglutide [Trulicity)
  - Example: exenatide 5 mcg subcutaneous (SC) BID (initial dose); after a month, may increase to 10 mcg SC BID.
  - Avoid exenatide with creatinine clearance under 30.
  - Carries a lower risk of hypoglycemia, however is costly.
  - May cause gastrointestinal adverse effects.

- Dipeptidyl peptidase 4 (DDP-4) inhibitors (e.g., linagliptin [Tradjenta], sitagliptin [Januvia], saxagliptin [Onglyza])
  - Example: sitagliptin 100 mg PO daily.
  - Dose adjustments may be necessary due to renal status (except linagliptin).
  - Carries a lower risk of hypoglycemia, however is costly.
- Sodium glucose cotransporter 2 (SGLT2) inhibitors (e.g., canagliflozin ([Invokana], empagliflozin [Jardiance])
  - Example: empagliflozin 10 mg PO daily (max: 25 mg/day).
  - Low risk of hypoglycemia and drug–drug interactions; may have mild blood pressure (BP) lowering effect.
  - Can be costly; carries an increased risk of urinary tract infection (UTI).
- Insulin (e.g., fast acting: lispro [Humalog], aspart [Novolog]; long acting: glargine [Lantus], detemir [Levemir])
  - Rapid-acting insulin analogs are superior to regular (more predictable).
  - Long-acting insulin analogs are superior to neutral protamine Hagedorn (NPH) (reduce risk of hypoglycemia and provide a fairly flat response for about 24 hours).
  - Moderate to high risk of hypoglycemia and needs frequent monitoring.
  - High likelihood of weight gain and fluid retention.

*Note: Monotherapy is appropriate with an A1C of under 7.5%; dual or triple therapy is appropriate with an A1C ≥ 7.5%, and insulin with other agents is appropriate in symptomatic individuals with an A1C above 9.0%.

The ADA and American Geriatric Society (AGS) recommend that glucose targets be individualized; AGS recommendations are shown below (ADA is slightly more stringent):

- A target HbA1C goal in older adults is 7.5%–8.0%.
  - Normal HbA1C is <5.7%; prediabetes is considered HbA1C 5.7%–6.4%.
- May consider goal of 7.0%–7.5% in healthier patients with few comorbidities

- In frail older adults with limited life expectancy or extensive comorbidities, an A1C goal of 8.0%–9.0% is appropriate.
- There is potential harm in lowering HbA1C to under 6.5% in older adults with type 2 diabetes.

- Monitoring
  - HbA1C frequency varies with control but can be done every 6–12 months, if stable.
  - HbA1C should be monitored every 3 months with medication changes.
  - Consider home glucose monitoring but must assess barriers including poor cognition, poor circulation, and financial issues.
- Screening for associated complications
  - Foot exam should be done at least annually.
  - Dilated eye exams every 1–3 years, depending on risk factors and symptoms.
  - Urine albumin to creatinine ratio (nephropathy) annually.
  - Monofilament testing (neuropathy) annually.
  - Blood pressure should be checked at every routine diabetes visit.
  - Lipid panel every 1–3 years (cardiovascular risk).
  - Screen for depression during the initial evaluation period (first 3 months); older adults with diabetes are at great risk for this.
- Dietitian referral (for individualized dietary plan)
- Endocrinology referral (if diabetes uncontrolled on multiple antidiabetic medications)

Note: Beers listed items, as mentioned above, include: sliding scale insulin/rapid-acting insulin, long duration sulfonylureas (chlorpropamide, glyburide) and thiazolidinediones (pioglitazone, rosiglitazone).

## Differential Diagnosis[9,10,11]

- Stroke or transient ischemic attack (TIA): Hypoglycemia can lead to a stroke-like presentation.
- Type 1 diabetes mellitus: Usually seen in young individuals (< age 35 years), whereas type 2 diabetes is more common in middle-aged or older adults. Urine ketones usually present in those with type 1 diabetes (not typical for type 2 diabetes unless there is severe volume depletion).

### CLINICAL PEARLS[3]

- Titrate medications slowly due to the risk of hypoglycemia in older adults.
- Older adults carry a higher risk of hypoglycemia due to decreased renal function, polypharmacy, and comorbidities. Most common symptoms include: confusion, delirium, dizziness, weakness, and falls.
- Consider poor eyesight, which may cause difficulty with giving injections in older adults.

## References

1. American Diabetes Association. (2016, January 6). Standards of medical care in diabetes – 2016. *Diabetes Care, 39*(Supp 1), S1–S81. Retrieved from http://care.diabetesjournals.org/content/suppl/2015/12/21/39.Supplement_1.DC2/2016-Standards-of-Care.pdf. Accessed January 13, 2018.
2. American Diabetes Association. (2002, January). Screening for diabetes. *Diabetes Care,* 25(Suppl 1), S21–S24. Retrieved from https://doi.org/10.2337/diacare.25.2007.
3. Bigelow, A., & Freeland, B. (2017). Type 2 diabetes care in the elderly. *Journal for Nurse Practitioners, 13*(3), 181–186. doi: http://dx.doi.org/10.1016/j.nurpra.2016.08.010
4. U.S. Preventive Services Task Force. (2008, June). Diabetes Mellitus (Type 2) in Adults: Screening. Retrieved from https://www.uspreventiveservicestaskforce.org/Page/Document/UpdateSummaryFinal/diabetes-mellitus-type-2-in-adults-screening. Accessed January 13, 2018.
5. U.S. Food and Drug Administration (FDA). (2016. April 8). FDA Revises Warnings Regarding Use of the Diabetes Medicine Metformin in Certain Patients with Reduced Kidney Function. Drug Safety and Availability: FDA Drug Safety Communication. Retrieved from https://www.fda.gov/Drugs/DrugSafety/ucm493244.htm. Accessed January 13, 2018.
6. Garber, A. J., Abrahamson, M. J., Barzilay, J. I., Blonde, L., Bloomgarden, Z. T., & Bush, M. A., . . . Davidson, M. H. (2015). AACE/ACE comprehensive diabetes management algorithm 2015. *Endocrine Practice, 21*(4), 438–447. doi:10.4158/ep15693.cs

7. Dinsmoor, R. S. (2014, May 6). Insulin analog. *Diabetes Self-Management*. Retrieved from https://www.diabetesselfmanagement.com/diabetes-resources/definitions/insulin-analog/. Accessed January 13, 2018.
8. American Geriatrics Society Expert Panel on Care of Older Adults with Diabetes Mellitus; Moreno, G., Mangione, C. M., Kimbro, L., & Valsberg, E. (2013, November). Guidelines abstracted from the American Geriatrics Society Guidelines for Improving the Care of Older Adults with Diabetes Mellitus: 2013 Update. *Journal of the American Geriatrics Society, 61*(11), 2020–2026. doi:10.1111/jgs.12514
9. Centers for Disease Control and Prevention. (2017). National Diabetes Statistics Report, 2017. Retrieved from https://www.cdc.gov/diabetes/pdfs/data/statistics/national-diabetes-statistics-report.pdf. Accessed January 13, 2018.
10. Jalili, M., & Niroomand, M. (2016). Type 2 diabetes mellitus. In Tintinalli, J. E., Stapczynski, J., Ma, O., Yealy, D. M., Meckler, G. D., & Cline, D. M. (Eds.) *Tintinalli's Emergency Medicine: A Comprehensive Study Guide* (8th ed.). New York, NY: McGraw-Hill. Retrieved from http://accessmedicine.mhmedical.com/content.aspx?bookid=1658&sectionid=109443625. Accessed January 13, 2018.
11. O'Connor, P. J., & Sperl-Hillen, J. M. (2017, November 13). Type 2 Diabetes Mellitus in Adults. Epocrates. Retrieved from https://online.epocrates.com/diseases/2411/Type-2-diabetes-mellitus-in-adults/Key-Highlights. Accessed January 13, 2018.
12. American Geriatrics Society 2015 Beers Criteria Update Expert Panel, Fick, D. M., Semla, T. P., Beizer, J., Brandt, N., & Dombrowski, R., . . . Steinman, M. (2015, October 8). American Geriatrics Society 2015 updated Beers criteria for potentially inappropriate medication use in older adults. *Journal of the American Geriatrics Society, 63*(11), 2227–2246. Retrieved from http://onlinelibrary.wiley.com/doi/10.1111/jgs.13702/abstract. Accessed October 3, 2017.

# Hyperthyroidism

## Definition

Hyperthyroidism is a form of thyrotoxicosis due to inappropriately high synthesis and secretion of thyroid hormone(s) by the thyroid.

## Categories[1,2,4,6]

**Subclinical hyperthyroidism:** subnormal thyroid-stimulating hormone (TSH) with normal T3 and T4.
**Overt hyperthyroidism:** subnormal TSH with elevated serum T3 and/or free T4.

## Causes[1,2,3,4,6]

- Grave's disease (most common cause in United States).
    - Autoimmune disorder in which thyrotropin receptor antibodies (TRAb) stimulate TSH receptor increasing thyroid hormone production and release.

- May have spontaneous remission in up to 30% of patients.
- Toxic nodular goiter
  - Related to dietary iodine deficiency.
  - May actually be more common than Grave's disease in older patients, especially in regions with iron deficiency.
- Painless thyroiditis (also known as subacute lymphocytic thyroiditis)
  - Inflammation of thyroid tissue with release of thyroid hormones.
  - Associated with some medications (e.g., lithium, amiodarone [Cordarone, Nexterone, Pacerone], cytokines, or tyrosine kinase inhibitors).
- Subacute thyroiditis
  - Caused by viral infection (associated with fever, painful and firm thyroid, and elevated erythrocyte sedimentation rate [ESR] above 50).

## Risk Factors[1]

- Autoimmune disease
- Some medications
- Viral infections

## Signs & Symptoms[1,2,3,4,6]

- Fatigue and weakness
- Weight loss
- Exophthalmos *(specific to Graves disease)*
- Osteoporosis
- Palpitations
- Atrial fibrillation or sinus tachycardia
- Embolic events
- Proximal muscular weakness
- Tremor
- Neuropsychiatric symptoms (e.g., anxiety)
- Poor concentration

## Tests[1,3,7]

- Serum TSH (initial screening test in hyperthyroidism), and free T4
  - TSH will be subnormal; in overt disease will be less than 0.01 mU/L.
  - Free T4 will be elevated in overt hyperthyroidism and normal in subclinical.
- Serum T3 *(not used much in clinical practice)*
  - Will be elevated in overt hyperthyroidism and normal in subclinical.
- Serum thyrotropin receptor antibody (TRAb)
  - Will be elevated in Grave's disease.
  - Should be ordered if unable to determine diagnosis clinically (e.g., lack of symmetrically enlarged thyroid, recent onset of orbitopathy, and moderate to severe hyperthyroidism).
  - May be best first test to determine etiology.
- Serum calcium, magnesium, liver enzymes, complete blood count (CBC)
  - Not uncommon to find hyper- or hypocalcemia, hypomagnesemia, increased liver enzymes, anemia, and/or decreased neutrophils in hyperthyroidism.
- Radioactive iodine uptake (RAIU)
  - Will be elevated in Grave's disease and toxic nodular goiter.
  - Near zero indicates subacute thyroiditis, factitious ingestion of thyroid hormone, or recent excess iodine intake.
  - Ordered if third-generation TRAb not available.
- Ultrasonography with color flow Doppler
  - Can distinguish thyroid hyperactivity (increased flow) from destructive thyroiditis.

## Treatment & Management[1,3,5,6,7,8]

- **Nonpharmacological and nursing interventions:**
  - In those with thyroiditis, support measures are adequate treatment.

- Monitor for weight changes.
  - Common to have a weight loss due to increased basal metabolic rate (BMP).
- Encourage patient to eat a balanced diet and to eat small meals, frequently throughout the day.
  - This approach will increase caloric intake and conserve energy.

- **Pharmacological and other interventions:**
  - If able, discontinue drugs associated with hyperthyroidism (benefit is not immediate in stopping amiodarone; half-life is about 100 days).
  - Beta-adrenergic receptor blockade (e.g., propranolol [Inderal], atenolol [Tenormin], metoprolol [Lopressor])
    - Example: atenolol 25–100 mg PO once to twice daily.
      - Increased compliance due to convenience of dosing
    - Recommended in all patients with symptomatic hyperthyroidism, especially elderly and patients with resting heart rate of 90 or coexistent cardiovascular disease.
    - Caution use in these agents in patients with heart failure, chronic obstructive pulmonary disease, or diabetes mellitus.
  - Antithyroid drugs (e.g., methimazole [Tapazole], propylthiouracil)
    - Example: methimazole 10–30 mg daily; TSH should be tested every 4 weeks until euthyroidism is achieved.
      - This is the preferred antithyroid drug due to longer half-life and few adverse effects.
      - Consult with endocrinologist for appropriate prescribing and monitoring.
    - Used in patients with mild thyrotoxicosis or small goiters; are used to prep older adults for surgery and radioactive iodine treatment.
    - Monitor for gastrointestinal effects, arthralgias, agranulocytosis, and pancytopenia.
- Dietitian consultation/referral
  - To assist in determining the patient's caloric needs.

- Endocrinology referral
  - Help decide which treatment options are most appropriate.
    - Patients with overt Grave's hyperthyroidism are treated with radioactive iodine therapy, antithyroid drugs, or thyroidectomy.
    - Surgery is recommended in patients with large toxic nodular goiter.

## Differential Diagnosis[5,7]

- Anxiety or depression: Severe cases of hyperthyroidism may cause anxiety, rapid speech, insomnia, and/or psychosis along with subnormal TSH and elevated levels of T4 or T3. Individuals with anxiety and/or depression will have normal thyroid levels.
- Malignancy: Will also have weight loss, fatigue, and higher risk of embolic events.

### CLINICAL PEARLS[1,2,6,8]

- The threshold is low to refer to endocrinologist for treatment options of hyperthyroidism.
- Untreated thyroid disease can lead to cardiac issues (e.g., atrial fibrillation, heart failure), along with bone mass loss and thyroid storm.

## References


1. Ross, D. S., Burch, H. B., Cooper, D. S., Greenlee, M. C., Laurberg, P., & Maia, A. L. . . . Walter, M. A. (2016). 2016 American Thyroid Association Guidelines for Diagnosis and Management of Hyperthyroidism and Other Causes of Thyrotoxicosis. *Thyroid*, *26*(10), 1343–1421. doi:10.1089/thy.2016.0229
2. Cappola AR. Thyroid diseases. In *Hazzard's Geriatric Medicine and Gerontology* (7th ed.). New York, NY: McGraw-Hill. Retrieved from http://accessmedicine.mhmedical.com/content.aspx?bookid=1923&sectionid=144561105. Accessed January 12, 2018.
3. Fitzgerald, P. A. Endocrine disorders. (2018). In *Current Medical Diagnosis & Treatment 2018*. New York, NY: McGraw-Hill. Retrieved from http://accessmedicine.mhmedical.com/content.aspx?bookid=2192&sectionid=167996562. Accessed January 12, 2018.

4. Gulanick, M., & Myers, J. L. (2017). *Nursing Care Plans: Diagnoses, Interventions, & Outcomes*. St. Louis, MO: Elsevier.
5. Gambert, S. R., Kant, R., & Miller, M. (2014). Thyroid, parathyroid, and adrenal gland disorders. In *Current Diagnosis & Treatment: Geriatrics* (2nd ed.). New York, NY: McGraw-Hill. Retrieved from http://accessmedicine.mhmedical.com/content.aspx?bookid=953&sectionid=53375665. Accessed January 12, 2018.
6. Skugor, M. (2014, August). Hypothyroidism and Hyperthryoidism. Cleveland Clinic Center for Continuing Education. Retrieved from http://www.clevelandclinicmeded.com/medicalpubs/diseasemanagement/endocrinology/hypothyroidism-and-hyperthyroidism/. Accessed January 13, 2018.
7. Kravets, I. (2016). Hyperthyroidism: Diagnosis and treatment. *American Family Physician*, 93(5), 363–370. Retrieved from https://www.aafp.org/afp/2016/0301/p363.html. Accessed January 13, 2018.
8. Endocrine Society. (n.d.). Value of an Endocrinologist. Hormone Health Network. Retrieved from https://www.hormone.org/you-and-your-endocrinologist/value-of-an-endocrinologist. Accessed January 18, 2018.

# Hypogonadism

## Definition

Hypogonadism is a clinical syndrome due to failure of testes to produce testosterone leading to decreased spermatozoa production and decrease in testosterone physiologic effects.

Note: 39% of men age 45 and older have hypogonadism leading to low testosterone.

## Classification[1,6,7,8,9]

Primary hypogonadism (or primary testicular failure): issue with testes.
Secondary hypogonadism: issue with hypothalamic axis.

## Causes[1,6,8,9]

- Testicular failure
  - Causes include Klinefelter syndrome; testicular trauma, torsion, or irradiation; environmental toxins (e.g., chemicals, pesticides); heavy alcohol consumption; human immunodeficiency virus (HIV); hemochromatosis; aging.
- Problem with the hypothalamic-pituitary axis

- Causes include pituitary tumor or other brain tumor located near the pituitary gland, some medications (e.g., opioids, steroids), severe systemic illness, head injury, radiation, obesity, stress; may be idiopathic.

## Risk Factors[1,3,5,7]

*Risk factors of hypogonadism coincide with causes.*

- Male sex
- Aging
- Associated with obesity, diabetes, chronic obstructive pulmonary disorder (COPD), hyperlipidemia, and hypertension; unclear if low testosterone is a cause or effect of these diseases.

## Signs & Symptoms[1,3,5,9]

- Decreased libido, spontaneous erections, shrinking testes
- Gynecomastia
- Loss of body hair
- Low trauma fracture, low bone mineral density
- Hot flashes/sweats
- Less specific symptoms: decreased muscle mass and strength, depressed mood, diminished energy, and increased fatigue

## Tests[1,3,4,5,7]

- Total testosterone (< 280–300 ng/dL is the normal lower limit range, per the Endocrine Society)
  - Should be obtained when patient is fasting, between 8–10 A.M. (peak testosterone levels).
  - If patient has condition that can affect sex hormone–binding globulin (SHBG) free testosterone should be obtained.
  - Levels must be checked on two separate days to confirm diagnosis.
  - Routine testing in older men for low testosterone is not recommended without clinical signs or symptoms.

- Gonadotropins (luteinizing hormone [LH] and follicle-stimulating hormone [FSH])
  - Low testosterone and low to normal LH and FSH implies secondary hypogonadism.
    - Consider checking prolactin, pituitary function test, iron saturation, and magnetic resonance imaging (MRI) of pituitary.
  - Low testosterone in the presence of high LH and FSH implies primary hypogonadism.

## Management & Treatment[1,2,3,4,7,8,10]

- **Nonpharmacological and nursing interventions:**
  - Encourage therapies to reduce stress: regular exercise, acupuncture, yoga.
    - Stress can depress testosterone levels.
  - Evaluate for depression as symptoms can often overlap.
- **Pharmacological and other interventions:**

*Treatment should be considered in older men with a testosterone level ≤ 200 ng/dL; the target level should be between 300–400 ng/dL.*

  - Intramuscular injections (e.g., testosterone enanthate [Delatestryl], cypionate [Depo-Testosterone])
    - Dosed 75–100 mg weekly or 150–200 mg q2 weeks.
    - Can be done at home, not as costly.
    - Testosterone levels may vary more than compared to transdermal form of replacement.
  - Transdermal testosterone patch (Androderm)
    - Androderm patch 2–4 mg applied q24 hours
      - Rotate sites with each application.
    - Therapy of choice in older men due to convenience and reversible action.
    - Monitor for skin irritation.

- Transdermal gels (available forms: gel packets, gel tubes, gel pump)
  - 50–100 mg daily (applied to upper arm/shoulder).
    - Allow the gel to air dry for about 10 minutes before dressing. Either wear a shirt or wash the area with soap and water to prevent spreading testosterone to others.
  - Easy to apply, flexible dosing, and decreased risk of skin irritation.
  - Important to educate patients that this medication may transfer to others via contact; has unpleasant odor.
- Buccal testosterone (Striant)
  - 30 mg tablet q12 hours (not to be chewed or swallowed).
  - May not be a preferred agent for some because it requires twice daily dosing.
  - Monitor for gum pain or irritation; causes ≥ 32.6% of gingivitis in patients.
- Subcutaneous pellets (Testopel)
  - Consider consultation with specialist.
  - These are difficult to reverse; should only be used in those in whom tolerance to testosterone therapy has been established. Duration of action can last up to 6 months.

Contraindications to the above treatment:

- Male breast cancer or prostate cancer
- Any patient with a prostate nodule, prostate-specific antigen (PSA) above 4 or above 3 in high-risk patients (i.e., black, first-degree relative with prostate cancer) should have evaluation by urology prior to starting replacement.
- Hematocrit (Hct) above 50%
  - Testosterone can cause increases in hematocrit leading to increased venous thromboembolism (VTE) risk.

    - Untreated obstructive sleep apnea (OSA)
    - Poorly controlled heart failure
    - International prostate symptoms score above 19

## Monitoring

- Prior to initiation:
    - PSA, CBC, liver function tests (LFTs), lipid panel, digital rectal exam (DRE)
- 3–6 months after initiation of testosterone:
    - Testosterone level
    - Hct (if > 54% therapy should be stopped)
    - DRE and PSA
        - This is due to prostate cancer concerns.
- Annually
    - Testosterone level
    - Hct
    - DRE and PSA

- Endocrinology consultation/referral (if therapy not working, Hct increasing, lipid abnormalities, and/or dose adjustments needed)
- Urology consultation/referral (if PSA increases or DRE abnormal)

Note: Beers listed items, as mentioned above, include: testosterone (avoid unless hypogonadism confirmed and with clinical symptoms).

## Differential Diagnosis[6,7]

- Depression: Consider this when evaluating a patient with hypogonadism; may include vague symptoms of mood changes and decreased energy.
- Pituitary macroadenoma or prolactinoma: Headache and visual changes would be noted; MRI of the pituitary would reveal lesion.

## CLINICAL PEARLS[1,2,4,7]

- Testosterone therapy is associated with drug–drug interactions. Caution use in men taking warfarin (Coumadin); the combination can increase the risk of bleeding. It can also produce hypoglycemia in men taking oral hypoglycemia agents and/or insulin.
- Men who are on testosterone replacement therapy may also require a bisphosphonate and vitamin D if they have severe osteoporosis.
- Benefits of testosterone replacement therapy: Improves mood, sexual desire, erectile function, muscle strength, exercise endurance, ability to climb stairs, weight loss (if used long term), bone mineral density, and quality of life, and may help support cardiovascular health (reduces cardiac events if serum testosterone is maintained between 212–742 ng/day). It may also improve obesity, type 2 diabetes mellitus, and exercise capacity.
  - Risks: It may worsen benign prostatic hyperplasia (BPH), sleep apnea, and increase risk for VTE.

# References


1. Tartavoulle, T. M., & Porche, D. J. (2012). Low testosterone. *Journal for Nurse Practitioners, 8*(10), 778–786. Retrieved from http://dx.doi.org/10.1016/j.nurpra.2012.05.004
2. Luthy, K. E., Williams, C., Freeborn, D. S., & Cook, A. (2017). Comparison of testosterone replacement therapy medications in the treatment of hypogonadism. *Journal for Nurse Practitioners, 13*(4), 241–249. doi:10.1016/j.nurpra.2016.11.016
3. Bhasin, S., Cunningham, G. R., Hayes, F. J., Matsumoto, A. M., Snyder, P. J., Swerdloff, R. S., & Montori, V. M. (2010). Testosterone therapy in men with androgen deficiency syndromes: An Endocrine Society clinical practice guideline. *Journal of Clinical Endocrinology & Metabolism,* 95(6), 2536–2559. doi:10.1210/jc.2009-2354
4. Fitzgerald, P. A. (2018). Endocrine disorders. In *Current Medical Diagnosis & Treatment 2018*. New York, NY: McGraw-Hill. Retrieved from http://accessmedicine.mhmedical.com/content.aspx?bookid=2192&sectionid=167996562. Accessed January 15, 2018.
5. Gruenewald, D. A., & Matsumoto, A. M. (2017). Aging of the endocrine system and selected endocrine disorders. In *Hazzard's Geriatric Medicine and Gerontology* (7th ed.). New York, NY: McGraw-Hill. Retrieved from http://accessmedicine.mhmedical.com/content.aspx?bookid=1923&sectionid=144560895. Accessed January 17, 2018.
6. Welliver, C. (2016, December 19). Hypogonadism in Males. Epocrates. Retrieved from https://online.epocrates.com/diseases/109311/Hypogonadism-in-males/Key-Highlights

7. Bhattacharya, R. K., & Bhattacharya, S. B. (2015). Late-onset hypogonadism and testosterone replacement in older men. *Clinics in Geriatric Medicine, 31*(4), 631–644. doi:10.1016/j.cger.2015.07.001 Accessed January 17, 2018.
8. Schieszer, J. (2016, January 15). Secondary Hypogonadism: Causes and Potential Treatment. Endocrinology Advisor. Retrieved from http://www.endocrinologyadvisor.com/androgen-and-reproductive-disorders/secondary-hypogonadism-causes-and-potential-treatment/article/465547/. Accessed January 17, 2018.
9. Kumar, P., Kumar, N., Thakur, D., & Patidar, A. (2010). Male hypogonadism: Symptoms and treatment. *Journal of Advanced Pharmaceutical Technology & Research, 1*(3), 297–301. doi:10.4103/0110-5558.72420
10. American Geriatrics Society 2015 Beers Criteria Update Expert Panel, Fick, D. M., Semla, T. P., Beizer, J., Brandt, N., & Dombrowski, R., . . . Steinman, M. (2015, October 8). American Geriatrics Society 2015 updated Beers criteria for potentially inappropriate medication use in older adults. *Journal of the American Geriatrics Society, 63*(11), 2227–2246. Retrieved from http://onlinelibrary.wiley.com/doi/10.1111/jgs.13702/abstract. Accessed October 3, 2017.

# Hypothyroidism

## Definition

Hypothyroidism is a condition when the thyroid underproduces thyroid hormones, which affects multiple organs; patients will have an elevated thyroid-stimulating hormone (TSH).

Note: TSH upper limit of normal is near 4.5.

## Categories[1,3,4,5]

**Subclinical hypothyroid:** TSH will be above normal with normal free T4 (thyroxine).
**Overt hypothyroid:** Hypothyroidism associated with TSH levels above 10 and with a low free T4.

## Causes[1,3,4,5]

- Most common cause outside the U.S. is iodine deficiency.
- The most common cause within the U.S.: chronic autoimmune thyroiditis (Hashimoto thyroiditis).
- Treatment of hyperthyroidism.
- Surgical thyroidectomy.
- Radiation therapy.
- Medications (e.g., amiodarone [Cordarone], lithium [Eskalith, Lithobid]).

## Risk Factor[3]

*Risk factors of hypothyroidism coincide with causes.*

- Female sex

## Signs & Symptoms[3,4,5]

- Nonspecific weakness
- Weight gain
- Decreased appetite
- Dry skin
- Cold sensitivity
- Fatigue
- Muscle cramps
- Voice changes
- Constipation
- Neurologic (e.g., carpal tunnel syndrome, dementia)
- Psychiatric/behavioral (e.g., apathy, depression, cognitive impairment)

## Tests[1,2,3,5]

- Serum TSH
  - May vary during the day (lowest in the afternoon, highest around time of sleep).
  - U.S. Preventive Services Task Force (USPSTF) recommends against routine screening in asymptomatic individuals.[2]
  - Upper limit of normal increases with age so mild elevation in older patients may not represent subclinical hypothyroidism.[1]
  - Levels are decreased in hospitalizations and in severe illness.
  - In patients with elevated TSH with normal free T4 (subclinical):
    - Free T4 (metabolically available form) is the test of choice over total T4.
    - Obtain thyroid peroxidase antibody (TPOAb); elevation can predict progression to overt hypothyroidism.

  - In patients with decreased free T4 (overt):
    - Obtain thyroid antibodies.
- Serum T3 (triiodothyronine)
  - Not much utility in ordering this; it is often normal due to hyperstimulation of remaining functioning thyroid disease.

## Treatment & Management[1,3,4,5,6]

- **Nonpharmacological and nursing interventions:**
  - Monitor for weight changes.
    - Common to have a weight gain due to slowing of metabolic processes.
  - Encourage a diet low in calories, cholesterol, and saturated fats.
    - Patients will require fewer calories to support metabolic activity.
    - Not atypical to have higher cholesterol levels in hypothyroidism.
    - Recommend six small meals throughout the day (this may improve energy levels).
  - Educate patient about sources of dietary fiber.
    - This will ease constipation (common symptom).
- **Pharmacological and other interventions:**
  - Levothyroxine (Unithroid, Tirosint, Synthroid, Levoxyl): Therapy is usually lifelong.
    - If decision is made to treat, start dose between 25 mcg and 50 mcg.
    - Use 1.6 mcg/kg for overt hypothyroidism (TSH > 10).
    - Doses of 25–75 mcg usually sufficient for subclinical (TSH 4.5–10).
    - Patients with cardiac disease should be started on lower doses of 12.5–25 mcg daily.
    - There are differing recommendations regarding treatment of subclinical hypothyroidism, but consider if symptoms consistent with hypothyroidism or high risk for cardiovascular disease.

        - Take medication 30–60 minutes before breakfast or 4 hours after last meal at night with water.
        - Monitor for drug effects such as arrhythmias (e.g., atrial fibrillation), palpitations, and bone loss in postmenopausal women.
    - Drug monitoring
        - Repeat TSH in 4–8 weeks (*except in cases of central hypothyroidism in which free T4 should be monitored*).
        - Small dose adjustments of 12–25 mcg are recommended.
        - Once adequate dosage determined, TSH should be monitored every 6–12 months.
        - Dosing requirements may change with some medications and aging.
            - Older adults often require 20%–25% less per kg daily due to decreased lean body mass.
- Dietitian consultation/ referral
    - To assist in determining the patient's caloric needs and achieve a stable weight.
- Endocrinology consultation/referral
    - Consider in patients with cardiac disease, structural changes in thyroid, presence of other endocrine disease, or unusual constellation of thyroid function tests.

## Differential Diagnosis[3,5]

- Depression: Symptoms present similarly to hypothyroidism; depression will however respond to behavioral therapy and/or antidepressants, not to thyroid hormone replacement therapy. Those with depression will have normal TSH.
- Alzheimer's dementia: Can be difficult to distinguish this from hypothyroidism in older adults (which is why a TSH is ordered in the workup of dementia); patients with Alzheimer's dementia will have normal TSH and will not respond to thyroid replacement therapy.
- Myxedema coma: Rare representation of hypothyroidism; symptoms may include altered mental state, hypothermia,

bradycardia, hypoventilation, hyponatremia, and hypoglycemia. This occurs almost exclusively in older patients, causing profound slowing across systems.

**CLINICAL PEARLS[1]**

- If TSH elevated during monitoring, make sure patient is taking the medication appropriately (as discussed above) before changing levothyroxine dose.
- Brand name may be more effective for some patients (brand name and generic name can have different absorption).

## References

1. Garber, J. R., Cobin, R. H., Gharib, H., Hennessey, J. V., Klein, I., & Mechanick, J. I. . . . Woeber, K. A.; American Association of Clinical Endocrinologists and American Thyroid Association Taskforce on Hypothyroidism in Adults. (2012, December). Clinical practice guidelines for hypothyroidism in adults: Cosponsored by the American Association of Clinical Endocrinologists and the American Thyroid Association. *Thyroid,* 22(12), 1200–1235. doi:10.1089/thy.2012.0205
2. U.S. Preventive Services Task Force (USPSTF). (2016, September). Final Update Summary: Thyroid Dysfunction: Screening. Retrieved from https://www.uspreventiveservicestaskforce.org/Page/Document/UpdateSummaryFinal/thyroid-dysfunction-screening. Accessed January 12, 2018.
3. Malaty, W. (2017, November 14). Primary Hypothyroidism. Epocrates. Retrieved from https://online.epocrates.com/diseases/53511/Primary-hypothyroidism/Key-Highlights. Accessed January 12, 2018.
4. Gulanick, M., & Myers, J. L. (2017). *Nursing Care Plans: Diagnoses, Interventions, & Outcomes*. St. Louis, MO: Elsevier.
5. Cappola, A. R. (2017). Thyroid diseases. In *Hazzard's Geriatric Medicine and Gerontology* (7th ed.). New York, NY: McGraw-Hill. Retrieved from http://accessmedicine.mhmedical.com/content.aspx?bookid=1923&sectionid=144561105. Accessed January 12, 2018.
6. Nelson, R. (2016, June 6). Subclinical hypothyroidism: Treat or not? *Clinical Endocrinology News.* Retrieved from https://www.mdedge.com/clinicalendocrinologynews/article/109445/pituitary-thyroid-adrenal-disorders/subclinical. Accessed January 12, 2018.

SECTION X

# Labs and Imaging

# Complete Metabolic Panel

| Measurement | Adult Reference Range *(Varies among laboratories)* | High Value Causes | Low Value Causes | Clinical Relevance/Notes |
|---|---|---|---|---|
| **Albumin**[1,9,10,17,23,28] | 3.5–5.5 g/dL or 35–55 g/L | Volume depletion, high protein consumption | Malnutrition, liver disease (e.g., cirrhosis), heart failure, nephrotic syndrome, protein-losing enteropathies | • Albumin maintains intravascular oncotic pressure; edema results with low levels.<br>• Aim at treating the underlying cause as opposed to replacing albumin (e.g., remove drugs that decrease appetite, treat the depression). |
| **Alkaline phosphatase (ALP)**[1,9,17,23,26,27] | 30–120 U/L | Liver disease, cirrhosis, hepatitis, biliary obstruction, renal and/or heart failure, diabetes, bacterial infections (e.g., osteomyelitis), hyperthyroidism, malignancy | Malnutrition, hypothyroidism, pernicious anemia, bisphosphonate treatment | • ALP helps detect liver disease or bone disorders.<br>• Often ordered with a gamma-glutamyl transpeptidase (GGTP) level; high GGTP indicates hepatobiliary disease, not a bone disorder.<br>• If ALP is elevated, along with AST and ALT, liver damage is suspected. |

| | | | | |
|---|---|---|---|---|
| | | (hepatic and/or bone), healing fractures, vitamin D deficiency, hepatotoxic medications | | |
| **Alanine transaminase (ALT) enzyme**[9,10,17,23,25] | 10–40 U/L | Liver disease, cirrhosis, hepatitis, biliary obstruction, alcohol abuse, hepatocellular carcinoma, hepatotoxic medications (e.g., acetaminophen, isoniazid [Nydrazid], nitrofurantoin [Macrobid], nonsteroidal anti-inflammatory drugs [NSAIDs], statins) | | • ALT is ordered to detect liver injury, along with an AST.<br>• ALT is more liver specific. The exception: ALT is often normal in alcoholic liver disease (AST is higher).<br>• ALT levels are not high with chronic hepatitis. |

(*Continues*)

| Measurement | Adult Reference Range *(Varies among laboratories)* | High Value Causes | Low Value Causes | Clinical Relevance/Notes |
|---|---|---|---|---|
| **Anion gap**[10,17,24] | 8–16 mEq/L | Ketoacidosis (alcoholic, diabetes, starvation), lactic acidosis, renal failure, toxic ingestions (e.g., salicylate, methanol) | Low albumin, multiple myeloma | • Anion gap calculator: ($Na^+$) minus ($Cl^-$ plus $HCO_3^-$). It is used for monitoring ill patients with expected elevated lactate levels (e.g., hypotension, shock, heart failure). |
| **Aspartate amino transferase (AST) enzyme**[1,9,10,17,23,25] | 10–40 U/L | Liver disease, cirrhosis, hepatitis, alcohol abuse, liver malignancy, acute renal failure, dehydration, muscle trauma, myocardial infarction, hepatotoxic medications | Chronic dialysis, severe liver disease | • AST is ordered to assess for liver disease; however ALT is more liver specific.<br>• ALT is usually higher with liver disease; the AST/ALT ratio is however increased with alcoholic liver disease. |

| | | | | |
|---|---|---|---|---|
| | | (e.g., acetaminophen, isoniazid, nitrofurantoin, NSAIDs, statins) | | |
| **Bilirubin, total**[1,9,10,17,21,22,23] | 0.3–1.0 mg/dL or 5.1–17 mmol/L | Liver disease, hepatitis, cholecystitis, sepsis, heart failure, biliary obstruction (i.e., stone, malignancies), hemolysis, ineffective erythropoiesis, medications (isoniazid, erythromycin, sulfa drugs, nitrofurantoin, NSAIDs, statins, acetaminophen) | Hypoalbuminemia | • Mild jaundice is noted once bilirubin levels reach 2–3 mg/dL.<br>• *Painless jaundice in older adults with weight loss is a sign of cancer.*<br>• Bilirubin can be measured into two forms: unconjugated or conjugated, which assists in diagnosing liver and bile duct diseases.<br>• Bilirubin is a component in the Model for End-Stage Liver Disease (MELD). |

(*Continues*)

| Measurement | Adult Reference Range *(Varies among laboratories)* | High Value Causes | Low Value Causes | Clinical Relevance/Notes |
|---|---|---|---|---|
| **Blood urea nitrogen (BUN)**[1,9,10,15,17,20] | 10–20 mg/dL or 3.6–7.1 mmol/L | Prerenal failure (e.g., gastrointestinal [GI] bleeding, volume depletion, heart failure, sepsis), intrarenal failure (e.g., acute tubular necrosis), obstructive uropathy, nephrotoxic medications | Malnutrition, muscle wasting, liver disease, overhydration | • Serum BUN is an unreliable indicator of renal function, as it can reflect other conditions.<br>• A high BUN with normal creatinine can aid in diagnosing gastrointestinal bleeding.<br>• BUN levels typically rise in those older than 60 years of age. |
| **Calcium**[1,9,10,17,18,19] | 8.8–10.5 mg/dL or 2.2–2.6 mmol/L | Medications (e.g., thiazide diuretics, excess vitamin D), primary hyperparathyroidism *(usually a single benign parathyroid tumor*), | Hypoalbuminemia (seen with liver disease or malnutrition), renal failure, low vitamin D or calcium intake, | • Corrected calcium equation: serum calcium + 0.8 (4-serum albumin) = corrected calcium.<br>• Calcium is monitored in those with kidney disease, cancers (such as multiple myeloma), and parathyroid disorder. |

| | | | | |
|---|---|---|---|---|
| | | malignancy, hyperthyroidism, prolonged immobilization, familial hypocalciuric hypercalcemia (FHH) | vitamin D and/or magnesium deficiency, some drugs (e.g., furosemide [Lasix], bisphosphonates) | The parathyroid hormone (PTH) and vitamin D assist in maintaining normal calcium levels. |
| **Carbon dioxide**[1,9, 10] | 23–29 mEq/L or 23–29 mmol/L | Lung disease, severe vomiting, diarrhea | Metabolic acidosis, malnutrition, renal failure, diarrhea, dehydration | • Ordered as part of the metabolic panel when acidosis or alkalosis suspected.<br>• For further evaluation of acid–base balance, obtain an arterial blood gas. |
| **Chloride**[1,9,10,17] | 96–106 mEq/L or 96–106 mmol/L | Dehydration, diarrhea, metabolic acidosis, hyperventilation (respiratory alkalosis) resuscitation with isotonic saline | Dehydration, heart failure, renal disease, syndrome of inappropriate antidiuretic hormone secretion (SIADH), | • Chloride works with other electrolytes (e.g., sodium) to regulate the amount of fluid in the body.<br>• Ordered as part of the metabolic panel when acidosis or alkalosis suspected. |

*(Continues)*

| Measurement | Adult Reference Range *(Varies among laboratories)* | High Value Causes | Low Value Causes | Clinical Relevance/Notes |
|---|---|---|---|---|
| | | | GI loss (e.g., vomiting, diarrhea), metabolic alkalosis, respiratory acidosis, diuretics | Treatment corresponds with that of abnormal sodium (e.g., diuresis, fluids). |
| **Creatinine**[1,9,10,15,16] | Males:<br>0.7–1.2 mg/dL or 60 to 110 mmol/L<br>Females:<br>0.5–1.0 mg/dL or 45 to 90 mmol/L | Prerenal failure (e.g., hypotension, volume depletion, heart failure, renal artery stenosis), intrarenal failure (e.g., acute tubular necrosis), obstructive uropathy (e.g., kidney stones, prostate hypertrophy), medications | Reduced muscle, severe liver disease | • Serum creatinine is an unreliable indicator of renal function in older adults; use estimate formulas instead, such as the Chronic Kidney Disease Epidemiology Collaboration (CKD-EPI) equation.<br>• Hypertension and diabetes are the most common causes of chronic kidney disease (CKD). |

| | | | | |
|---|---|---|---|---|
| | | (angiotensis-converting enzyme inhibitors [ACEIs], diuretics, NSAIDs, contrast dye) | | |
| **Glucose**[1,9,10,13,14] | • 70–99 mg/dL or 3.9–5.5 mmol/L<br>• 100–125 mg/dL or 5.6–6.9 mmol/L indicates prediabetes.<br>• ≥ 126 mg/L (on more than one occasion) indicates diabetes. | Diabetes, medications (e.g., steroids, antipsychotics, thiazide diuretics, statins), acute stress (e.g., heart attack, stroke, surgery), pancreatitis, hyperthyroidism | Malnutrition, hypoglycemic agents (e.g., insulin), severe illness, hypothyroidism, severe liver disease, kidney and heart failure, excessive alcohol intake | • HbA1C is most convenient when diagnosing diabetes. |
| **Potassium**[1,6,9,12] | 3.5–5.3 mEq/L | Medications (ACEIs, angiotensis-receptor blockers [ARBs], potassium-sparing diuretics, | Medications (e.g., loop and thiazide diuretics, insulin, steroids), | • Potassium is ordered to monitor or evaluate kidney disease (especially in those on dialysis), diuretic therapy, and metabolic acidosis. |

*(Continues)*

| Measurement | Adult Reference Range *(Varies among laboratories)* | High Value Causes | Low Value Causes | Clinical Relevance/Notes |
|---|---|---|---|---|
| | | potassium supplements, NSAIDs), kidney disease, increased intake (e.g., dietary salt substitutes) | GI loss (vomiting, diarrhea, malabsorption), poor intake, low magnesium | • Hypokalemia can be treated with 10–20 meQ at a time; hyperkalemia is treated with diuresis (loop), sodium polystyrene sulfonate (Kayexalate), +/– dialysis. |
| **Protein, total**[1,2,9,10,11] | 6.0–8.3 gm/dL or 60 to 80 g/L | Dehydration, chronic inflammation (e.g., hepatitis B or C), multiple myeloma | Malnutrition, liver disease, nephrotic syndrome | • Ordered when assessing a patients' overall health, such as nutritional status. |
| **Sodium**[1,2,3,4,5,6,7,8] | 135–145 mEq/L | Water loss (e.g., diarrhea, vomiting, diuretics especially loops), decreased oral intake | Hypovolemic → volume depletion (e.g., diarrhea or vomiting), diuretics, severe hypoalbuminemia | • Sodium imbalance is especially common in older adults residing in nursing facilities.<br>• Treatment options vary and it's important to determine patient's volume status. |

| | | | | |
|---|---|---|---|---|
| | | Others: sodium chloride tablets, hypertonic saline administration | Hypervolemic → heart failure, cirrhosis, kidney disease (acute and chronic)<br>Euvolemic → medications (diuretics especially thiazides, antidepressants), SIADH, severe hypothyroidism | • Treatment for hyponatremia may include isotonic saline and/or stopping the diuretic for hypovolemic causes; diuresis, salt and/or fluid restrictions for hypervolemia; discontinuing the offending medication, fluid restriction, and/or oral sodium chloride for euvolemic causes.<br>• Hypernatremia management involves treating the underlying cause and water replacement. |

# References


1. Gomella, L. G., & Haist, S. A. (Eds.). (2007). *Clinician's Pocket Reference: The Scut Monkey* (11th ed.). New York, NY: McGraw-Hill; Chapter 4. Laboratory Diagnosis: Chemistry, Immunology, Serology. Retrieved from http://accessmedicine.mhmedical.com/content.aspx?bookid=365&sectionid=43074913. Accessed October 8, 2017.
2. Simon, E. E. (2017, June 21). Hyponatremia. Medscape. Retrieved from http://emedicine.medscape.com/article/242166-overview. Accessed October 9, 2017.
3. Berl, T. (2013, March 7). An elderly patient with chronic hyponatremia. *Clinical Journal of the American Society of Nephrology*, 8(3), 469–475. Retrieved from http://cjasn.asnjournals.org/content/8/3/469.full. Accessed October 9, 2017.
4. Veis, J. H. (2017, April 26). Hyponatremia. Epocrates. Retrieved from https://online.epocrates.com/diseases/1214/Hyponatremia. Accessed October 8, 2017.
5. Sam, R., & Ing, T. S. (2017, May 4). Hypernatremia. Epocrates. Retrieved from https://online.epocrates.com/diseases/1215/Hypernatremia. Accessed October 8, 2017.
6. Lederer, E., & Nayak, V. Disorders of fluid and electrolyte balance. In *Hazzard's Geriatric Medicine and Gerontology* (7th ed.). New York, NY: McGraw-Hill. Retrieved from http://accessmedicine.mhmedical.com/content.aspx?bookid=1923&sectionid=144526158. Accessed October 9, 2017.
7. Shah, M. K., Workeneh, B., & Taffet, G. E. (2014). Hypernatremia in the Geriatric Population. National Center for Biotechnology Information, U.S. National Library of Medicine, National Institutes of Health. Retrieved from https://www.ncbi.nlm.nih.gov/pmc/articles/PMC4242070/. Accessed October 10, 2017.
8. Lukitsch, I. (2017, August 17). Hypernatremia. Medscape. Retrieved from http://emedicine.medscape.com/article/241094-overview. Accessed October 10, 2017.
9. American Association for Clinical Chemistry (AACC). (2017). Lab Tests Online for Health Professionals. Retrieved from https://labtestsonline.org/for-health-professionals/. Accessed October 10, 2017.
10. U.S. National Library of Medicine, National Institutes of Health. (2017, September). Databases. Retrieved from https://www.nlm.nih.gov/?_ga=2.63715881.769328030.1507665199-1049439008.1471202369. Accessed October 10, 2017.
11. Mayo Clinic. (2017, October 4). High Blood Protein Causes. Retrieved from http://www.mayoclinic.org/symptoms/high-blood-protein/basics/causes/SYM-20050599. Accessed October 10, 2017.
12. Lederer, E. (2017, August 17). Hyperkalemia. Medscape. Retrieved from http://emedicine.medscape.com/article/240903-overview#a5. Accessed October 10, 2017.
13. Bigelow, A., & Freeland, B. (2017, March). Type 2 diabetes care in the elderly. *Journal for Nurse Practioners, 13*(3), 181–186. Retrieved from http://www.npjournal.org/article/S1555-4155(16)30445-7/fulltext. Accessed October 11, 2017.
14. Rivera, J. A., Conell-Price, J., & Lee, S. (2014). Diabetes. In *Current Diagnosis & Treatment: Geriatrics* (2nd ed.). New York, NY: McGraw-Hill. Retrieved from http://accessmedicine.mhmedical.com/content.aspx?bookid=953&sectionid=53375666. Accessed October 11, 2017.
15. Shimada, M., Dass, B., & Ejaz, A. (2016, September 15). Evaluation of Creatinine. Epocrates. Retrieved from https://online.epocrates.com/diseases/935/Evaluation-of-elevated-creatinine. Accessed October 11, 2017.
16. Bowling, C. B., & Booth, K. Chronic kidney disease. In *Current Diagnosis & Treatment: Geriatrics* (2nd ed.). New York, NY: McGraw-Hill. Retrieved from http://

accessmedicine.mhmedical.com/content.aspx?bookid=953&sectionid=53375662. Accessed October 11, 2017.

17. LeBlond, R. F., Brown, D. D., Suneja, M., & Szot, J. F. (Eds.) (2014). *DeGowin's Diagnostic Examination,*(10th ed.). New York, NY: McGraw-Hill. Retrieved from http://accessmedicine.mhmedical.com/content.aspx?bookid=1192&sectionid=68671769. Accessed October 11, 2017.
18. Gambert, S. R., Kant, R., & Miller, M. (2014). Thyroid, parathyroid, & adrenal gland disorders. In *Current Diagnosis & Treatment: Geriatrics* (2nd ed.). New York, NY: McGraw-Hill. Retrieved from http://accessmedicine.mhmedical.com/content.aspx?bookid=953&sectionid=53375665. Accessed October 11, 2017.
19. McAuley, D. (2017, October 11). Corrected Calcium Calculator. Global RPh. Retrieved from http://www.globalrph.com/calcium.cgi. Accessed October 11, 2017.
20. Lerma, E. V. (2017, September 20). Blood Urea Nitrogen (BUN). Medscape. Retrieved https://emedicine.medscape.com/article/2073979-overview#a2. Accessed October 13, 2017.
21. Wehbi, M. (2015, January 14). Bilirubin. Medscape. Retrieved from https://emedicine.medscape.com/article/2074068-overview#a2. Accessed October 13, 2017.
22. Herrine, S. K., & Kimmel, S. (2016, May). Jaundice – Hepatic and Biliary Disorders. Merck Manuals: Professional. Retrieved from http://www.merckmanuals.com/professional/hepatic-and-biliary-disorders/approach-to-the-patient-with-liver-disease/jaundice. Accessed October 13, 2017.
23. Pratt, D. S. (2015). Evaluation of liver function. In Kasper, D., Fauci, A., Hauser, S., Longo, D., Jameson, J., & Loscalzo, J. *Harrison's Principles of Internal Medicine* (19th ed.). New York, NY: McGraw-Hill. Retrieved from http://accessmedicine.mhmedical.com/content.aspx?bookid=1130&sectionid=79748389. Accessed October 13, 2017.
24. DuBose, T. D., Jr. (2015). Acidosis and alkalosis. In Kasper, D., Fauci, A., Hauser, S., Longo, D., Jameson, J., & Loscalzo, J. *Harrison's Principles of Internal Medicine* (19th ed.). New York, NY: McGraw-Hill. Retrieved from http://accessmedicine.mhmedical.com/content.aspx?bookid=1130&sectionid=79726883. Accessed October 13, 2017.
25. Amirana, S., & Babby, J. (2015, February). A review of drug-induced liver injury. *Journal for Nurse Practitioners, 11*(2), 270–271. Retrieved from http://www.npjournal.org/article/S1555-4155(14)00804-6/fulltext. Accessed October 14, 2017.
26. Mukaiyama, K., Kamimura, M., Uchiyama, S., Ikegami, S., Nakamura, Y., & Kato, H. (2015, August). Elevation of serum alkaline phosphatase (ALP) level in postmenopausal women is caused by high bone turnover. *Aging Clinical and Experimental Research,* 27(4), 413–418. Retrieved from https://doi.org/10.1007/s40520-014-0296-x. Accessed October 14, 2017.
27. Siddique, A., & Kowdley, K. V. (2012, May). Approach to a Patient with Elevated Serum Alkaline Phosphatase. National Center for Biotechnology Information, U.S. National Library of Medicine, National Institutes of Health. Retrieved from https://www.ncbi.nlm.nih.gov/pmc/articles/PMC3341633/. Accessed October 14, 2017.
28. Purelta, R. (2017, September 29). Hypoalbuminemia. Medscape. Retrieved from https://emedicine.medscape.com/article/166724-overview. Accessed October 14, 2017.

# Complete Blood Count with Differential

| Measurement | Adult Reference Range *(Varies among laboratories)* | High Value Causes | Low Value Causes | Clinical Relevance/ Notes |
|---|---|---|---|---|
| **Hematocrit (Hct)**[1,2,3,4,5,6,8] | Male: 42%–52%<br>Female: 37%–48% | Dehydration, chronic hypoxia (from lung disease), smoking, living in higher altitudes | Iron deficiency, anemia of chronic disease (e.g., rheumatoid arthritis, malignancy, long-term infection such as human immunodeficiency virus (HIV), hepatitis B and C), chronic kidney disease, acute or chronic blood loss, marrow failure (e.g., chemotherapy), myelodysplastic syndrome, nutritional (e.g., vitamin B12 deficiency), unexplained | • Anemia is characterized by low Hct levels.<br>• Anemia of chronic disease is especially common in older adults, given the higher rate of chronic disease.<br>• *Anemia is not a diagnosis; it develops from an underlying disorder.*<br>• About one-third of older adults have unexplained anemias. |

| | | | | |
|---|---|---|---|---|
| **Hemoglobin (Hgb)**[1,2,3,4,5,6,8] | Male: 13–18 g/dL<br>Female: 12–16 g/dL | Dehydration, chronic hypoxia (from lung disease), smoking, living in higher altitudes | Iron deficiency, anemia of chronic disease (e.g., rheumatoid arthritis, malignancy, long-term infection such as HIV, hepatitis B and C), chronic kidney disease, acute or chronic blood loss, marrow failure (e.g., chemotherapy) myelodysplastic syndrome, nutritional (e.g., vitamin B12 deficiency), unexplained | • Anemia is characterized by low hemoglobin levels.<br>• Anemia of chronic disease is especially common in older adults, given the higher rate of chronic disease.<br>• Transfusion may be beneficial when the Hgb is < 6–7 g/dL.<br>• *Anemia is not a diagnosis; it develops from an underlying disorder.*<br>• About one-third of older adults have unexplained anemias. |

(*Continues*)

| Measurement | Adult Reference Range *(Varies among laboratories)* | High Value Causes | Low Value Causes | Clinical Relevance/ Notes |
|---|---|---|---|---|
| **Mean corpuscular hemoglobin (MCH)**[1,2,3,7,9] | 28–33 pg/cell | Megaloblastic anemia, (i.e., vitamin B12 *[more common]* or folate deficiency), hypothyroidism, liver disease, alcohol abuse, chemotherapy | Anemia of chronic disease, iron deficiency anemia, thalassemia | • The MCH is part of the red blood cell (RBC) indices, which aids in diagnosing underlying causes of anemia. It parallels with MCV results. |
| **Mean corpuscular hemoglobin concentration (MCHC)**[1,2,3,7] | 32–36 g/dL or 334–355 g/L | Megaloblastic anemia (i.e., vitamin B12 *[more common]* or folate deficiency), chemotherapy | Anemia of chronic disease, iron deficiency, thalassemia | • MCHC is part of the RBC indices; knowing if the MCHC is high (hyperchromia) or low (hypochromia) is helpful in the differential diagnosis of anemia.<br>• Normochromic anemia can be seen with acute hemorrhage, chronic disease, or renal failure. |

| | | | | |
|---|---|---|---|---|
| **Mean corpuscular volume (MCV)**[1,3,6,7,8] | 80–100 fL | Megaloblastic anemia (i.e., vitamin B12 *[more common]* or folate deficiency), medications (e.g., chemotherapy, trimethoprim [Primsol]), alcohol abuse, liver disease, myelodysplasia, hypothyroidism | Anemia of chronic disease, iron deficiency, thalassemia | • MCV is part of the RBC indices; knowing if the MCV is high (macrocytic) or low MCV (microcytic) is helpful in the differential diagnosis of anemia.<br>• Normocytic anemia can result from acute hemorrhage, chronic disease, or renal failure. |
| **Mean platelet volume (MPV)**[10] | 6–10 fL | Megaloblastic anemia (i.e., vitamin B12 *[most common]* myelodysplastic syndrome, idiopathic thrombo-cytopenia purpura (ITP) | Aplastic anemia | • MPV can be useful in the workup of platelet disorders. |
| **Platelet (Plt) count**[3,10,11,12,13] | 150,000–400,000 cells/$mm^3$ or 150–400 K/uL | Chronic myeloid leukemia, chronic iron deficiency, post-splenectomy; | Vitamin B12 deficiency, myelodysplastic syndrome, alcohol abuse, liver disease, infection (acute or chronic), | • High platelet count is known as thrombocytosis, whereas a low platelet count is known as thrombocytopenia. |

*(Continues)*

| Measurement | Adult Reference Range *(Varies among laboratories)* | High Value Causes | Low Value Causes | Clinical Relevance/ Notes |
|---|---|---|---|---|
| | | common following surgery, infection, trauma | medications (e.g., heparin, aspirin, NSAIDs), pulmonary embolism, immune thrombocytopenia purpura | • A count below 10,000 can lead to spontaneous bleeding. |
| **Red blood cell (RBC) count**[1,2,3,4,5,6,7,8,10] | Male: 4.7–6.1 million cells/mcL or 4.7–6.1 million cells/uL<br>Female: 4.2–5.4 million cells/mcL or 4.2–5.4 million cells/uL | Dehydration, chronic hypoxia (from lung disease), smoking, living in higher altitudes, medications (e.g., gentamicin, methyldopa) | Iron deficiency, anemia of chronic disease (e.g., rheumatoid arthritis, malignancy, long-term infection such as HIV, hepatitis B and C), chronic kidney disease, acute or chronic blood loss, marrow failure (e.g., chemotherapy), myelodysplastic syndrome, vitamin B12 deficiency, unexplained | • RBC count is parallel to the Hgb and Hct count; when it is low, the patient is considered anemic. When levels go above the normal range, this is considered polycythemic. |

| | | | | |
|---|---|---|---|---|
| **Red cell distribution width (RDW)**[3,10,14] | 11.5%–14.5% | Iron deficiency, vitamin B12 or folate deficiency, liver disease | | • RDW is used along with the MCV to determine underlying cause of anemia (e.g., high RDW with low MCV is associated with iron deficiency). |
| **White blood cell (WBC) count**[3,10,16,17] | 4,500–10,500 cells/$mm^3$ or 4.5–10.5 K/uL | Infections (bacterial more so than viral), corticosteroids, stressful stimulus (e.g., following surgery, heart attack, seizures, infarction) inflammatory conditions (e.g., rheumatoid arthritis), allergic response (allergies, asthma), malignancy (leukemia), splenectomy | Medications (e.g., chemotherapy, psychotropic agents, anti-inflammatory agents, some antibiotics and diuretics), vitamin B12 or folate deficiency, viral or bacterial infections *(self-limited in viral infections; if due to bacterial, from overworked bone marrow)*, malignancy | • A high WBC is called leukocytosis, whereas a low WBC is called leukopenia.<br>• Not uncommon for older adults to have an impaired response to infection, therefore may not see leukocytosis and/or fever.<br>• Older adults have atypical presentations; therefore, important to not focus solely on lab results. |

*(Continues)*

| Types of WBC | Adult Reference Range *(Varies among laboratories)* | High Value Causes | Low Value Causes | Clinical Relevance/ Notes |
|---|---|---|---|---|
| **Basophil**[3,7,10,15,17] | 0.5%–1%<br>Absolute count: 15–100 cells/$mm^3$ or 1.5–10.0 K/uL | Inflammatory conditions (e.g., rheumatoid arthritis, ulcerative colitis), chronic myelogenous leukemia, post-splenectomy, hypothyroidism | Acute infection, hyperthyroidism, drugs (e.g., chemotherapy, glucocorticoids) | • Is the least common leukocyte.<br>• Elevated basophils (basophilia) most commonly associated with leukemia and myeloproliferative disorders. |
| **Eosinophil**[3,7,10,15,17] | 1%–4%<br>Absolute count: < 450 cells/$mm^3$ or < 0.45 K/uL | Allergic disorder, reaction from medications, infection (e.g., parasitic) malignancies, inflammatory bowel disease | Bone marrow failure, corticosteroids | • Known for its increased response to hypersensitivity reactions and parasitic infections.<br>• High levels are called eosinophilia. |

| | | | | |
|---|---|---|---|---|
| **Lympho-cyte**[3,7,10,15,17] | 20%–40%<br>Absolute count:<br>1,000–4,000 cells/$mm^3$ or 1–4 K/uL | Infections (acute viral or some bacterial), lymphocytic leukemia, lymphoma, multiple myeloma | HIV/acquired immunodeficiency syndrome (AIDS) infection, medications (e.g., corticosteroids, chemotherapy), rheumatoid arthritis, sepsis, leukemia | • Elevated lymphocytes are termed lymphocytosis, whereas a low level is lymphocytopenia. |
| **Mono-cyte**[3,7,10,15,17] | 2%–8%<br>Absolute count:<br>$<$ 500 cells/$mm^3$ or $<$ 0.5 K/uL | Infections (viral, parasitic, bacterial), inflammatory bowel disease, rheumatoid arthritis, numerous malignancies | Aplastic anemia, bone marrow failure | • Elevated levels are termed monocytosis.<br>• Monocytes can be elevated with chronic infections. |
| **Neutro-phil**[3,7,10,15,17] | 40%–60%<br>Absolute count:<br>3,000–7,000 cells/$mm^3$ or 3–7 K/uL | Infections (mainly bacterial), stressful stimulus (e.g., surgery, emotional distress, seizures, myocardial infarction), rheumatoid arthritis, gout, malignancies (e.g., myelocytic leukemia), corticosteroids | Viral or bacterial infections, dietary deficiencies (e.g., vitamin B12, folate), medications (e.g., chemotherapy, analgesics, psychotropics), radiation therapy or exposure, malignancies, rheumatoid arthritis | • A high neutrophil count is termed neutrophilia, whereas a low count is neutropenia.<br>• Higher risk of infection when count is $<$ 500 cells/$mm^3$. |

# References

1. Braunstein, E. M. (2017, February). Evaluation of Anemia – Hematology and Oncology. Merck Manuals: Professional. Retrieved from http://www.merckmanuals.com/professional/hematology-and-oncology/approach-to-the-patient-with-anemia/evaluation-of-anemia. Accessed October 15, 2017.
2. LeBlond, R. F., Brown, D. D., Suneja, M., & Szot, J. F. (Eds.). (2014). *DeGowin's Diagnostic Examination,*(10th ed.); Common Laboratory Tests. New York, NY: McGraw-Hill. Retrieved from http://accessmedicine.mhmedical.com/content.aspx?bookid=1192&sectionid=68671769. Accessed October 11, 2017.
3. American Association for Clinical Chemistry (AACC). (2017). Lab Tests Online for Health Professionals. Retrieved from https://labtestsonline.org/for-health-professionals/. Accessed October 10, 2017.
4. National Institute of Diabetes and Digestive and Kidney Diseases. (2013, September 1). Anemia of Inflammation & Chronic Disease. National Institutes of Health. Retrieved from https://www.niddk.nih.gov/health-information/blood-diseases/anemia-inflammation-chronic-disease. Accessed October 15, 2017.
5. Vanasse, G. J. (2014). Anemia. In *Current Diagnosis & Treatment: Geriatrics* (2nd ed.). New York, NY: McGraw-Hill. Retrieved from http://accessmedicine.mhmedical.com/content.aspx?bookid=953&sectionid=53375667. Accessed October 15, 2017.
6. Goodnough, L. T., & Schrier, S. L. (2014, January). Evaluation and Management of Anemia in the Elderly. National Center for Biotechnology Information, U.S. National Library of Medicine, National Institutes of Health. Retrieved from https://www.ncbi.nlm.nih.gov/pmc/articles/PMC4289144/. Accessed October 15, 2017.
7. National Library of Medicine, National Institutes of Health. (2017, September). Databases. Retrieved from https://www.nlm.nih.gov/?_ga=2.63715881.769328030.1507665199-1049439008.1471202369. Accessed October 10, 2017.
8. Artz, A. S. (2015, November 26). Anemia in Elderly Persons. Medscape. Retrieved from https://emedicine.medscape.com/article/1339998-overview?pa=qo4lBmMsrlq5cs%2Bw81Z4hWTA5jNaPrA3caSB%2FmIXLD0GxgaME81lshl60Kq35m1PNFsYxDuz%2Fz2hge3aAwEFsw%3D%3D#a1. Accessed October 15, 2017.
9. Merritt, B. Y. (2017, January 6). Mean Corpuscular Hemoglobin (MCH) and Mean Corpuscular Hemoglobin Concentration (MCHC). Medscape. Retrieved from https://emedicine.medscape.com/article/2054497-overview#a2. Accessed October 15, 2017.
10. Epocrates. (n.d.). Retrieved from https://www.epocrates.com (Lab section). Accessed October 15, 2017.
11. Coagulation disorders. In *Hazzard's Geriatric Medicine and Gerontology* (7th ed.). New York, NY: McGraw-Hill. Retrieved from http://accessmedicine.mhmedical.com/content.aspx?bookid=1923&sectionid=144560586. Accessed October 17, 2017.
12. Imashuku, S., Kudo, N., Kubo, K., Takahashi, N., & Tohyama, K. (2012, April 24). Persistent thrombocytosis in elderly patients with rare hyposplenias that mimic essential thrombocythemia. *International Journal of Hematology,* 95(6), 702–705. Retrieved from https://link.springer.com/article/10.1007/s12185-012-1082-1. Accessed October 17, 2017.
13. Izak, M., & Bussel, J. B. (2014). Management of Thrombocytopenia. National Center for Biotechnology Information, U.S. National Library of Medicine, National Institutes of Health. Retrieved from https://www.ncbi.nlm.nih.gov/pmc/articles/PMC4047949/. Accessed October 17, 2017.

14. Curry, C. V. (2015, January 13). Red Cell Distribution Width (RDW). Medscape. Retrieved from https://emedicine.medscape.com/article/2098635-overview#a2. Accessed October 18, 2017.
15. LeBlond, R. F., Brown, D. D., Suneja, M., & Szot, J. F. (Eds.). (2014). *DeGowin's Diagnostic Examination,* (10th ed.); Common Laboratory Tests. New York, NY: McGraw-Hill. Retrieved from http://accessmedicine.mhmedical.com/content.aspx?bookid=1192&sectionid=68671769. Accessed October 18, 2017.
16. Atypical presentations of illness in older adults. In *Current Diagnosis & Treatment: Geriatrics* (2nd ed.). New York, NY: McGraw-Hill. Retrieved from http://accessmedicine.mhmedical.com/content.aspx?bookid=953&sectionid=53375629. Accessed October 18, 2017.
17. White cell disorders. In *Hazzard's Geriatric Medicine and Gerontology* (7th ed.). New York, NY: McGraw-Hill. Retrieved from http://accessmedicine.mhmedical.com/content.aspx?bookid=1923&sectionid=144560220. Accessed October 18, 2017.

# Urinalysis

| Measurement | Reference Range *(Varies among laboratories)* | Interpretation | Clinical Relevance/ Notes |
|---|---|---|---|
| **Appearance, urine**[1,2,3] | Clear | Cloudy urine can come from cells from the skin, contaminants (e.g., lotions), diet, and/or bacterial infections. | • The appearance is impacted by urinary substance, such as vaginal discharge, debris, and/or bacteria. |
| **Bilirubin, urine**[1,3] | Negative | Positive bilirubin in the urine suggests early sign of liver disease, biliary obstruction, hepatitis. | • Positive results imply impaired hepatic function; liver function tests are ordered to establish diagnosis. |
| **Blood, urine**[1,2,3,4] | Negative | Positive results suggest infection, gross hematuria includes coagulation defects, renal infarction, renal stones, renal or bladder carcinoma, prostatitis, trauma (e.g., indwelling catheter), medications. | • Positive dipstick results should be confirmed with microscopic exam. |
| **Color, urine**[1,2,3,4,6,7] | Light/pale yellow to deep amber | *Blue-green:* indomethacin (Indocin), amitriptyline (Elavil), urinary tract infection (UTI) caused by *Pseudomonas aeruginosa.* | • Gives an idea of hydration status, presence of infection, and/or use of medications. |

| | | | |
|---|---|---|---|
| | | *Bright yellow:* multivitamins.<br>*Brown:* myoglobinuria, medications (metronidazole [Flagyl]), levodopa [Sinemet]).<br>*Cloudy white:* urinary tract infection.<br>*Dark yellow:* dehydration.<br>*Orange:* vitamin C, medications (rifampin [Rifadin], phenazopyridine [Pyridium]).<br>*Red:* infections, hemoglobinuria, food (e.g., beets or blackberries). | |
| **Glucose, urine**[1,2,3,4,6,7,8] | Negative | Glucosuria can indicate hyperglycemia in uncontrolled diabetes. Other causes: renal disease (e.g., acute tubular damage), liver disease, medications (e.g., steroids, tetracycline). | • Glucosuria seen with serum glucose above 180 mg/dL.<br>• Not to be used as a diagnostic tool for monitoring/testing diabetes.<br>• Dipsticks exposed to air for prolonged periods can result in false positive glucosuria. |

(*Continues*)

| Measurement | Reference Range *(Varies among laboratories)* | Interpretation | Clinical Relevance/ Notes |
|---|---|---|---|
| **Ketones, urine**[1,2,3,4,8,9] | None | Positive results can indicate acute illness, starvation, or fasting; low carbohydrate intake; diabetic ketoacidosis (DKA); prolonged vomiting. | • A positive result does not ensure a diagnosis of diabetic ketoacidosis (DKA).<br>• If concerned for DKA, check a plasma glucose for hyperglycemia and an arterial blood gas (ABG) for acidosis. |
| **Leukocyte esterase, urine**[1,2,3,4,6,7,9] | Negative | Positive results (pyuria) can indicate urinary tract infection, contamination (vaginal flora), nephrolithiasis. | • Aids in the diagnosis of a UTI (should be confirmed with microscopic exam). |
| **Nitrite, urine**[1,2,3,6] | Negative | Positive results can indicate urinary tract infection. | • Some bacteria are unable to convert nitrate to nitrite (e.g., *Pseudomonas*, enterococci); therefore a negative result does not rule out a UTI. |

| | | | |
|---|---|---|---|
| **pH, urine**[1,3,4] | 4.5–8.0 | Urine is usually acidic, *(pH of about 6)*. Acidic urine is affected by high protein diet, cranberries, uric acid, or cystine calculi. Alkaline urine: presence of UTI, calcium oxalate calculi, renal tubular acidosis (RTA). | • Knowing urine pH assists with diagnosis of UTI, nephrolithiasis, and renal tubular acidosis (RTA). |
| **Protein, urine**[1,2,3,4,10,11,12] | Negative | Positive results (proteinuria) can be benign (e.g., fever, heart failure, dehydration).<br>Glomerular damage (e.g., hypertension, diabetes, glomerulonephritis).<br>Nephrotoxic agents (NSAIDs). | • Proteinuria is not a normal part of the aging process and should be investigated. It is usually benign and self-limited.<br>• Persistent proteinuria carries an increased risk of progressive renal disease and death. |
| **Specific gravity, urine**[1,3,4,6,7] | 1.003–1.030 | Low results can indicate excessive hydration, renal failure.<br>High results can indicate dehydration, contrast media, heart failure, SIADH. | • Gives an idea of hydration status.<br>• It is often low in older adults and those with renal impairment due to inability to concentrate urine. |
| **Urobilinogen, urine**[1,3,8] | 0.5–1 mg/dL | Increased urobilinogen in the urine can suggest liver disease, constipation, hepatotoxic medications, hyperthyroidism, heart failure. | • Positive results imply impaired hepatic function; liver function tests are ordered to establish diagnosis. |

(*Continues*)

| Microscopic Urinalysis | Reference Range *(Varies among laboratories)* | Interpretation | Clinical Relevance/ Notes |
|---|---|---|---|
| **Bacteria, urine**[1,2,6] | None | Can indicate infection or contamination *(especially in the presence of multiple organisms)*. | • The presence of bacteriuria and no symptoms represents asymptomatic bacteruria, which does not require antibiotic therapy. |
| **Casts, urine**[1,4,5,6] | 0–5 hyaline casts/lpf | Abnormal results can include fatty casts (seen with nephrotic syndrome), granular casts (seen with multiple types of renal diseases), red blood cell casts (seen with glomerulonephritis), renal tubular epithelial cell casts (seen with renal tubular necrosis, renal transplant rejection), waxy casts (seen with chronic renal disease).<br>WBC casts indicate acute renal infection (e.g., pyelonephritis). | • Depending on the type of casts, gives an idea of associated conditions.<br>• Presence of hyaline cast is *nonspecific* (noted in those without renal disease).<br>• Results can be affected by specimen processing and/or clinical laboratory not identifying urinary casts; therefore the absence of casts does not rule out a presumed diagnosis. |
| **Crystals, urine**[1,3,13] | Occasionally | If positive, may include the following types of stones: uric acid, struvite, calcium oxalate, cystine. | • Can indicate stone formation; stones can occur in older adults as a result of poor hydration. |

| | | | |
|---|---|---|---|
| **RBC, urine**[1,2,3] | 0–4 RBCs/hpf | Nephrolithiasis, urinary tract infections, prostatitis, benign prostatic hypertrophy, malignancies (e.g., renal, bladder, prostate), glomerular causes, urological trauma (e.g., indwelling catheter or procedure), medications (e.g., anticoagulants, NSAIDs). | • Microscopic hematuria can be a number of etiologies, ranging from benign to life threatening.<br>• If unsure of the cause, especially with persistent hematuria, workup advised (e.g., BUN and creatinine levels, urinary tract imaging, cystoscopy). |
| **Squamous epithelial cells, urine**[1,2,3,6] | None to few (≤ 15–20 squamous epithelial cells/hpf) | Contamination. | • Presence of squamous epithelial cells should raise suspicion for urinary specimen contamination. |
| **White blood cells (WBCs), urine**[1,2,3,4,6,7] | 0–5 WBCs/hpf | High amount is seen in those with a urinary tract infection, contamination (vaginal flora), infection or inflammation in the genitourinary tract. | • Presence of nitrites, leukocyte esterase, WBCs, and an isolated organism aid in diagnosing a urinary tract infection (UTI). |
| **Yeast, urine**[1,3] | None | Positive results indicate either infection (e.g., *Candida* species) or contamination. | • Indicator of underlying infection or contamination. |

# References

1. Lerma, E. V. (2015, December 16). Urinalysis. Medscape. Retrieved from https://emedicine.medscape.com/article/2074001-overview#showall. Accessed October 18, 2017.
2. Sharp, V. J., Lee, D. K., & Askeland, E. J. (2014, October 15). Urinalysis: Case presentations for the primary care physician. *American Family Physician, 90*(8), 542–547. Retrieved from http://www.aafp.org/afp/2014/1015/p542.html. Accessed October 18, 2017.
3. American Association for Clinical Chemistry (AACC). (2017). Lab Tests Online for Health Professionals. Retrieved from https://labtestsonline.org/for-health-professionals/. Accessed October 10, 2017.
4. LeBlond, R. F., Brown, D. D., Suneja, M., & Szot, J. F. (Eds.). (2014). *DeGowin's Diagnostic Examination,*(10th ed.). Common Laboratory Tests. New York, NY: McGraw-Hill. Retrieved from http://accessmedicine.mhmedical.com/content.aspx?bookid=1192&sectionid=68671769. Accessed October 18, 2017.
5. Penn State Hershey Medical Center. (2015, August 29). Urinary Casts. Retrieved from http://pennstatehershey.adam.com/content.aspx?productid=117&pid=1&gid=003586. Accessed October 19, 2017.
6. Schaffer, A. C. (2016). Urinalysis and urine electrolytes. In *Principles and Practice of Hospital Medicine* (2nd ed.). New York, NY: McGraw-Hill. Retrieved from http://accessmedicine.mhmedical.com/content.aspx?bookid=1872&sectionid=146978210. Accessed October 18, 2017.
7. Shah, A. P. (2016, November). Evaluation of the Renal Patient – Genitourinary Disorders. Merck Manuals: Professional. Retrieved from http://www.merckmanuals.com/professional/genitourinary-disorders/approach-to-the-genitourinary-patient/evaluation-of-the-renal-patient#v1152664. Accessed October 21, 2017.
8. *Clinician's Pocket Reference: The Scut Monkey* (11th ed.). New York, NY: McGraw-Hill; Chapter 6. Laboratory Diagnosis: Urine Studies..Retrieved from http://accessmedicine.mhmedical.com/content.aspx?bookid=365&sectionid=43074915. Accessed October 21, 2017.
9. Kitabchi, A. E., & Nematollahi, L. R. (2017, April 04). Diabetic Ketoacidosis. Epocrates. Retrieved from https://online.epocrates.com/diseases/162/DKA-diabetic-ketoacidosis. Accessed October 21, 2017.
10. Wiggins, J., & Patel, S. R. (2017). Aging of the kidney. In *Hazzard's Geriatric Medicine and Gerontology* (7th ed.). New York, NY: McGraw-Hill. Retrieved from http://accessmedicine.mhmedical.com/content.aspx?bookid=1923&sectionid=144525776. Accessed October 21, 2017.
11. Bowling, C. B., & Booth, K. (2014). Chronic kidney disease. . In *Current Diagnosis & Treatment: Geriatrics* (2nd ed.). New York, NY: McGraw-Hill. Retrieved from http://accessmedicine.mhmedical.com/content.aspx?bookid=953&sectionid=53375662. Accessed October 21, 2017.
12. Akbarian, F., Lawati, H. A., & Shafiee, M. A. (2011, September–October). Approach to proteinuria in adults and elderly. *Journal of Current Clinical Care,* 45–56. Retrieved from https://www.healthplexus.net/files/content/2011/August/0104Proteinuria.pdf. Accessed October 21, 2017.
13. Pierorazio, P. (2014, March 7). Kidney Stones in the Elderly. Brady Urology at Johns Hopkins Hospital. Retrieved from http://bradyurology.blogspot.com/2014/03/kidney-stones-in-elderly.html. Accessed October 21, 2017.

# Common Labs Ordered

| Measurement | Adult Reference Range *(Varies among laboratories)* | High Value Causes | Low Value Causes | Clinical Relevance/ Notes |
|---|---|---|---|---|
| **Acute phase reactant serum:** C-reactive protein (CRP)[1,2,3,4,5,6] | < 1 mg/L | Infections (mostly bacterial), tissue injury (e.g., following surgery, myocardial infarction). inflammatory disorders (e.g., gout, rheumatoid arthritis, giant cell arteritis (GCA), polymyalgia rheumatica (PMR), renal and/or thyroid disease, malignancy, advanced age | Statins, weight loss, alcohol, and/or appropriate response to therapy | • Acute phase reactants offer guidance in monitoring the severity of various conditions.<br>• CRP and ESR are nonspecific markers of acute or chronic inflammation.<br>• They rise with a variety of similar conditions; CRP however rises faster than the ESR. |

*(Continues)*

| **Measurement** | **Adult Reference Range *(Varies among laboratories)*** | **High Value Causes** | **Low Value Causes** | **Clinical Relevance/ Notes** |
|---|---|---|---|---|
| Acute phase reactant serum: Erythrocyte sedimentation rate (ESR)[1,2,3,4,5,6] | Male < 20 mm/hr<br>Female < 30 mm/hr | Infections, tissue injury, inflammatory disorders, anemia, renal and/or thyroid disease, malignancy, high cholesterol, advanced age | Leukocytosis, renal failure, heart failure, cachexia, steroids, and/or appropriate response to therapy | See above. |
| Acute phase reactant serum: Procalcitonin[1,2,3,4,5,6] | < 0.3 ng/ml | Severe bacterial infection, major surgery | Viral infection, and/or appropriate response to therapy | • Elevated procalcitonin is specific to bacterial infections and correlates with severity; it helps differentiate from noninfectious conditions. |
| Ammonia, serum[1,4,5,7] | 15–45 mcg/dL or 8.8–26.4 mmol/L | Liver disease, gastrointestinal bleeding, renal failure, medications (e.g., narcotics, diuretics, valproic acid), cigarette smoking | Medications (e.g., lactulose, some antibiotics such as neomycin) | • Ordered often in the setting of hepatic encephalopathy.<br>• How high the ammonia is does not correlate to severity of liver disease. |

| | | | | |
|---|---|---|---|---|
| Amylase, serum[1,4,5,8] | 23–140 units/L | Pancreatitis, following surgery, malignancies (e.g., pancreatic, lung), renal failure, liver disease, gastroenteritis, obstructed bowel, perforated ulcer, medications (e.g., aspirin, thiazide diuretics, some antibiotics, cholinergics) | Renal disease, chronic pancreatitis | • Ordered with a lipase to aid in the diagnosis and monitoring of acute pancreatitis.<br>• High levels do not correlate with disease severity. |
| Anemia workup: Iron studies (Serum Iron, Transferrin Saturation, Total Iron Binding Capacity [TIBC], Serum Ferritin), Vitamin B12, Folate[1,4,5,9,10,11,12,13,14,15] | | | | • Workup is required once anemia has been confirmed on the CBC.<br>• The red cell indices, along with the results of the anemia workup give an idea to the underlying cause. |

(*Continues*)

| Measurement | Adult Reference Range *(Varies among laboratories)* | High Value Causes | Low Value Causes | Clinical Relevance/ Notes |
|---|---|---|---|---|
| Anemia workup: (*continued*) | | | | • Other tests to consider: **occult blood** *(check for underlying GI blood loss)*, **peripheral blood smear** *(can diagnose a variety of conditions, such as MDS)*, **renal function** *(check for renal disease)*, **bone marrow biopsy** *(can be used to diagnose MDS)*, **reticulocyte count** *(used to reflect bone marrow activity and response to anemia treatment)*. |
| Serum Iron | 60–170 mcg/dL or 10.74–30.43 mcmol/L | Iron overload, liver disease | Iron deficiency, anemia of chronic disease, GI blood loss | See above. |

| | | | | |
|---|---|---|---|---|
| Transferrin saturation | 20%–50% | Iron overload | Iron deficiency, anemia of chronic disease | See above. |
| Total iron-binding capacity (TIBC) | 240–450 mcg/L or 42.96–80.55 mcmol/L | Iron deficiency | Anemia of chronic disease *(results can be normal)*, gastrointestinal blood loss, iron overload | See above. |
| Serum ferritin | Male: 20–250 ng/ml (20–250 g/L)<br>Female: 10–120 ng/ml (10–120 g/L) | Anemia of chronic disease *(results can be normal)*, advanced age, iron overload | Iron deficiency, GI blood loss | See above. |
| Vitamin B12 | 200–900 ng/ml or 453–2,039 nmol/L | Chronic renal failure, heart failure, liver disease, diabetes | Malnutrition, malabsorption, medications (e.g., proton pump inhibitors, metformin), chronic alcoholism | See above. |

(*Continues*)

| Measurement | Adult Reference Range *(Varies among laboratories)* | High Value Causes | Low Value Causes | Clinical Relevance/ Notes |
|---|---|---|---|---|
| Folate | 2.7–17 ng/ml or 6.12–38.52 nmol/L | Hyperthyroidism, pernicious anemia, dietary intake (vegetarianism), bacterial overgrowth syndrome | Malnutrition, malabsorption, chronic alcoholism | See above. |
| B-type natriuretic peptide (BNP), serum[1,5,16,17] | < 100 pg/ml or 28.9 pmol/L | Heart failure *(especially with levels above 400 pg/ml)*, renal failure, advanced age, hypertension, acute coronary syndrome | Medications (e.g., ACEIs, beta blockers), obesity | • BNP is ordered when the underlying diagnosis is unclear; validates symptoms such as acute dyspnea due to heart failure as opposed to COPD.<br>• Is ordered for the monitoring of heart failure severity. |

| | | | | |
|---|---|---|---|---|
| D-dimer, serum[1,4,5,17,18,19,20] | < 0.5 mcg/ml or < 0.5 mg/L | Thrombus formation (seen with deep vein thrombosis and pulmonary embolism), recent surgery, sepsis, liver disease, malignancy, cardiovascular disease, advanced age, trauma | | • Test is useful when the clinical suspicion for thrombus is **low** and needing to exclude VTE as the underlying diagnosis.<br>• Advanced age (≥ 80 years) is associated with higher false positives. |
| Gamma-glutamyl transpeptidase (GGTP or GTP), serum[1,4,5] | 7–51 units/L | Liver disease, hepatitis, cirrhosis, alcohol abuse, liver carcinoma, liver metastasis, bile duct obstruction, acute pancreatitis, heart failure, hepatotoxic medications, smoking | Bone disease, renal failure | • Useful when investigating an elevated alkaline phosphatase (ALP).<br>• If GGT is also elevated, this implies disease of the bile ducts and/or liver *(will be decreased in bone disease)*. |

(*Continues*)

| Measurement | Adult Reference Range *(Varies among laboratories)* | High Value Causes | Low Value Causes | Clinical Relevance/ Notes |
|---|---|---|---|---|
| Hemoglobin A1c (HbA1C), serum[1,4,5,21,32] | • < 5.7% (39 mmol/mol)<br>• 5.7%–6.4% (39–46 mmol/mol) indicates prediabetes.<br>• ≥ 6.5% (48 mmol/mol) indicates diabetes. | Diabetes, iron deficiency anemia | Acute blood loss, chronic renal failure | • The American Geriatric Society (AGS) recommends a target HbA1C of:<br>• 7.5%–8% in older adults.<br>• 7.0%–7.5% in healthier patients with few comorbidities.<br>• 8%–9% with limited life expectancy. |
| Lipase, serum[1,4,5,8] | 0–160 U/L or 0–2.67 microkat/L | Pancreatitis, pancreatic tumors, peptic ulcer, cholecystitis, diabetic ketoacidosis, biliary disease, renal failure, HIV, medications (e.g., indomethacin, narcotics, valproic acid, furosemide, thiazide diuretics) | Cystic fibrosis, medications (e.g., hydroxyurea, somatostatin) | • Ordered with a serum amylase to diagnose acute pancreatitis; lipase is more specific than amylase in acute pancreatitis.<br>• High levels do not correlate with disease severity. |

| | | | | |
|---|---|---|---|---|
| Magnesium, serum[1,4,5,22] | 1.8–3.0 mg/dL or 0.74–1.23 mmol/L | Renal failure, hypothyroidism, volume depletion, medications (e.g., antacids, milk of magnesia, aminoglycosides, calcitriol) | Alcoholism, malnutrition, malabsorption, severe diarrhea, hypercalcemia, uncontrolled diabetes, medications (e.g., diuretics, PPIs, insulin) | • If taking a PPI and/or diuretic (loop or thiazide) for long periods, check magnesium periodically.<br>• Chronic hypomagnesemia is associated with hypocalcemia and hypokalemia. |
| Parathyroid hormone (PTH) intact[1,4,5,23] | 10–55 pg/mL or 10–55 ng/L | Primary hyperparathyroidism (e.g., adenoma), secondary hyperparathyroidism (e.g., renal failure, vitamin D deficiency), thiazide diuretics, immobilization | Following neck surgery, malignancy, hypomagnesemia, excess vitamin D | • Commonly ordered in those with renal disease and/or a calcium imbalance. |

(*Continues*)

| Measurement | Adult Reference Range *(Varies among laboratories)* | High Value Causes | Low Value Causes | Clinical Relevance/ Notes |
|---|---|---|---|---|
| Phosphorus, serum[1,4,5,24] | 2.4–4.1 mg/dL or 0.78–1.34 mmol/L | Renal disease, hypoparathyroidism, diabetic ketoacidosis, rhabdomyolysis, laxatives containing phosphorus | Alcoholism, malnutrition, vitamin D deficiency, hyperparathyroidism, medications (e.g., insulin, antacids, niacin, thiazide diuretics) | • Commonly ordered in those with chronic renal disease. |
| Prealbumin, serum[1,5,25] | 16–35 mg/dL or 160–350 g/L | Renal failure, iron deficiency, medications (e.g., steroids) | Malnutrition, liver disease, states of inflammation or infections, medications (e.g., amiodarone) | • Is an indicator of inflammation and disease severity, however not a reliable marker of nutritional status. |

| | | | | |
|---|---|---|---|---|
| Prostatic-specific antigen (PSA), serum[1,4,5,25,33] | • < 4 n/ml or < 4 g/L<br>• 4–10 ng/mL or 4–10 g/L is borderline.<br>• 10 ng/mL or > 10 g/L is high. | Benign prostatic hypertrophy, prostate cancer *(especially if level > 10)*, prostatitis, or urinary tract infection | Statin medications | • U.S. Preventive Services Task Force (USPSTF) recommends against PSA-based screening.<br>• American Urological Association (AUA) recommends screening in those age 55–69 every 2 years with life expectancy of at least 10 years. |
| Thyroid function tests:[1,4,5,30,31] Thyroid-stimulating hormone (TSH) and free T4 | **TSH:** 0.4–4 mIU/ml or 0.4–4 IU/L<br>4.5–10 is subclinical.<br>> 10 is overt.<br>**Free T4:** 0.9–2.4 mcg/dL or 11.7–33.2 nmol/L | **TSH:** hypothyroidism, recovery from illness (transient), pituitary tumor, medications (e.g., amiodarone, sulfonylureas, lithium)<br>**Free T4:** hyperthyroidism, some medications | **TSH:** hyperthyroidism, acute illness, medications (levothyroxine, aspirin, corticosteroids)<br>**Free T4:** hypothyroidism, acute illness (transient), some medications | • In the setting of a high TSH and normal free T4, this is subclinical hypothyroidism (treatment is controversial).<br>• Most experts agree treatment (levothyroxine) should be initiated with a TSH ≥10, with target serum TSH of 3–6.<br>• Not much clinical utility in checking T3 (triiodothyronine). |

*(Continues)*

| Measurement | Adult Reference Range *(Varies among laboratories)* | High Value Causes | Low Value Causes | Clinical Relevance/ Notes |
|---|---|---|---|---|
| Uric acid[1,4,5,27,28] | 3–7 mg/dL or 178–416 mcmol/L | Renal failure, alcoholism, gout, volume depletion, purine-rich diet, hypothyroidism, medications (e.g., low-dose aspirin, diuretics, chemotherapeutic agents) | Medications (e.g., allopurinol, enalapril, high-dose aspirin), liver disease, SIADH | • Older adults with hyperuricemia should be advised on limiting purine-rich foods and alcohol intake.<br>• Avoid agents that promote hyperuricemia, such as thiazide or loop diuretics.<br>• Uric acid goal: < 6 mg/dL. |
| Vitamin D, 25-OH[1,4,5,29] | • 30–40 ng/mL or 75–100 nmol/L<br>• 21–29 ng/mL or 52.5–72.5 nmol/L is insufficient.<br>• < 20 ng/mL or 50 mnol/L is deficiency. | Oversupplementation of vitamin D *(leads to hypercalcemia)* | Reduced intake of vitamin D, staying indoors, malabsorption, chronic kidney disease | • Targeting levels to 28–40 ng/mL reduces fracture risk.<br>• Supplementing with vitamin D (800–1,000 IU daily) reduces falls and fractures in those ≥ 65 years old. |

## References


1. American Association for Clinical Chemistry (AACC). (2017). Lab Tests Online for Health Professionals. Retrieved from https://labtestsonline.org/for-health-professionals/. Accessed October 10, 2017.
2. RheumaKnowledgy. (2014, November 25). Acute Phase Reactants (ESR, CRP). Retrieved from http://www.rheumaknowledgy.com/acute-phase-reactants/. Accessed October 22, 2017.
3. Kushner, I. (2017, July 12). Acute Phase Reactants. UpToDate. Retrieved from https://www.uptodate.com/contents/acute-phase-reactants?source=search_result&search=acute phase reactants&selectedTitle=1~150#H22. Accessed October 22, 2017.
4. National Library of Medicine, National Institutes of Health. (2017, September). Databases. Retrieved from https://www.nlm.nih.gov/?_ga=2.63715881.769328030.1507665199-1049439008.1471202369. Accessed October 10, 2017.
5. Epocrates. (n.d.). Retrieved from https://www.epocrates.com. Accessed October 22, 2017.
6. PulmCCM. (2014, March 29). Can Procalcitonin Help Guide Therapy for Suspected Pneumonia & Other Infections? (Review). Retrieved from https://pulmccm.org/review-articles/can-procalcitonin-help-guide-antibiotic-therapy-for-suspected-pneumonia-review-chest/?utm_source=TrendMD&utm_medium=cpc&utm_campaign=PulmCCM_TrendMD_0. Accessed October 22, 2017.
7. Ferenci, P. (2015, September 23). Hepatic Encephalopathy in Adults: Clinical Manifestations and Diagnosis. UpToDate. Retrieved from https://www.uptodate.com/contents/hepatic-encephalopathy-in-adults-clinical-manifestations-and-diagnosis?source=search_result&search=ammonia level adult&selectedTitle=1~150#H152815085. Accessed October 22, 2017.
8. Gelrud, D., & Gress, F. G. (2017, February 3). Approach to the Patient with Elevated Serum Amylase or Lipase. UpToDate. Retrieved from https://www.uptodate.com/contents/approach-to-the-patient-with-elevated-serum-amylase-or-lipase?source=search_result&search=amylase elevation&selectedTitle=1~150. Accessed October 22, 2017.
9. Melbourne Haematology. (2014, January 4). A Guide to Interpretation of Iron Studies. Retrieved from http://www.melbournehaematology.com.au/pdfs/guidelines/melbourne-haematology-guidelines-iron-studies.pdf. Accessed October 22, 2017.
10. Maakaron, J. E. (2016, September 24). Anemia Workup. Medscape. Retrieved from https://emedicine.medscape.com/article/198475-workup#showall. Accessed October 22, 2017.
11. Price, S. A., & Schrier, S. L. (2017, September 11). Anemia in the Older Adult. UpToDate. Retrieved from https://www.uptodate.com/contents/anemia-in-the-older-adult?source=see_link. Accessed October 22, 2017.
12. Kane, R. L., Ouslander, J. G., Resnick, B., & Malone, M. L. (Eds.). (2013). *Essentials of Clinical Geriatrics* (8th ed.). New York, NY: McGraw-Hill; Chapter 3. Evaluating the Geriatric Patient. Retrieved from http://accessmedicine.mhmedical.com/content.aspx?bookid=678&sectionid=44833880. Accessed October 22, 2017.
13. Vanasse, G. J. (2014). Anemia. In *Current Diagnosis & Treatment: Geriatrics* (2nd ed.). New York, NY: McGraw-Hill. Retrieved from http://accessmedicine.mhmedical.com/content.aspx?bookid=953&sectionid=53375667. Accessed October 22, 2017.

14. Chapter 41: Hematologic emergencies. In Stone, C., & Humphries, R. L. (Eds.). *CURRENT Diagnosis & Treatment Emergency Medicine* (7th ed.). New York, NY: McGraw-Hill. Retrieved from http://accessmedicine.mhmedical.com/content.aspx?bookid=385&sectionid=40357257. Accessed October 22, 2017.
15. D'Amora, J., & Boshra, S. S. (2014). Anemia and leukemia. In Burggraf, V., Kim, K. Y., & Knight, A. L. (Eds.). *Healthy Aging: Principles and Clinical Practice for Clinicians* (pp. 367–382). Philadelphia, VA: Lippincott Williams & Wilkins.
16. Mangla, A. (2014, May 23). Brain-Type Natriuretic Peptide (BNP). Medscape. Retrieved from https://emedicine.medscape.com/article/2087425-overview#showall. Accessed October 23, 2017.
17. Bowers, M. T. (2013). Managing patients with heart failure. *Journal for Nurse Practitioners, 9*(10), 634–642. Retrieved from http://dx.doi.org/10.1016/j.nurpra.2013.08.025. Accessed October 23, 2017.
18. Szigeti, R. G. (2014, December 10). D-Dimer. Medscape. Retrieved from https://emedicine.medscape.com/article/2085111-overview#showall. Accessed October 22, 2017.
19. Peripheral arterial disease & venous thromboembolism. In *Current Diagnosis & Treatment: Geriatrics* (2nd ed.). New York, NY: McGraw-Hill. Retrieved from http://accessmedicine.mhmedical.com/content.aspx?bookid=953&sectionid=53375656. Accessed October 23, 2017.
20. Schouten, H. J., Geersing, G. J., Koek, H. L., Zuithoff, N. P., Janssen, K. J., & Douma, R. A., . . . Reitsma, J. B. (2013, May 3). Diagnostic accuracy of conventional or age adjusted D-dimer cut-off values in older patients with suspected venous thromboembolism: Systematic review and meta-analysis. *BMJ, 346,* f2492. Retrieved from http://www.bmj.com/content/346/bmj.f2492. Accessed October 23, 2017.
21. Rivera, J. A., Conell-Price, J., & Lee, S. (2014). Diabetes. In *Current Diagnosis & Treatment: Geriatrics* (2nd ed.). New York, NY: McGraw-Hill. http://accessmedicine.mhmedical.com/content.aspx?bookid=953&sectionid=53375666. Accessed October 23, 2017.
22. Yu, A. S. (2016, February 4). Causes of Hypomagnesemia (Goldfarb, S., & Lam, A. Q., Eds.). UpToDate. Retrieved from https://www.uptodate.com/contents/causes-of-hypomagnesemia?source=see_link#H8658137. Accessed October 24, 2017.
23. Michels, T. C., & Kelly, K. M. (2013, August 15). Parathyroid disorders. *American Famiy Physician, 88*(4), 249–257. Retrieved from http://www.aafp.org/afp/2013/0815/p249.html. Accessed October 24, 2017.
24. Lewis, J. L. (2016, April). Hyperphosphatemia – Endocrine and Metabolic Disorders. Merck Manuals: Professional. Retrieved from https://www.merckmanuals.com/professional/endocrine-and-metabolic-disorders/electrolyte-disorders/hyperphosphatemia. Accessed October 24, 2017.
25. Sullivan, D. H., & Johnson, L. E. (2017). Nutrition and obesity. In *Hazzard's Geriatric Medicine and Gerontology* (7th ed.). New York, NY: McGraw-Hill. Retrieved from http://accessmedicine.mhmedical.com/content.aspx?bookid=1923&sectionid=144520120. Accessed October 24, 2017.
26. Hamilton, R. J., Goldberg, K. C., Platz, E. A., & Freedland, S. J. (2008, November 5). Influence of statin medications on prostate-specific antigen levels. *Journal of the National Cancer Institute, 100*(21), 1511–1518. Retrieved from https://academic.oup.com/jnci/article/100/21/1511/2519184/The-Influence-of-Statin-Medications-on-Prostate. Accessed October 22, 2017.
27. Becker, M. A. (2017, September 19). Urate Balance (Dalbeth, N., & Romain, P. L., Eds.). UpToDate. Retrieved from https://www.uptodate.com/contents/urate-balance

?source=search_result&search=causes of high uric acid&selectedTitle=2~150. Accessed October 25, 2017.

28. Strano-Paul, L. (2014). Managing joint pain in older adults. In *Current Diagnosis & Treatment: Geriatrics* (2nd ed.). New York, NY: McGraw-Hill. Retrieved from 2014. http://accessmedicine.mhmedical.com/content.aspx?bookid=953&sectionid=53375690. Accessed October 25, 2017.
29. Dawson-Hughes, B. (2017, October 2). Vitamin D Deficiency in Adults: Definition, Clinical Manifestations, and Treatment (Drezner, M. K., & Mulder. J. E., Eds.). UpToDate. Retrieved from https://www.uptodate.com/contents/vitamin-d-deficiency-in-adults-definition-clinical-manifestations-and-treatment?source=search_result&search=causes of low vitamin d&selectedTitle=1~150. Accessed October 25, 2017.
30. Ross, D. S. (2017, April 13). Sublinical Hypothyroidism in Nonpregnant Adults (Cooper, D. S., & Mulder, J. E., Eds.). UpToDate. Retrieved from https://www.uptodate.com/contents/subclinical-hypothyroidism-in-nonpregnant-adults?source=search_result&search=subclinical hypothyroidism&selectedTitle=1~81. Accessed October 25, 2017.
31. Aytug, S. (2017, August 27). Euthyroid Sick Syndrome. Medscape. Retrieved from https://emedicine.medscape.com/article/118651-overview. Accessed October 25, 2017.
32. American Geriatrics Society Expert Panel on Care of Older Adults with Diabetes Mellitus; Moreno, G., Mangione, C. M., Kimbro, L., & Valsberg, E. (2013, November). Guidelines abstracted from the American Geriatrics Society Guidelines for Improving the Care of Older Adults with Diabetes Mellitus: 2013 update. *Journal of the American Geriatrics Society*, *61*(11), 2020–2026. doi:10.1111/jgs.12514.
33. American Urological Association (AUA). (2015). Early Detection of Prostate Cancer. Retrieved from http://www.auanet.org/guidelines/early-detection-of-prostate-cancer-(2013-reviewed-and-validity-confirmed-2015). Accessed February 17, 2018.

# Imaging Tests

| Imaging Type | Indications | Clinical Notes |
|---|---|---|
| **Computed tomography (CT)**[1,2,3,4,5,6]<br>• Patient will be exposed to radiation (carries small risk of cancer).<br>• Contrast is used to better visualize the area being examined.<br>• Check for contrast allergies; diphenhydramine (Benadryl) and corticosteroids can be given prior to imaging for history of mild allergic response to contrast (e.g., anxiety, flushing, rash, hives). Avoid contrast with a history of contrast-induced anaphylaxis.<br>• Renal failure is usually reversible following contrast administration; caution contrast use in age > 70 years, volume depletion, chronic kidney disease, heart failure, and diabetes. | **Head:** acute stroke, head injuries, severe headache, tumors, hydrocephalus<br>**Chest:** chest pain or dyspneic complaints, tumors, pneumonia, interstitial lung disease, evaluation of chest abnormalities detected on X-ray, yearly lung cancer screening.<br>**Abdomen/pelvis:** abdominal or pelvic pain of unknown etiology, infections (e.g., abscesses), diverticulitis, inflammatory bowel disease, cirrhosis, malignancies, nephrolithiasis, pancreatitis, abdominal aortic aneurysm<br>**Extremities:** soft tissue swelling, infection, trauma; peripheral arterial disease | • Will need CT perfusion or non-contrast enhanced CT of the head in acute stroke.<br>• CT angiography (CTA) ordered when evaluating for brain tumors.<br>• Order an annual low-dose chest CT when screening individuals for lung cancer.<br>• Angiography ordered if pulmonary embolism suspected.<br>• CT enterography is useful when identifying disorders of the small bowel, such as tumors, abscesses or fistulas, or bowel obstruction; used to diagnose inflammatory bowel disease. Angiography is needed with cancer staging. Order a CT colonography to screen for colon cancer. |

| | | |
|---|---|---|
| • Metformin should be discontinued on the day contrast is administered, up to 48 hours afterwards, and ensuring renal function stable. | **Spine:** spinal pain, measures bone density, vertebral metastases, spinal stenosis, infections, vertebral fracture | • When CT of an extremity is ordered, angiography is ordered in peripheral arterial disease.<br>• MRI offers more detail on the spinal cord compression than a CT scan. |
| **Magnetic resonance imaging (MRI)**[1,3,4,5,6]<br>• Does not use radiation; takes longer than CT examinations.<br>• Contraindications: pacemaker or implantable cardioverter defibrillator (ICD), clips for brain aneurysms, certain implants.<br>• The contrast used (gadolinium) is unlikely to cause an allergic reaction.<br>• Evaluate renal function prior to test (although rare, nephrogenic systemic fibrosis occurs with severely impaired function).<br>• MR angiography (MRA) is ordered over CTA if unable to tolerate contrast media. | **Head:** acute stroke, infections, tumors, hydrocephalus<br>**Chest:** detect tumors, evaluation of cardiac and vascular structures, heart valve abnormalities<br>**Abdomen/pelvis:** abdominal or pelvic pain, evaluation of blood flow and lymph nodes, tumors, abscesses, liver disease<br>**Musculoskeletal system:** degenerative arthritis, tumors involving bones and joints, herniated disk, joint abnormalities (e.g., ligament or cartilage tears), spinal back pain, fractures, osteomyelitis | • MRI imaging of the brain offers more anatomy detail than CT (greater sensitivity in early brain metastases).<br>• CT of chest is typically preferred over MRI when evaluating for lung abnormalities.<br>• MRI of the abdomen/pelvis assists in staging cancers and clarifying findings from CT scan.<br>• For most musculoskeletal concerns, MRI is the procedure of choice. |

(Continues)

| Imaging Type | Indications | Clinical Notes |
|---|---|---|
| **X-ray (radiography)**[1,3,4,6]<br>• The radiation associated with X-rays is minimal.<br>• Accuracy of diagnosis is limited. | **Bone:** fractures, joint dislocation, arthritis<br>**Chest:** chest pain or dyspneic complaints, pneumonia, heart failure<br>**Abdomen:** abdominal pain or nausea/vomiting with unknown etiology, ensure placement of feeding tube, intestinal obstruction, constipation, nephrolithiasis | • Quickest imaging test that can determine bone injury.<br>• An X-ray is often times ordered first with indications seen next to the chest.<br>• If more detail is needed after abdominal X-ray ordered, order further imaging such as CT of the abdomen and pelvis. |
| **Ultrasound**[1,3,4,6]<br>Ultrasound is a safe procedure with no known harmful effects (no radiation). | **Abdomen:** abdominal pain, acute cholecystitis, elevated liver enzymes, obstructive biliary disease, abdominal aorta, cirrhosis<br>**Heart** (echocardiography): evaluates the valves and blood flow; post stroke, myocardial infarctions, heart failure<br>**Extremities:** deep vein thrombosis, peripheral arterial disease | • After initial ultrasound, order CT and/or MRI for further visualization.<br>• Transthoracic echocardiography (TTE) is the most common type of echocardiography ordered.<br>• Order a vascular ultrasound of the affected extremity. |

# References


1. American College of Radiology. (n.d.). Retrieved from https://www.acr.org/. Accessed October 26, 2017.
2. Rawson, J. V., & Pelletier, A. L. (2013, September 1). When to order contrast-enhanced CT. *American Family Physician, 88*(5), 312–316. Retrieved from http://www.aafp.org/afp/2013/0901/p312.html. Accessed October 26, 2017.
3. Ilasan, H. (n.d.). Overview of Imaging Tests – Special Subjects. Merck Manuals: Professional. Retrieved from https://www.merckmanuals.com/home/special-subjects/common-imaging-tests/overview-of-imaging-tests. Accessed October 26, 2017.
4. Gastrointestinal imaging. In *Introduction to Diagnostic Radiology.* New York, NY: McGraw-Hill. Retrieved from http://accessmedicine.mhmedical.com/content.aspx?bookid=1562&sectionid=95877120. Accessed October 25, 2017.
5. Jacobson, F. L., & McKean, S. C. (2016). Introduction to radiology. In *Principles and Practice of Hospital Medicine* (2nd ed.). New York, NY: McGraw-Hill. Retrieved from http://accessmedicine.mhmedical.com/content.aspx?bookid=1872&sectionid=146978297. Accessed October 25, 2017.
6. National Library of Medicine, National Institutes of Health. (2017, September). Databases. Retrieved from https://www.nlm.nih.gov/?_ga=2.63715881.769328030.1507665199-1049439008.1471202369. Accessed October 26, 2017.

SECTION XI

# Beers List

These are medications that should be used with caution in adults $\geq 65$ years of age due to potentially harmful effects. The decision to use these drugs should be tailored to the individual patient and circumstances.

| Drug Type or Class and Example(s) | Clinical Relevance |
|---|---|
| **ALLERGY** | |
| **First-generation antihistamines:** diphenhydramine (Benadryl), [1,6] hydroxyzine (Vistaril), [1,6] promethazine (Phenergan), [1,6] | They have significant anticholinergic properties.*[1,3,6,16] Avoid especially in those with delirium, dementia, or cognitive impairment.[1,6] Alternatives: nasal lavage with intranasal saline rinses,[6] nasal steroids,[6] or nonsedating second-generation antihistamine (e.g., cetirizine [Zyrtec]).[6] |
| **ANTIBIOTIC** | |
| Nitrofurantoin (Macrobid)[1] | Risk of peripheral neuropathy, liver impairment, and/or pulmonary fibrosis when used long term; should be avoided for creatinine clearance (CrCl) $\leq$ 30 ml/min.[1,16] |
| **CARDIOVASCULAR** | |
| **Antiarrhythmics:** | |
| • Amiodarone[1] (Pacerone, Cordarone) | Carries high potential for toxicities, QT prolongation, arrhythmias, severe bradycardia, lung toxicity.[1] *Avoid as primary agent unless presence of heart failure or significant left ventricular hypertrophy.*[1,16] |
| • Digoxin (Lanoxin)[1,3,6] | Renal insufficiency leads to toxic effects (e.g., fatal arrhythmias).[1,7] Doses are not to exceed $\geq$ 125 mcg.[1,16] *Avoid as primary agent in atrial fibrillation or heart failure.*[1,7,16] |
| • Disopyramide (Norpace) immediate release | Has significant anticholinergic properties; caution use in those with heart failure.[1] Alternative: nondihydropyridines calcium channel blocker (CCB) or a beta blocker.[6,16] |
| • Dronedarone (Multaq) | Avoid in those with persistent atrial fibrillation or severe heart failure (associated with poor outcomes and heart failure exacerbation).[1] |

| | |
|---|---|
| **Anticoagulants:** | |
| • Dabigatran (Pradaxa)[1] | Higher risk of bleeding compared with other anticoagulants[1]; caution use if CrCl < 30 mL/min or age ≥ 75 years.[1] |
| • Others: apixaban (Eliquis), enoxaparin (Lovenox)[1] | Risk of bleeding; may need to avoid completely or reduce dose, depending upon renal function[1] (apixaban requires evaluation of renal impairment, age, and weight).[1] |
| **Antiplatelets:** | |
| • Aspirin (Bufferin, Ecotrin)[1] | Risk of bleeding; insufficient evidence to support its use for primary prevention in those ≥ age 80 years old.[1] |
| • Dipyridamole (Persantine)[1,6] | Severe hypotension.[1] Alternative: clopidogrel (Plavix) or aspirin/dipyridamole (Aggrenox) for secondary prevention of noncardioembolic stroke.[6] |
| **Dihydropyridine calcium channel blockers (CCBs):** nifedipine (Procardia)[6] | Risk of severe hypotension and myocardial infarction.[1] Alternative: Switch to a long-acting dihydropyridine CCB (e.g., amlodipine [Norvasc], felodipine [Plendil]).[6] |
| **Nondihydropyridine CCBs:** diltiazem (Cardizem) and verapamil (Calan) | Can exacerbate heart failure.[1] |
| **Peripheral alpha blockers:** doxazosin (Cardura), terazosin (Hytrin), prazosin (Minipress)[1] | Risk of postural hypotension,[1] dizziness; caution taking these medications in combination with loop diuretics (urinary incontinence is increased in females).[1] |
| **Potassium-sparing diuretics:** spironolactone (Aldactone),[1] triamterene (Dyrenium)[1] | Avoid use with CrCl < 30 mL/min; risk of hyperkalemia and renal injury,[1] especially if also taking a nonsteroidal anti-inflammatory drug (NSAID), angiotensin-converting enzyme (ACE) inhibitor or angiotensin-receptor blocker (ARB), potassium supplement. |

| Drug Type or Class and Example(s) | Clinical Relevance |
|---|---|
| **ENDOCRINE** | |
| **Corticosteroids:** | |
| oral methylprednisolone (Medrol), prednisone (Rayos), dexamethasone | Can cause psychosis, worsens heart failure; can cause or worsen delirium.[1] Use lowest dose and duration for chronic conditions, such as asthma or chronic obstructive pulmonary disease.[1] |
| **Diabetic agents:** | |
| Thiazolidinediones: pioglitazone (Actos), rosidglitazone (Avandia)[1] | Can exacerbate heart failure.[1] |
| Sliding scale insulin, fast-acting: lispro (Humalog)[1,8] | Is more of a reactive approach to glycemic control; does not effectively treat hyperglycemia and results in more hypoglycemic events.[1,8,16] |
| Sulfonylurea: chlorpropamide and glyburide (DiaBeta)[6] | Prolonged hypoglycemia.[1,16] Alternative: glipizide (Glucotrol) or metformin (Glucophage, Glumetza).[6] |
| **Estrogens:** | |
| (PO or transdermal), with or without progestin[1,6] | Carry risk of breast, ovarian, and endometrial cancer, and thromboembolism.[1,6] Alternative: vasomotor symptoms → escitalopram (Lexapro), venlafaxine (Effexor), and/or or gabapentin (Neurontin, Gralise).[6] Alternative: vulvovaginal atrophy → over-the-counter (OTC) vaginal lubricants or moisturizers; vaginal estrogen (e.g., Premarin Vaginal).[1,6] |
| **Megestrol (Megace)** | Not very effective[1]; carries risk of thromboembolic events.[1,10,16] Alternatives: nutritional supplements (e.g., shakes, puddings), flavor enhancers; if depression present, consider mirtazapine (Remeron).[10] |
| **Androgens:** | |
| testosterone (Striant)[1] | Carry risk of venous thromboembolism and myocardial infarction.[1] Exception: symptomatic hypogonadism.[1] |

| | |
|---|---|
| **GASTROINTESTINAL** | |
| **Antiemetics:** | |
| prochlorperazine and promethazine (Phenergan,)[1] | Have significant anticholinergic properties.*[1,18] Can cause or worsen delirium; avoid especially in those with dementia or cognitive impairment.[1] |
| Metoclopramide (Reglan)[1] | Risk of extrapyramidal symptoms, dystonia, tardive dyskinesia.[1] Caution use in Parkinson's disease. Exception: gastroparesis.[11] Alternative to antiemetics: ondansetron (Zofran).[18] |
| **Antispasmodics:**[1] dicyclomine (Bentyl)[1], hyoscyamine (Levsin,[1] Levbid), scopolamine *(excluding ophthalmic)*[1] | |
| **Histamine-2 (H2) blockers:** ranitidine (Zantac), famotidine (Pepcid)[1,6] | Can cause or worsen delirium; avoid especially in those with dementia or cognitive impairment.[1] Caution use with impaired renal function.[1] Alternative: proton pump inhibitor (PPI) (generally are well tolerated; try and use for under 2 months).[6,19] |
| **Laxative:** oral mineral oil[1] | Risk of aspiration.[1] Alternatives: behavioral interventions (e.g., scheduled toileting), increased fluid and fiber intake, bulking agents (e.g., psyllium [Metamucil], polyethylene glycol, docusate sodium, linaclotide [Linzess], lubiprostone [Amitiza]).[11] |

| Drug Type or Class and Example(s) | Clinical Relevance |
| --- | --- |
| **Proton pump inhibitors (PPIs):** omeprazole (Prilosec), pantoprazole (Protonix), esomeprazole (Nexium) | Using beyond 2 months is associated with *Clostridium difficile* infection, bone fracture, vitamin B12 deficiency, hypomagnesemia.[1,12,19,20] Exception: can use if indicated (e.g., ongoing NSAID use, erosive esophagitis).[1] Use lowest effective dose.[19] |
| <u>**GOUT**</u> Probenecid and colchicine (Colcrys, Mitigare)[1] | Increased risk of gastrointestinal symptoms (e.g., nausea), aplastic anemia. Avoid or reduce dose for CrCL $< 30$.[1] |
| <u>**PAIN RELIEVING**</u> **Muscle relaxants:** cyclobenzaprine (Flexeril),[1] metaxalone (Skelaxin),[1] methocarbamol (Robaxin),[1] orphenadrine (Norflex[1])[1,6] | Have significant anticholinergic properties* (especially cyclobenzaprine and orphenadrine)[1]; risk of fractures.[1,16] |
| **NSAIDs:** ibuprofen (Advil, Motrin), meloxicam (Mobic, Vivlodex), naproxen (Naprosyn)[1] | Risk of gastrointestinal bleeding with chronic use (use of PPI decreases this risk).[1,6] Can exacerbate heart failure and worsen renal function.[1,6] |
| Indomethacin (Indocin)[1,6] | More adverse effects than the other NSAIDs; risk of bleeding. Can worsen heart failure.[1] |

| | |
|---|---|
| **Opioids:** meperidine (Demerol)[1,6] and pentazocine (Talwin)[6] | Carry central nervous system (CNS) adverse effects, especially in those with renal impairment;[1] risk of orthostatic hypotension, syncope, ataxia.[1] Associated with falls, drug diversion, and misuse.[2] Evidence is lacking on long-term use of opioids in the setting of noncancerous pain.[2] Caution use in those with history of falls or fractures.[1,2]<br>Exception: prior joint replacement surgery or fractures.[1]<br>Alternative pain medications: acetaminophen (Tylenol),[1,2,6] salicylates (e.g., choline magnesium trisalicylate),[1,6] topical NSAID[2,6] (e.g., Voltaren gel), tramadol[2,6] (ConZip, Ultram), oral NSAID (*avoid long term given gastrointestinal, cardiac, and renal risks*),[2,6] topical lidocaine.[2,16] Opioids if the above fail and pain interferes with physical functioning: oxycodone, morphine, hydrocodone.[2,6] Pregabalin, gabapentin, serotonin, and norepinephrine reuptake inhibitor (SNRI) for neuropathic pain.[1,2,6]<br>Nonpharmacological interventions: physical and occupational therapy referral, professional cognitive-behavioral therapy, acupuncture, massage, involvement in exercise program.[2] |
| **PARKINSONISM**<br>Benztropine (Cogentin) oral form[1,6]<br>Trihexyphenidyl[1,6] | Has significant anticholinergic properties.*[1] Can cause or worsen delirium; avoid especially in those with dementia or cognitive impairment.[1]<br>Alternative: carbidopa-levodopa (Sinemet).[6] |

| Drug Type or Class and Example(s) | Clinical Relevance |
| --- | --- |
| **PSYCHOTROPIC** | |
| **Antidepressants:**<br>SSRI → paroxetine (Paxil)[1]<br>Tricyclics → amitriptyline (Elavil), nortriptyline (Pamelor)[1,6,16] | Have significant anticholinergic properties.[1,13,16] Risk of postural hypotension, syncope, ataxia, hyponatremia.[1,13] Can cause or worsen delirium; avoid especially in those with dementia or cognitive impairment, history of falls or fractures.[1,6]<br>Alternatives: a selective serotonin reuptake inhibitor (SSRI) with fewer adverse effects and drug–drug interactions (e.g., citalopram [Celexa], escitalopram [Lexapro], sertraline [Zoloft]),[13] SNRI (e.g., venlafaxine [Effexor]), mirtazapine (Remeron) or bupropion (Wellbutrin).[6,13] |
| **Anticonvulsants:**<br>carbamazepine (Tegretol), phenytoin (Dilantin, Phenytek)[1,6] | Carry CNS adverse effects; use with caution in those with a history of unsteady gait, falls, or fractures.[6]<br>Alternatives: lamotrigine (Lamictal), levetiracetam (Keppra).[6] |
| **Antipsychotics:**<br>first-generation (e.g., haloperidol [Haldol], chlorpromazine [Thorazine], fluphenazine [Prolixin])[1] or second-generation (e.g., risperidone [Risperdal], aripiprazole [Abilify], clozapine [Clozaril])[1] | Some have significant anticholinergic properties.*[1] Cause somnolence, dizziness, postural hypotension, ataxia, hyponatremia; can worsen parkinsonian symptoms.[1]<br>Limited effectiveness;[1,6] associated with increased mortality, strokes, falls, and fractures.[1,6,16]<br>Avoid use in dementia-related psychosis.[1,16]<br>Exception: can use in behavioral problems of dementia or delirium if nondrug measures were unsuccessful and patient is a harm to self or others.[1,6]<br>Use for short term.[6]<br>To learn more about nondrug measures in effort to avoid antipsychotics, go to www.nursinghometoolkit.com.[1] |

| | |
|---|---|
| **Barbituates:**<br>phenobarbital (Solfoton), butalbital (Fioricet)[6] | Risk of dependency, abuse;[1] sedation, ataxia; can cause or worsen delirium.[1]<br>Alternative: If used for epilepsy, switch to levetiracetam (Keppra) or lamotrigine (Lamictal).[6] |
| **Benzodiazepines:**<br>lorazepam (Ativan)[1], alprazolam (Xanax)[1], clonazepam (Klonopin)[1], diazepam (Valium)[1] | Increase risk of CNS adverse effects, falls, and fractures;[1,6,16] avoid especially in those with delirium, dementia, or cognitive impairment.[1,16]<br>Alternative: buspirone (Buspar), SSRI, or SNRI.[6] |
| **Hypnotics/Insomnia:**<br>eszopiclone (Lunesta), zolpidem (Ambien), zaleplon (Sonata) | Increase risk of CNS adverse effects, falls, and fractures[1,6,16] and are minimally effective.[1,14]<br>Avoid especially in those with delirium, dementia, or cognitive impairment.[1]<br>Alternatives: psychological interventions (e.g., sleep restrictions), melatonin.[6,14,15] |
| **Stimulants:**<br>amphetamines (Adderall), methylphenidate (Ritalin, Concerta)[1] | Increase risk of CNS adverse effects; dependency, abuse; psychosis, aggressive behavior; prevents sleep.[1] |

| Drug Type or Class and Example(s) | Clinical Relevance |
|---|---|
| **URINARY INCONTINENCE** | |
| oxybutynin (Ditropan XL), tolterodine (Detrol)[1] | Have significant anticholinergic properties.*[1] Can cause or worsen delirium; avoid especially in those with dementia or cognitive impairment, history of falls or fractures.[1]<br>Alternatives: behavioral interventions (e.g., avoiding caffeine and alcohol, bladder training, consultation with pelvic floor physical therapist).[1,17] |

* Anticholinergic properties include, but are not limited to, mental or behavioral changes (e.g., nervousness, disorientation, hallucinations, delirium), dizziness, dry mouth, urinary retention, constipation, and visual changes.[3,6]

# References


1. American Geriatrics Society 2015 Beers Criteria Update Expert Panel, Fick, D. M., Semla, T. P., Beizer, J., Brandt, N., & Dombrowski, R., . . .Steinman, M. (2015, October 8). American Geriatrics Society 2015 updated Beers criteria for potentially inappropriate medication use in older adults. *Journal of the American Geriatrics Society, 63*(11), 2227–2246. Retrieved from http://onlinelibrary.wiley.com/doi/10.1111/jgs.13702/abstract. Accessed October 3, 2017.
2. Makris, U. E., Abrams, R. C., Gurland, B., & Reid, M. C. (2014, August 27). Management of persistent pain in the older patient: A clinical review. *JAMA, 312*(8), 825–836. Retrieved from https://www.ncbi.nlm.nih.gov/pmc/articles/PMC4372897/. Accessed October 7, 2017.
3. Gray, S. L., & Hanlon, J. T. (2016, October). Anticholinergic medication use and dementia: Latest evidence and clinical implications. *Therapeutic Advances in Drug Safety,* 7(5), 217–224. Retrieved from https://www.ncbi.nlm.nih.gov/pmc/articles/PMC5014048/. Accessed October 3, 2017.
4. Kumar, K., & Manning, W. J. (2016, October 10). Rhythm Control versus Rate Control in Atrial Fibrillation. UpToDate. Retrieved from https://www.uptodate.com/contents/rhythm-control-versus-rate-control-in-atrial-fibrillation. Accessed October 3, 2017.
5. Coggins, M. D. (2012). Sliding-scale insulin: An ineffective practice. *Aging Well,* 5(6), 8. Retrieved from http://www.todaysgeriatricmedicine.com/archive/110612p8.shtml. Accessed October 3, 2017.
6. Hanlon, J. T., Semla, T. P., & Schmader, K. E. (2015). Alternative Medications for Medications in the Use of High-Risk Medications in the Elderly and Potentially Harmful Drug-Disease Interactions in the Elderly Quality Measures. American Geriatrics Society. Retrieved from http://micmrc.org/system/files/AGS%202015%20Beers%20Criteria%20Alternative%20Medications%20List.pdf. Accessed October 3, 2017.
7. Pincus, M. (2016, February). Management of digoxin toxicity. *Australian Prescriber, 39*(1), 18–20. Retrieved from https://www.ncbi.nlm.nih.gov/pmc/articles/PMC4816869/. Accessed October 7, 2017.
8. Moses, M. S. (2017, October 4). Insulin Sliding Scale. Family Practice Notebook. Retrieved from http://www.fpnotebook.com/Endo/Pharm/InslnSldngScl.htm. Accessed October 7, 2017.
9. North American Menopause Society (NAMS). (2013, September). Management of symptomatic vulvovaginal atrophy: 2013 position statement of The North American Menopause Society. *Menopause, 20*(9), 888–902. Retrieved from https://www.ncbi.nlm.nih.gov/pubmed/23985562. Accessed October 7, 2017.
10. Gaddey, H. L., & Holder, K. (2014, May 1). Unintentional weight loss in older adults. *American Family Physician,* 89(9), 718–722. Retrieved from http://www.aafp.org/afp/2014/0501/p718.html. Accessed October 7, 2017.
11. Mounsey, A., Raleigh, M. F., & Wilson, A. (2015, September 15). Management of constipation in older adults. *American Family Physician,* 92(6), 500–504. Retrieved from http://www.aafp.org/afp/2015/0915/p500.html. Accessed October 7, 2017.
12. Lam, J. R., Schneider, J. L., Zhao, W., & Corley, D. A. (2013, December 11). Proton pump inhibitor and histamine 2 receptor antagonist use and Vitamin B12 deficiency. *JAMA, 310*(22), 2435–2442. Retrieved from https://jamanetwork.com/journals/jama/fullarticle/1788456. Accessed October 7, 2017.

13. Wiese, B. S. (2011, September). Geriatric depression: The use of antidepressants in the elderly. *British Columbia Medical Journal,* 53(7), 341–347. Retrieved from http://www.bcmj.org/articles/geriatric-depression-use-antidepressants-elderly. Accessed October 7, 2017.
14. Rodriguez, J. C., Dzierzewski, J. M., & Alessi, C. A. (2015, March). Sleep problems in the elderly. *Medical Clinics of North America,* 99(2), 431–439. Retrieved from https://www.ncbi.nlm.nih.gov/pmc/articles/PMC4406253/. Accessed October 7, 2017.
15. Xiong, G. L. (2017, September 25). Geriatric Sleep Disorder Medication. Medscape. Retrieved from http://emedicine.medscape.com/article/292498-medication. Accessed October 7, 2017.
16. Terrery, C. L., & Nicoteri, J. L. (2016, March). The 2015 American Geriatric Society Beers criteria: Implications for nurse practitioners. *Journal for Nurse Practioners, 12*(3), 192–200. Retrieved from http://www.npjournal.org/article/S1555-4155(15)01124-1/fulltext. Accessed October 7, 2017.
17. Ellsworth, P. I. (2017, September 19). Overactive Bladder Treatment & Management. Medscape. Retrieved from http://emedicine.medscape.com/article/459340-treatment. Accessed October 7, 2017.
18. Brainard, A. (2017, July 19). Motion Sickness Medication. Medscape. Retrieved from http://emedicine.medscape.com/article/2060606-medication. Accessed October 7, 2017.
19. Vaezi, M. F., Yang, Y., & Howden, C. W. (2017). Complications of proton pump inhibitor therapy. *Gastroenterology, 153*(1), 35–48. doi:10.1053/j.gastro.2017.04.047
20. Therapeutic Research Center. (2015, December). PL Detail-Document, Potentially Harmful Drugs in the Elderly: Beers List. Pharmacist's Letter/Prescriber's Letter.
21. Epocrates. (n.d.). Retrieved from https://www.epocrates.com (used for brand and generic names, along with a few adverse effects [benzodiazapines, hypnotics, testosterone, Reglan, indomethacin, peripheral alpha blockers, antipsychotics, Sudafed, tegretol, gabapentin, Lyrica, amiodarone, dipyradamole, dronedarone, dabigatran, apixaban, nifedipine, alternative long-acting dihydropyridine CCBs, steroids, PPIs], vitamin B12 deficiency, and gout information). Accessed October 7, 2017.

SECTION XII

# Common Presentations

## Dizziness

### Definition[1,2,3,4,5,6,7,8,9,10,12]

Dizziness is a nonspecific term used by patients to describe a sensation. Symptoms lasting less than 2 months is acute dizziness or chronic for symptoms beyond 2 months.

Sensation is classified as vertigo (i.e., sense of spinning), disequilibrium (i.e., sense of imbalance or gait abnormality), presyncope (i.e., sense of an impending faint), and/or light headedness.

- Differentiating between the four categories of dizziness is of low clinical significance given patients have difficulty explaining their symptoms.

### Causes[1,2,3,4,5,6,7,8,9,10,11,12]

| Causes | Medical Condition |
|---|---|
| **Peripheral causes** | • Benign paroxysmal positional vertigo (BPPV)<br>• Meniere's disease |
| **Central causes** | • Vertebrobasilar insufficiency or infarction<br>• Posterior fossa tumor |
| **Other causes** | • Medication effects (e.g., antihypertensives, diuretics, anticholinergics, antipsychotics)<br>• Orthostatic hypotension<br>• Psychogenic (anxiety, depression)<br>• Acute anemia<br>• Hypoglycemia<br>• Dehydration<br>• Sensory impairment (visual, hearing)<br>• Parkinson's disease<br>• Peripheral neuropathy<br>• Vitamin B12 deficiency<br>• Cardiac arrhythmia |

## Tests[1,5,6,8,9,12]

- Orthostatic vital sign measurement
    - Helps to identify orthostatic hypotension.
- Dix-Hallpike maneuver
    - Used to diagnose BPPV.
- Reasonable to order a complete blood count (CBC), glucose, basic metabolic panel (BMP), thyroid-stimulating hormone (TSH), vitamin B12
    - Evaluate for anemia, diabetes, metabolic impairment, azotemia, hypothyroidism, vitamin B12 deficiency.
- Electrocardiogram and/or Holter monitor
    - If abnormal cardiac rhythm suspected.
- Neuroimaging (e.g., brain magnetic resonance imaging [MRI])
    - If concern for central pathology.

## Treatment & Management[5,6,8,9,10,12,13,14]

- **Identify and treat the underlying issue(s),** such as:
  *(The etiology of dizziness in older adults is multifactorial.)*
    - Correction of anemia, metabolic derangements, vitamin B12 deficiency, thyroid disease.
    - Correction of sensory impairments (vision and hearing).
    - Treat anxiety and depression.
    - Reduce or stop the offending medication.
    - Epley maneuver: used to treat BPPV.
    - Salt restriction recommended for treatment of Meniere's disease.
- **Nonpharmacological and nursing interventions:**
    - Focus on the impact of dizziness.
        - Safety measures for prevention of falls
    - Educate about the adverse effects of medications.
- **Pharmacological and other interventions:**
    - Drugs are used to treat acute onset nausea, vomiting, vertigo, and anxiety for short term.

    - Meclizine (Antivert), scopolamine, or diazepam (Valium)
        - Meclizine and scopolamine are highly anticholinergic.
        - Diazepam increases risk of falls, delirium, and fractures.
- Vestibular rehabilitation
    - Recommended for chronic dizziness.

Note: Beers listed items, as mentioned above, include meclizine, scopolamine, and diazepam.

## CLINICAL PEARLS[1,3,4,5,6,8,9,10,11,12]

- Perform a full exam to guide diagnosis and treatment plan (e.g., check for irregular cardiac rhythm, ear cerumen, gait pattern, nystagmus).
- BPPV, which accounts for half of all vertigo in older adults, is best managed with repositioning maneuvers. Medications, such as meclizine (Antivert), have no role in BPPV and have unfavorable adverse effects and prolong recovery.
- Watch for red flags, such as acute onset vertigo and neurological findings (e.g., vertical nystagmus, diplopia, hearing loss, headache), which are signs of central etiology.
    - Will need immediate neuroimaging and treatment.

## References

1. Marill, K. A. (2017, August 29). Central Vertigo. Medscape. Retrieved from http://emedicine.medscape.com/article/794789-overview. Accessed September 30, 2017.
2. Conde, M. V., Wang, E., & Henderson, M. C. (2012). Chapter 6. Dizziness. In Henderson, M. C., Tierney, L. M., Jr., & Smetana, G. W. (Eds.). *The Patient History: An Evidence-Based Approach to Differential Diagnosis*. New York, NY: McGraw-Hill. Retrieved from http://accessmedicine.mhmedical.com/content.aspx?bookid=500&sectionid=41026549. Accessed September 30, 2017.
3. Thompson, T. L., & Amedee, R. (2009, Spring). Vertigo: A review of common peripheral and central vestibular disorders. *Ochsner Journal*, 9(1), 20–26. Retrieved from https://www.ncbi.nlm.nih.gov/pmc/articles/PMC3096243/. Accessed September 30, 2017.
4. Shaia, W. T. (2017, September 21). Dizziness Evaluation. Medscape. Retrieved from http://emedicine.medscape.com/article/1831429-overview#a1/. Accessed September 30, 2017.

5. Douglas, S. A., & Gibson, W. (2016, October 24). Evaluation of Dizziness. Epocrates. Retrieved from https://online.epocrates.com/diseases/71/Evaluation-of-dizziness/. Accessed September 30, 2017.
6. Vestibular Disorders Association (VeDA). (2016, April 18). About Vestibular Disorders. Retrieved from http://vestibular.org/understanding-vestibular-disorder/. Accessed September 30, 2017.
7. Collie, M. J., & Ramsey, A. R. (2014). Differentiating benign paroxysmal positional vertigo from other causes of dizziness. *Journal for Nurse Practitioners, 10*(6), 393–400. doi:10.1016/j.nurpra.2014.03.008
8. Dizziness. In *Hazzard's Geriatric Medicine and Gerontology* (7th ed.). New York, NY: McGraw-Hill. Retrieved from http:/accessmedicine.mhmedical.com/content.aspx?bookid=1923&sectionid=144522011. Accessed September 30, 2017.
9. Buttaro, T. M., Trybulski, J., Bailey, P. P., & Sandberk-Cook, J. (2008).Dizziness and vertigo. In McQueen, N. L. (Ed.). *Primary Care A Collaborative Practice* (pp. 1045–1049). St. Louis, MO: Mosby Elsevier.
10. Watford, K. E. (2013). 5-minute diagnosis of dizziness. *Journal for Nurse Practitioners,* 9(10), 712–713. doi:10.1016/j.nurpra.2013.07.010
11. Kaski, D. (2015, May 20). Understanding and managing the dizzy patient. *Nursing in Practice.* Retrieved from https://www.nursinginpractice.com/article/understanding-and-managing-dizzy-patient. Accessed October 1, 2017.
12. Muncie, H. L., Sirmans, S. M., & James, E. (2017). Dizziness: Approach to evaluation and management. *American Family Physician,* 95(3), 154–161.
13. Nettina, S. M. (2001). Comprehensive Management of Dizziness in Elderly Clients. Medscape. Retrieved from https://www.medscape.com/viewarticle/408404_1. Accessed October 29, 2017.
14. American Geriatrics Society 2015 Beers Criteria Update Expert Panel, Fick, D. M., Semla, T. P., Beizer, J., Brandt, N., & Dombrowski, R., . . . Steinman, M. (2015, October 8). American Geriatrics Society 2015 updated Beers criteria for potentially inappropriate medication use in older adults. *Journal of the American Geriatrics Society,* 63(11), 2227–2246. Retrieved from http://onlinelibrary.wiley.com/doi/10.1111/jgs.13702/abstract. Accessed October 3, 2017.


# Headache

## Definition[1,2,4,5,7]

Headaches *(i.e., any part of the head that causes discomfort)* after the age of 50 are typically secondary, which means they occur from an underlying condition.

Chronic headache: headaches occurring ≥ 15 times per month, for a minimum of 3 months.

## Signs & Symptoms[1,2,3,4,5,6,7,8,10]

Although not exhaustive, below are signs and symptoms of secondary headaches encountered in older adults:

| Secondary Headache | Typical Features |
|---|---|
| Temporal arteritis or giant cell arteritis (GCA) | Throbbing temple pain, temporal artery tenderness, visual changes, myalgias, weight loss, fatigue, jaw claudication. |
| Trigeminal neuralgia (TN) | Sudden, severe, unilateral facial pain that feels like an electrical shock; exacerbated by chewing or talking. |
| Intracranial tumor | Generalized headache, change in mental state, focal neurological deficits, nausea, vomiting, visual changes, ataxia. |
| Intracranial hemorrhage (e.g., subdural, subarachnoid) | Sudden, severe headache (subarachnoid hemorrhage), changes in mental state (e.g., confusion, loss of alertness). |
| Cerebrovascular accident (i.e., hemorrhagic or ischemic strokes) | Sudden or insidious headache, focal neurological deficits. |
| Uncontrolled arterial hypertension | Chronic morning headache, severe, sudden headaches, angina, dizziness. |
| Medication related (i.e., overuse or side effects) | Headache worsens after taking offending medication; headache frequency worsens with time, variable location and intensity. |

## Tests[1,2,3,4,7]

- Head computed tomography (CT) and/or magnetic resonance imaging (MRI)
    - Recommended especially with acute focal neurological deficits, severe headache, headache following trauma, mental status changes, presumed brain lesion.
    - Brain MRI is *more sensitive* over CT. CT is however more widely used and is quicker than MRI.
- Erythrocyte sedimentation rate (ESR) and C-reactive protein (CRP)
    - If GCA suspected.

- Temporal artery biopsy
  - Diagnostic for GCA.

## Treatment & Management[2,3,6,7,8,9,11,12,13,14,15]

- **Identify and treat the underlying issue:**
  - GCA responds well to corticosteroids such as prednisone; treatment is required to prevent blindness.
  - Trigeminal neuralgia responds well to low-dose carbamazepine (Tegretol, Carbatrol, Equetro); other options: topiramate (Topamax), lamotrigine (Lamictal).
    - Carbamazepine may cause hyponatremia.
  - Brain tumor treatment should be individualized; consider performance status, comorbidities, and life expectancy. Treatment can range from surgical, medical, and/or palliative care.
  - Acute onset headache from intracranial hemorrhage and/or stroke should be managed in hospital for appropriate treatment.
  - Treat the hypertension.
  - Discontinue or taper the medication causing the headaches. Medications that can cause headaches include:
    - Analgesics (e.g., caffeine, nonsteroidal anti-inflammatory drugs [NSAIDs], aspirin), estrogens/progestin, opioids, selective serotonin reuptake inhibitors (SSRIs), triptans, nitrates.
- **Nonpharmacological and nursing interventions:**
  - Implement strategies to decrease intracranial pressure (e.g., maintain head of bed elevation, maintain normal oxygen levels and body temperature).
  - Encourage use of a headache diary (*offers clues on potential triggers*).
- **Pharmacological interventions:**

  *As mentioned above, depends on the underlying cause.*
  - Avoid opioids.
- Referral to appropriate specialists (e.g., ophthalmologist for GCA)

Note: Beers listed items, as mentioned above, include opioids, carbamazepine, and oral corticosteroids.

**CLINICAL PEARL[1,2]**

- New onset headache after the age of 50 warrants investigation (usually from a critical underlying condition).

## References


1. Silberstein, S. D. (2016, July). Approach to the Patient With Headache – Neurologic Disorders. Merck Manuals: Professional. Retrieved from https://www.merckmanuals.com/professional/neurologic-disorders/headache/approach-to-the-patient-with-headache. Accessed October 27, 2017.
2. Anderson, K., & Wold, J.Treating headaches in older adults. In *Current Diagnosis & Treatment: Geriatrics* (2nd ed.). New York, NY: McGraw-Hill. Retrieved from http://accessmedicine.mhmedical.com/content.aspx?bookid=953&sectionid=53375685. Accessed October 27, 2017.
3. Hainer, B. L., & Matheson, E. (2013, May 15). Approach to acute headache in adults. *American Family Physician,* 87(10), 682–687. Retrieved from http://www.aafp.org/afp/2013/0515/p682.html. Accessed October 27, 2017.
4. Green, M. W. (2012). Secondary Headaches. Lebanese Society of Neurology. Retrieved from http://www.lsneuro.org/files/c/headache/Secondary%20Headaches.pdf. Accessed October 27, 2017.
5. National Institute of Neurological Disorders and Stroke (NINDS). (n.d.). Headache Information Page. National Institutes of Health. Retrieved from https://www.ninds.nih.gov/Disorders/All-Disorders/Headache-Information-Page. Accessed October 28, 2017.
6. Beck, E. (2013, May 15). Hard-to-diagnose headache: Practical tips for diagnosis and treatment. *American Family Physician,* 87(10), 672–673. Retrieved from http://www.aafp.org/afp/2013/0515/p672.html. Accessed October 28, 2017.
7. Halker, R. B., Hastriter, E. V., & Dodick, D. W. (2011, February 15). Chronic daily headache: An evidence-based and systematic approach to a challenging problem. *Neurology,* 76(7 Suppl 2), S37–43. Retrieved from http://www.neurology.org/content/76/7_Supplement_2/S37.full#T1. Accessed October 28, 2017.
8. Neblett, M. T. (2017, August 04). Evaluation of Acute Headache in Adults. Epocrates. Retrieved from https://online.epocrates.com/diseases/9/Headache-acute-adult-evaluation-of. Accessed October 28, 2017.
9. Eighth Joint National Committee (JNC 8) Hypertension Guideline Algorithm. (2014). Retrieved from http://www.nmhs.net/documents/27JNC8HTNGuidelinesBookBooklet.pdf. Accessed October 28, 2017.
10. Headache. In Kasper, D., Fauci, A., Hauser, S., Longo, D., Jameson, J., & Loscalzo, J. *Harrison's Principles of Internal Medicine* (19th ed.). New York, NY: McGraw-Hill. Retrieved from http://accessmedicine.mhmedical.com/content.aspx?bookid=1130&sectionid=79724323. Accessed October 28, 2017.

11. Mayo Clinic. (2014, December 2). Rebound Headaches Follow Pain-Medication Overuse. Retrieved from https://www.mayoclinic.org/diseases-conditions/rebound-headaches/basics/definition/con-20024096. Accessed October 28, 2017.
12. Reuben, D. B., Herr, K. A., Pacala, J. T., Pollock, B. G., Potter, J. F., & Semia, P. T. (2016). *Geriatrics at Your Fingertips* (18th ed.). New York, NY: American Geriatrics Society (AGS).
13. Bell, L. (2009). Nursing care and intracranial pressure monitoring. *American Journal of Critical Care, 18*(4), 338. Retrieved from http://ajcc.aacnjournals.org/content/18/4/338.full.pdf html. Accessed October 28, 2017.
14. Sippel, R. E. (2011, November 22). EMS Recap: Intracranial Pressure and the Cushing Reflex. EMSWorld. Retrieved from https://www.emsworld.com/article/10453662/ems-recap-intracranial-pressure-and-cushing-reflex. Accessed October 28, 2017.
15. American Geriatrics Society 2015 Beers Criteria Update Expert Panel, Fick, D. M., Semla, T. P., Beizer, J., Brandt, N., & Dombrowski, R., . . . Steinman, M. (2015, October 8). American Geriatrics Society 2015 updated Beers criteria for potentially inappropriate medication use in older adults. *Journal of the American Geriatrics Society, 63*(11), 2227–2246. Retrieved from http://onlinelibrary.wiley.com/doi/10.1111/jgs.13702/abstract. Accessed October 3, 2017.

# Pruritus

## Definition[3,4,5,6]

Pruritus is a common symptom, rather than a specific disease. Chronic pruritus is defined as itching that lasts longer than 6 weeks.

## Causes[1,2,3,4,5,6,7]

When the cause of pruritus is known, pruritus can be divided into the following categories:

- Dermatologic (pruritus resulting from primary skin disorders)
  - Examples: xerosis, atopic dermatitis, psoriasis, scabies, cutaneous infections
- Systemic (occurs without skin eruption)
  - Examples: drug-induced pruritus, chronic renal failure, liver disease, hematologic or lymphoproliferative disorders, malignancy
- Neurologic (pruritus due to disorders of the peripheral or central nervous system)
  - Examples: notalgia paresthetica, brachioradial pruritus, multiple sclerosis

- Psychogenic
  - Examples: depression, anxiety, psychogenic excoriation, delusional infestation (also called delusional parasitosis)
- Mixed (pruritus attributed to more than one cause)

## Risk Factors[1,2,3,4,5,6,7,8]

- Dry skin
- Autoimmune disease
- Viral illnesses
- Allergies
- Advanced age
- Multiple drug use
- Sex (influences susceptibility to certain forms of pruritus. As an example, vulvar pruritus is a common symptom in females that can occur as a feature of a wide variety of cutaneous disorders.)
- Burns and scars (common in adults and are associated with significant pruritus)

## Signs & Symptoms[1,2,3,4,5,6,7]

The clinical presentation of pruritus is divided into three groups:

- Group I: Pruritus on diseased (inflamed) skin; dermatological causes most common.
- Group II: Pruritus on nondiseased (noninflamed skin); seen in neurologic or psychiatric origin.
- Group III: Pruritus presenting with severe chronic secondary scratch lesions; includes patients with excoriations, crusts, papules, and nodules.

Signs of systemic disease are as follows:

- Renal pruritus: Diffuse xerosis and half-and-half nails may be seen. The patient may have signs of peripheral neuropathy and uremia.
- Cholestatic pruritus: Signs of liver disease include jaundice, spider angioma, Dupuytren contractures, white nails, gynecomastia (in men), xanthelasma, splenomegaly, and ascites.

- Endocrine pruritus: Patients with hypothyroidism have brittle nails and dry, course skin and hair. Patients with hyperthyroidism may have warm, smooth, and fine skin. They may also have chronic urticaria and angioedema. Other signs are fever, tachycardia, exophthalmos (associated with Grave's disease), and atrial fibrillation.
- Hematologic pruritus: Patients with iron deficiency may have pallor if they have anemia; they might also have glossitis and angular cheilitis. Polycythemia vera may result in a ruddy complexion around the lips, cheeks, nose, and ears, along with hypertension and splenomegaly.
- Pruritus and malignancy: Patients with Hodgkin's disease may have ill-defined hyperpigmentation of the skin, ichthyosis, nontender lymphadenopathy, and splenomegaly.

## Tests[1,2,3,4,5,6,8]

- Skin biopsy
  - To determine if a drug reaction is the cause or another etiology.
- Skin scraping: potassium hydroxide (KOH)
  - To determine if dermatophyte is the cause of pruritus.
- Chest X-ray
  - To check for adenopathy.
- Serum CBC, complete metabolic panel (CMP), thyroid panel, human immunodeficiency virus (HIV) antibody, and hepatitis B and C serologies
  - Helpful in determining for underlying malignancy, anemia, renal or liver disease, or thyroid disease. HIV and hepatitis testing should be performed if risk factors present.

## Treatment & Management[1,2,3,4,5,6,8,12]

- **Nonpharmacological and nursing interventions:**
  - Identify and treat underlying issues, such as evaluating bathing habits, chemical exposures, hobbies, home

exposures, and incidence of family members having pruritus.
  - Encourage therapeutic measures (e.g., use of skin moisturizers and lubricants, humidify indoor environment, avoidance of skin irritants, stress reduction, keep fingernails trimmed, use of mild, unscented soaps and limited bathing to brief exposure, pat skin dry).
  - Occlusion of localized areas of pruritus with Unna boots or occlusive dressings.
  - Encourage loose clothing and avoid clothing made of wool. Wear smooth cotton clothing.
  - Avoid/limit caffeine, alcohol, intake of hot and spicy foods. Avoid heat, dry climates, and excessive sweating.
- **Pharmacological and other interventions:**
  *Treatment varies depending upon underlying etiology.*
  - Topical therapies (e.g., capsacin, steroids, anesthetics, and antihistamines)
    - Temporarily reduces pruritus.
  - Antihistamines, oral (e.g., first-generation hydroxyzine [Vistaril], diphenhydramine [Benadryl])
    - Are sedating; however can be effective in those with nighttime pruritus.
    - Second-generation antihistamines are not as effective at relieving itch compared to first-generation antihistamines, however are less sedating.
  - Tricyclic antidepressant, such as doxepin (Silenor)
    - Dosages of 25–50 mg at bedtime are helpful at relieving itch.
    - May cause ataxia and contribute to falls.
  - Antidepressant: mirtazapine (Remeron)
    - Used at dosages of 15–30 mg at bedtime.
    - Consider antidepressants when pruritus does not respond to other therapies.
    - Use with caution, may lower sodium levels.
  - Gabapentin (Neurontin)

- Efficacious in treating neurogenic pruritus and more recently has demonstrated effectiveness in uremic, hematologic, and idiopathic pruritus.
- Associated with central nervous system (CNS) adverse effects; dosage may need to be changed based off renal function.

- Antinausea neurokinin receptor 1 antagonist: aprepitant (Emend)
  - Highly effective in reducing pruritus in a group of patients with various skin disorders. Patients with atopic dermatitis and prurigo nodularis seemed to respond best.

- Dermatology consultation/referral (assists in effective management of pruritus)

Note: Beers listed items, as mentioned above, include gabapentin, mirtazapine, tricyclic antidepressants, and oral antihistamines.

## CLINICAL PEARLS[8,9,10,11]

- A systemic disorder should be considered in older adults with a generalized itch without clinical evidence of primary skin lesions. Malignancies can present with a generalized itch and be present before the malignancy is noticed.
- Chronic pruritus significantly impacts quality of life and is associated with a diverse possibility of underlying diseases. In older adults, it is often related to dryness, cold weather, and constant use of hot foot soaks. It is therefore important to focus on nonpharmacological interventions to alleviate symptoms.

## References

1. Butler, D. F. (2017, June 23). Pruritus and Systemic Disease Treatment & Management. Medscape. Retrieved from http://emedicine.medscape.com/article/1098029-treatment#d6. Accessed January 10, 2018.
2. Frazio, S. B. (2017, November 20). Pruritus: Overview of Management. UpToDate. Retrieved from http://www.uptodate.com/contents/pruritus-overview-of-management. Accessed January 10, 2018.
3. Frazio, S. B., & Yosipovitch, G. (2016, September 23). Pruritus: Etiology and Patient Evaluation. UpToDate. Retrieved from http://www.uptodate.com/contents/pruritis-etiology-and-patient-evaluation. Accessed January 10, 2018.

4. Garcia-Albea, V., & Limaye, K. (2012, March–April). The clinical conundrum of pruritus. *Journal of the Dermatology Nurses' Association*, 4(2), 106–107.
5. Lyons, F., & Ousley, L. (2015). *Dermatology for the Advanced Practice Nurse*. New York, NY: Springer Publishing Company.
6. Moses, S. (2003, September 15). Pruritus. *American Family Physician*, 68(6), 1135–1142.
7. Grundmann, S., & Ständer, S. (2011). Chronic pruritus: Clinics and treatment. *Annals of Dermatology*, 23(1), 1–11. doi:10.5021/ad.2011.23.1.1
8. Rajagopalan, M., Saraswat, A., Godse, K., Shankar, D. K., Kandhari, S., & Shenoi, S., . . . Zawar, V. (2017). Diagnosis and management of chronic pruritus: An expert consensus review. *Indian Journal of Dermatology*, 62(1), 7–17. doi:10.4103/0019-5154.198036
9. Helfand, A. E., & Robbins, J, M. (2017). Foot problems. In *Hazzard's Geriatric Medicine and Gerontology* (7th ed.). New York, NY: McGraw-Hill. Retrieved from http://accessmedicine.mhmedical.com/content.aspx?bookid=1923&sectionid=144563300. Accessed January 10, 2018.
10. Fett, N., Haynes, K., Propert, K. J., & Margolis, D. J. (2014). Five-year malignancy incidence in patients with chronic pruritus: A population-based cohort study aimed at limiting unnecessary screening practices. *Journal of the American Academy of Dermatology*, 70(4), 651–658. doi:10.1016/j.jaad.2013.11.045
11. Johannesdottir, S., Farkas, D., Vinding, G., Pedersen, L., Lamberg, A., Sørensen, H., & Olesen, A. (2014). Cancer incidence among patients with a hospital diagnosis of pruritus: A nationwide Danish cohort study. *British Journal of Dermatology*, 171(4), 839–846. doi:10.1111/bjd.13157
12. American Geriatrics Society 2015 Beers Criteria Update Expert Panel, Fick, D. M., Semla, T. P., Beizer, J., Brandt, N., & Dombrowski, R., . . . Steinman, M. (2015, October 8). American Geriatrics Society 2015 updated Beers criteria for potentially inappropriate medication use in older adults. *Journal of the American Geriatrics Society*, 63(11), 2227–2246. Retrieved from http://onlinelibrary.wiley.com/doi/10.1111/jgs.13702/abstract. Accessed October 3, 2017.

# Syncope

## Definition[1,2,4,5,6]

Syncope is a sudden and temporary loss of consciousness due to impaired cerebral perfusion.

## Causes[1,2,3,4,5,6]

- Neurally mediated syncope
  - Includes carotid sinus hypersensitivity, vasovagal (e.g., due to fear, pain, stress), situational (e.g., due to coughing, defecation).
- Orthostatic hypotension
  - Includes medications (e.g., diuretics, tricyclic agents, antihypertensives, antianginal agents), volume depletion

(includes blood loss and hot weather), autonomic dysfunction (e.g., Parkinson's disease), deconditioning due to prolonged bed rest, postprandial.
- Arrhythmias
  - Includes brady- and tachyarrythmias, implanted device malfunction (e.g., implantable cardioconverter defribrillator [ICD]), medication induced (e.g., sotalol [Betapace], quinidine).
- Valvular disease (e.g., aortic stenosis)
- Stroke or transient ischemic attack (TIA), vertebral basilar artery
- Seizures
- Hypoglycemia
- Massive pulmonary embolism
- Hypertrophic and other cardiomyopathies
- Myocardial infarction or ischemia
- Psychiatric disorders
  - Includes anxiety, major depression, conversion disorder.

## Tests[1,2,3,4,5,6]

- 12-lead ECG, Holter monitor, or loop recorders
  - ECG recommended in all individuals with syncope to evaluate for underlying arrhythmia or cardiac disease. Holter monitor should be ordered when syncope occurs frequently (≥ 1/week). Loop recorder reserved in those with infrequent syncopal episodes and low risk of sudden cardiac death.
- Orthostatic vital signs
  - Useful in neurally mediated and orthostatic hypotension syncope.
- Serum electrolytes, blood urea nitrogen (BUN) and creatinine, blood glucose, complete blood count
  - Ordered only if clinically suspicious (e.g., volume depletion or blood loss anemia, hypoglycemia). Blood tests are otherwise of little to no benefit.

- Echocardiography
  - Ordered when ECG is not diagnostic, in individuals with history of cardiac disease, or presence of a cardiac murmur. Aids in the diagnosis of hypertrophic cardiomyopathy, aortic stenosis, and others.
- Exercise testing
  - Used to investigate cardiac disease; ordered in individuals with exercise-induced syncope.
- Tilt-table test
  - Ordered when neurally mediated syncope suspected, recurrent unexplained falls, and psychiatric disorders.
- Carotid sinus massage
  - Reserved in individuals when carotid sinus hypersensitivity suspected and/or recurrent syncope with unknown etiology.
- Electroencephalography (EEG)
  - If seizure disorder suspected.
- Brain imaging (CT or MRI)
  - Not recommended in asymptomatic adults with syncope or in the setting of a normal neurological evaluation.

## Treatment & Management[2,4,5,6,7]

- **Nonpharmacological and nursing interventions:**
  - In the setting of orthostatic hypotension, educate patient to change positions slowly, encourage sodium and water intake, and avoidance of triggers (e.g., eating large meals).
  - Prevent injury (e.g., wear nonskid socks, keep bed in low position, items needed within close reach).
  - Encourage avoidance of the trigger in vasovagal events.
  - Encourage use of compression stockings and relaxation techniques for vasovagal syncope.
  - Instruct patient to avoid driving if syncope cause unknown.

- **Pharmacological and other interventions:**
  - Reduce or stop the offending medication.
  - Paroxetine (Paxil).
    - Can be used in adults with recurrent vasovagal syncope and concurrent psychiatric disorder.
    - Highly anticholinergic.
  - Midodrine (Amatine), fludrocortisone (Florinef), and desmopressin (DDAVP).
    - Used in orthostatic hypotension.
  - Indomethacin (Indocin), ocreotide (Sandostatin), or caffeine.
    - Effective in postprandial syncope.
- Cardiology consultation/referral
  - When syncope is due to cardiac etiology (treatment may include antiarrhythmics, pacing, ablation, and/or implantable device).
- Psychiatry consultation/referral
  - To evaluate for underlying psychiatric illness, especially if syncopal episodes are recurrent and unexplained.
- Physical therapy consultation/referral
  - Useful in the treatment of neurally mediated syncope.

Note: Beers listed items, as mentioned above, include indomethacin, caffeine, desmopressin, oral corticosteroids, and paroxetine.

## CLINICAL PEARLS[2,4,5,6]

- Syncope in older adults is usually multifactorial. Reviewing the past medical history and performing a full history and physical examination assists in determining the etiology. The presence of cardiovascular disease implies the syncopal episode(s) are most likely due to a cardiac etiology.
- Syncope due to an underlying cardiac arrhythmia, hypoglycemia, and/or vasovagal etiology are transient, whereas syncope due to seizures will have prolonged recovery period.
- Medications contribute to 5%–15% of syncope cases.

## References


1. Wasson, S. (2017, June 26). Evaluation of Syncope. Epocrates. Retrieved from https://online.epocrates.com/diseases/248/Evaluation-of-syncope. Accessed November 16, 2017.
2. Freeman R. Syncope. In Kasper, D., Fauci, A., Hauser, S., Longo, D., Jameson, J., & Loscalzo, J.*Harrison's Principles of Internal Medicine* (19th ed.). New York, NY: McGraw-Hill. Retrieved from http://accessmedicine.mhmedical.com/content.aspx?bookid=1130&sectionid=79724617. Accessed November 15, 2017.
3. Assessing older adults for syncope following a fall. In *Current Diagnosis & Treatment: Geriatrics* (2nd ed.). New York, NY: McGraw-Hill. Retrieved from http://accessmedicine.mhmedical.com/content.aspx?bookid=953&sectionid=53375684. Accessed November 15, 2017.
4. Runser, L. A., Gauer, R. L., & Houser, A. (2017, March 1). Syncope: Evaluation and differential diagnosis. *American Family Physician,* 95(5), 303–312B. Retrieved from http://www.aafp.org/afp/2017/0301/p303.html. Accessed November 16, 2017.
5. Higginson, L. A. (2016, October). Syncope – Cardiovascular Disorders. Merck Manuals: Professional. Retrieved from https://www.merckmanuals.com/professional/cardiovascular-disorders/symptoms-of-cardiovascular-disorders/syncope. Accessed November 16, 2017.
6. .(2017). In *Hazzard's Geriatric Medicine and Gerontology* (7th ed.). New York, NY: McGraw-Hill. Retrieved from http://accessmedicine.mhmedical.com/content.aspx?bookid=1923&sectionid=144522113. Accessed November 19, 2017.
7. American Geriatrics Society 2015 Beers Criteria Update Expert Panel, Fick, D. M., Semla, T. P., Beizer, J., Brandt, N., & Dombrowski, R., . . . Steinman, M. (2015, October 8). American Geriatrics Society 2015 updated Beers criteria for potentially inappropriate medication use in older adults. *Journal of the American Geriatrics Society,* 63(11), 2227–2246. Retrieved from http://onlinelibrary.wiley.com/doi/10.1111/jgs.13702/abstract. Accessed October 3, 2017.


# Tremor

## Definition[4,7,8]

Tremor is an involuntary twitching movement of one or more body parts.

It is classified as an action tremor (i.e., tremor occurs with voluntary movement) or a rest tremor (i.e., tremor occurs with relaxed muscles).

## Types[1,2,3,5,7,8]

| Type | Tremor Classification | Typical Features |
|---|---|---|
| **Essential tremor (ET)** | Action | • Family history is common.<br>• Affects bilateral hands, head, voice.<br>• Absence of other neurological findings.<br>• Exacerbating factors: caffeine, stress; relieved with alcohol. |
| **Parkinsonian tremor** | Rest | • Rarely due to family history.<br>• Asymmetric tremor; involves distal extremities; tremor has a gradual onset.<br>• Presents with other neurological findings (e.g., bradykinesia, rigidity, postural instability).<br>• Exacerbating factor: stress. |
| **Psychogenic tremor** | Action and rest | • Psychiatric history.<br>• Tremor has a sudden onset and resolves spontaneously.<br>• Tremor can affect all body parts.<br>• Absence of other neurological findings.<br>• Exacerbating factors: caffeine, stress. |
| **Enhanced physiologic tremor** | Action and rest | • Tremor reverses once the cause is corrected, such as medications (e.g., stimulants, antipsychotics), alcohol withdrawal, or metabolic causes (e.g., overactive thyroid, hypoglycemia).<br>• Tremor is high frequency, low amplitude. |

## Tests[4,6,7,8]

*Not typically ordered; diagnosis can be made based off a thorough history and physical examination.*

- CMP, magnesium, glucose, TSH, vitamin B12 level
  - Assess for metabolic causes such as liver or renal failure, electrolyte imbalance, hypoglycemia, hyperthyroidism, and vitamin B12 deficiency.
- Plain CT or MRI
  - Consider to evaluate for secondary causes (e.g., stroke, tumor).

## Treatment & Management[1,2,3,4,5,6,7,8,9,10,11,13]

- **Identify and treat the type of tremor accordingly**.
  - Diagnosis is based off the history and physical and neurological exam.
  - Determine tremor classification and location, which will offer guidance on the appropriate treatment.
- **Nonpharmacological and nursing interventions:**
  - Educate patient on the adverse effects of medication therapy.
  - Alcohol should be used with caution.
    - Can worsen essential tremor (ET) in some patients.
    - Avoid with tremor related to Parkinson's disease.
  - Offer emotional support (e.g., remind patient that ET is common and shouldn't be embarrassed).
  - Encourage involvement in support group, such as the National Tremor Foundation.
  - Encourage lifestyle interventions to reduce anxiety (e.g., limiting caffeine intake with ET and psychogenic tremor).
- **Pharmacological interventions:**
  - Essential tremor
    - Propranolol (Inderal) and/or primidone (Mysoline)
  - Parkinsonian tremor
    - Anticholinergics (e.g., trihexyphenidyl [Artane], benztropine [Cogentin])
    - Dopamine agonists

- Psychogenic tremor
  - Treatment of depression and anxiety, options include but not limited to: citalopram (Celexa), sertraline (Escitalopram), venlafaxine (Effexor).
- Enhanced physiological tremor
  - Removal of the offending medication

Note: Beers listed items, as mentioned above, include SSRIs, serotonin-norepinephrine reuptake inhibitors (SNRIs), benztropine, and trihexyphenidyl.

## CLINICAL PEARLS[1,2,5,7,8]

- Screen for alcohol abuse, caffeine use, and perform a thorough medication review.
- If tremor occurs *suddenly*, the cause is probably medication or psychogenic related.
- Parkinson's disease is the most common cause of parkinsonism.
- Refer to neurology when the above interventions fail or unsure of underlying etiology.

## References

1. Galifianakis, N. B., & Ghazinouri, A. A. (2014). Parkinson disease & essential tremor. In *Current Diagnosis & Treatment: Geriatrics* (2nd ed.). New York, NY: McGraw-Hill. Retrieved from http://accessmedicine.mhmedical.com/content.aspx?bookid=953&sectionid=53375648. Accessed October 1, 2017.
2. Aminoff, M. J., & Douglas, V. C. (2018). Nervous system disorders. In *Current Medical Diagnosis & Treatment 2018*. New York, NY: McGraw-Hill. Retrieved from http://accessmedicine.mhmedical.com/content.aspx?bookid=2192&sectionid=168019736. Accessed October 1, 2017.
3. Kriebel-Gasparro, A. (2016). Parkinon's disease: Update on medication management. *Journal for Nurse Practitioners, 12*(3), 81–89. Retrieved from http://dx.doi.org/10.1016/j.nurpra.2015.10.020. Accessed October 1, 2017
4. Olanow, C., Schapira, A. V., & Obeso, J. A. (2015). Parkinson's disease and other movement disorders. In Kasper, D., Fauci, A., Hauser, S., Longo, D., Jamesom, J., & Loscalzo, J. (Eds.). *Harrison's Principles of Internal Medicine* (19th ed.). New York, NY: McGraw-Hill. Retrieved from http://accessmedicine.mhmedical.com/content.aspx?bookid=1130&sectionid=79755616. Accessed October 1, 2017.
5. Parkinson's Disease Foundation (PDF). (n.d.). Understanding Parkinson's. Retrieved from http://www.pdf.org/about_pd. Accessed October 1, 2017.

6. Burke, D. A. (2017, July 19). Essential Tremor. Medscape. Retrieved from http://emedicine.medscape.com/article/1150290-overview#a1. Accessed October 1, 2017.
7. Crawford, P., & Zimmerman, E. E. (2011). Differentiation and diagnosis of tremor. *American Family Physician, 83*(6), 697–702. Retrieved from http://www.aafp.org/afp/2011/0315/p697.html. Accessed October 1, 2017.
8. National Institute of Neurological Disorders and Stroke (NINDS). (n.d.). Tremor Fact Sheet. National Institutes of Health. Retrieved from https://www.ninds.nih.gov/Disorders/Patient-Caregiver-Education/Fact-Sheets/Tremor-Fact-Sheet. Accessed October 1, 2017.
9. Wall, A. (2016, February 9). Caring for the patient with essential tremor. Retrieved from https://www.nursinginpractice.com/article/caring-patient-essential-tremor. *Nursing in Practice*. Accessed October 29, 2017.
10. RNpedia. (2017, July 24). Parkinson's Disease Nursing Care Plan & Management. Nursing Notes. Retrieved from https://www.rnpedia.com/nursing-notes/medical-surgical-nursing-notes/parkinsons-disease/. Accessed October 29, 2017.
11. Jankovic, J., Vuong, K. D., & Thomas, M. (2006, July). Psychogenic tremor: Long-term outcome. *CNS Spectrums, 11*(7), 501–508 (published online November 1, 2014). Retrieved from https://doi.org/10.1017/S1092852900013535. Accessed October 29, 2017.
12. Frank, C. (2014, February). Pharmacologic treatment of depression in the elderly. *Canadian Family Physician, 60*(2), 121–126. Retrieved from https://www.ncbi.nlm.nih.gov/pmc/articles/PMC3922554/. Accessed October 29, 2017.
13. American Geriatrics Society 2015 Beers Criteria Update Expert Panel, Fick, D. M., Semla, T. P., Beizer, J., Brandt, N., & Dombrowski, R., . . . Steinman, M. (2015, October 8). American Geriatrics Society 2015 updated Beers criteria for potentially inappropriate medication use in older adults. *Journal of the American Geriatrics Society, 63*(11), 2227–2246. Retrieved from http://onlinelibrary.wiley.com/doi/10.1111/jgs.13702/abstract. Accessed October 3, 2017.

# Unintentional Weight Loss

## Definition[1,2,5,6]

Unintentional weight loss is defined as the loss of 10 pounds or at least 5% of the patient's usual body weight over 6 months to a year.

## Causes[1,2,5,6]

- Changes associated with aging
  - Declining chemosensory function, reduced effectiveness of chewing, slowed gastric emptying, changes in hormones and peptides
- Malignancy
  - Gastrointestinal, hepatobiliary, lymphomas, breast, lung, bladder

- Gastrointestinal
  - Malabsorption, peptic ulcer, constipation, inflammatory bowel disease, chronic pancreatitis
- Psychological
  - Depression, anxiety, paranoia, alcoholism
- Oral and dental problems
  - Poor fitting dentures, poor dentition
- Endocrinopathies
  - Hyperthyroidism, diabetes
- Neurological related
  - Dementia, Parkinson's disease, stroke, multiple sclerosis
- Heart failure
- Infections
- End-stage kidney or liver failure
- Rheumatoid arthritis
- Medication side effects
  - Antibiotics (e.g., erythromycin), opiates, NSAIDs, benzodiazepines, antihistamines, anticholinergics, dopamine agonists, angiotensin-converting enzyme (ACE) inhibitors
- Social factors
  - Low income, inadequate access to food, social isolation
- Unknown

## Tests[1,2,6]

- Reasonable to order basic labs, such as: CBC, CMP, TSH, stool hemoccult, chest radiograph, urinalysis, ESR and CRP.
  - Used to evaluate for underlying infection or anemia; liver and renal impairment; thyroid disease.
  - Positive focal occult blood can be seen with gastrointestinal malignancies.
  - Chest radiograph can show infection or heart failure exacerbation.
  - Urinalysis to evaluate for underlying urinary tract infection.
  - ESR/CRP are nonspecific; however are elevated with inflammation and infections.

## Treatment & Management[1,2,3,4,5,6]

- **Nonpharmacological and nursing interventions:**
  - Monitor weights while investigating the underlying cause.
  - Dietary modification:
    - Use nutritional supplements (recommended between meals) and flavor enhancers.
    - Provide frequent, small meals and high-calorie snacks.
    - Offer feeding assistance, if needed (patients eat more when fed by family members).
    - Minimize dietary restrictions.
    - Focus on the patient's food preferences.
  - Encourage increased physical activity (e.g., daily walking).
    - Helps to maintain lean body mass, while improving appetite and functional status.
- **Pharmacological and other interventions:**
  - Decrease or discontinue medications that can cause nausea or anorexia.
  - Use of an appetite stimulant:
    - Antidepressant: mirtazapine (Remeron)
      - An appropriate choice, especially if depression is thought to be the underlying cause of poor intake and weight loss. It leads to more weight gain than SSRI antidepressants. Evidence is lacking on using this medication to promote weight gain in the absence of depression.
      - May decrease sodium levels, cause dizziness and/or orthostatic hypotension.
    - Megestrol (Megace)
      - Not been shown to be effective in older adults and has significant side effects.
      - Increased risk of thrombotic events and associated with fluid retention and mortality.
    - Dronabinol (Marinol)
      - Not been shown to be effective in older adults and has significant side effects.

    - Cyproheptadine (Periactin)
        - Not been shown to be effective in older adults.
        - Highly anticholinergic.
- Can be complicated, therefore a multidisciplinary approach is recommended (consulting dentistry, dietitian, gastroenterology, psychiatry, social worker).
- Surgical or gastroenterology consultation/referral (for percutaneous tube placement)
    - Enteral nutrition should be considered in those who cannot meet their nutritional requirements by oral intake.
        - When to provide this type of nutrition is not well established; consider first the patients prognosis and preferences.
        - Educate patient and family about the risk of pulmonary aspiration or pneumonia.
        - The use of tube feeds is *not* recommended in patients with advanced dementia (i.e., does not improve pressure sores, infections, functional status or quality of life).

Note: Beers listed items, as mentioned above, include cyproheptadine, megestrol, and mirtazapine.

## CLINICAL PEARLS[1,2,5,6]

- The cause of weight loss is multifactorial; the three most common causes in older adults are depression, gastrointestinal disorders, and malignancy. Overall, nonmalignant diseases are more common.
- Most of the time, the underlying diagnoses of unintentional weight loss can be made with a thorough history, physical examination, and basic lab work.
- Involuntary weight loss has no identifiable cause in about 25% of adults, despite extensive workups. Prognosis is usually better when the cause is not known compared to when it is known (particularly malignancy).
- Weight loss in older adults is associated with functional decline, pressure ulcers, hip fracture, increased infection risk, and overall mortality.
- Oral and dental problems are easily overlooked as causes of involuntary weight loss in older adults; they may present as halitosis, dry mouth, difficulty chewing, and/or poor oral hygiene.

## References


1. Robertson, R. G., & Jameson, J. (2015). Involuntary weight loss. In Kasper, D., Fauci, A., Hauser, S., Longo, D., Jamesom, J., & Loscalzo, J. (Eds.) *Harrison's Principles of Internal Medicine* (19th ed.). New York, NY: McGraw-Hill. Retrieved from http://accessmedicine.mhmedical.com/content.aspx?bookid=1130&sectionid=79726329. Accessed January 27, 2018.
2. Wallace, J. I. (2017). Malnutrition and enteral/parenteral alimentation. In *Hazzard's Geriatric Medicine and Gerontology* (7th ed.). New York, NY: McGraw-Hill. Retrieved from http://accessmedicine.mhmedical.com/content.aspx?bookid=1923&sectionid=144520275. Accessed January 27, 2018.
3. American Geriatrics Society 2015 Beers Criteria Update Expert Panel, Fick, D. M., Semla, T. P., Beizer, J., Brandt, N., & Dombrowski, R., . . . Steinman, M. (2015, October 8). American Geriatrics Society 2015 updated Beers criteria for potentially inappropriate medication use in older adults. *Journal of the American Geriatrics Society, 63*(11), 2227–2246. Retrieved from http://onlinelibrary.wiley.com/doi/10.1111/jgs.13702/abstract. Accessed October 3, 2017.
4. Kane, R. L., Ouslander, J. G., Resnick, B., & Malone, M. L. (Eds.) (2017). *Essentials of Clinical Geriatrics* (8th ed.); Pallative Care. New York, NY: McGraw-Hill. Retrieved from http://accessmedicine.mhmedical.com/content.aspx?bookid=2300&sectionid=178120780. Accessed January 27, 2018.
5. Yukawa M. (2014). Defining adequate nutrition for older adults. In *Current Diagnosis & Treatment: Geriatrics* (2nd ed.). New York, NY: McGraw-Hill. Retrieved from http://accessmedicine.mhmedical.com/content.aspx?bookid=953&sectionid=53375693. Accessed January 27, 2018.
6. Gaddey, H. L., & Holder, K. (2014). Unintentional weight loss in older adults. *American Family Physician, 89*(9), 718–722. Retrieved from https://www.aafp.org/afp/2014/0501/p718.html. Accessed January 27, 2018.

SECTION XIII

# Topics of Discussion

## Driving

- Compared to younger drivers, older adults are more likely to be wearing seat belts, recognize danger zones, obey the speed limit, avoid driving in bad weather, and aren't under the influence of alcohol.[1,2]
- Following accidents, given age and comorbid conditions, older adults take longer to recover and are more likely to suffer mortality (17 times more likely than their younger counterparts).[1] Fatal crash rates increase dramatically from age 75 to 80 years old and older.
- Conditions most frequently affecting driving abilities:
  - Arthritis with painful joints and reduced ability to twist, turn, grip the steering wheel and pump the brake.[1]
  - Medications impairing driving abilities (dizziness, sleepiness).[1]
  - Parkinson's disease.[3]
  - Dementia or impaired memory.[3]
- Preventive measures for elderly drivers to avoid injury/accidents:[4]
  - Have routine eye and hearing examinations.
  - Routine physician/pharmacist discussions about medications for possible interactions and side effects that could impair driving abilities.
  - Exercise to remain fit and active.
  - Drive in optimal driving conditions (avoid rain, wind, snow, fog).
  - Avoid driving distractions (cell phone, radio, extra passengers).

  - Leave extra distance between your vehicle and the one in front.
  - Plan the route of travel before leaving home.
- Warning signs it may be time to consider restricting or revoking a driver's license:[3]
  - Forgetting to use turn signals.
  - Drifting into other lanes.
  - Difficulty changing lanes.
  - Getting lost/forgetting route of travel.
  - Minor fender benders/finding damage to vehicle.
  - Difficulty judging braking distance.
  - Family is noticing driving abilities have changed.
- There is no single point in time or age requirement that determines when a license is to be revoked.[3]
- The Department of Motor Vehicles (DMV) offers an elderly driving course for geriatric patients to help with aging concerns and driving.[3] There is no evidence that supports these courses as beneficial in older adults with neurodegenerative diseases.[5]
- It is recommended that each practitioner familiarize him or herself with state laws mandating elderly driving restrictions/recertification.[4]

## References


1. AAA. (n.d.). Senior Driving: Facts & Research. Retrieved from https://seniordriving.aaa.com/resources-family-friends/conversations-about-driving/facts-research/. Accessed February 22, 2018.
2. Centers for Disease Control and Prevention (CDC). (2017, November 30). Motor Vehicle Safety: Older Adult Drivers. Retrieved from https://www.cdc.gov/motorvehiclesafety/older_adult_drivers/index.html. Accessed February 22, 2018.
3. Department of Motor Vehicles (DMV). (n.d.). Seniors: When to Turn Over the Car Keys. Retrieved from https://www.dmv.org/how-to-guides/senior-driving.php. Accessed February 22, 2018.
4. Department of Motor Vehicles (DMV). (n.d.). Senior Drivers in Virginia. Retrieved from https://www.dmv.com/va/virginia/senior-drivers. Accessed February 25, 2018.
5. Aminoff M. J., Douglas V. C. Nervous System Disorders. In: Papadakis M. A., McPhee S. J., Rabow M. W. eds. *Current Medical Diagnosis & Treatment 2018* New York, NY: McGraw-Hill; . http://accessmedicine.mhmedical.com/content.aspx?bookid=2192&sectionid=168019736. Accessed July 23, 2018.

## Elder Abuse

- Elder abuse is experienced by 1 out of every 10 elder Americans who still live at home.[1]
- The most commonly abused are geriatric women and those with cognitive issues (i.e., dementia, memory disorders).[1] Abuse could be from family, staff in a long-term care facility, or another patient.[2]
- Elder abuse is defined as a purposeful act, or failure to act, by a direct caregiver or another person in a trusting relationship that causes harm or creates a risk of harm to an older adult (defined as someone age 60 years old or older).[2]
- Types of abuse:[1,2]
  - Physical: hitting, slapping, pushing
  - Emotional: preventing the person from seeing loved ones, name calling
  - Neglect: failure to respond to the elder's needs
  - Abandonment: leaving the individual alone without means to care for self
  - Sexual: forced to take part in or watch sexual acts
  - Financial: forging checks, misusing benefits, changing names on will/banking accounts
  - Health care: by doctors, hospital staff, or other workers; includes overcharging, billing twice for the same service, or billing for services not rendered
- Risk factors include a diagnosis of mental illness, current alcohol abuse, high levels of hostility or agitation, history of abuse as a child, poor coping skills, lack of social support, among others.[2]
- Signs of neglect:[1,2]
  - Recurrent sleeping difficulties
  - New depression/confusion; becomes withdrawn
  - Malnutrition or dehydration
  - Signs of trauma (e.g., welts, wounds, injuries, including bruising)

  - Acts agitated or violent
  - Unkempt with dirty clothing or unwashed hair
  - Increased susceptibility to new infections including sexually transmitted infections
  - Persistent physical pain
- Long-term effects from elder abuse include post-traumatic stress disorder, fear and anxiety, and learned helplessness.[2]
- It is recommended, as his or her practitioner, to discuss your concerns with the individual about possible abuse, if he or she is mentally capable. If abuse is suspected, it is required to be reported. Long-term care facilities are required to have an ombudsman available who is an advocate for patients' rights and who is trained in managing concerns of abuse.[1,3]
- There are national hotlines available for reporting, as well as various state options available. It is recommended to research what is available in your respective state.[2]
- The Centers for Disease Control and Prevention (CDC) provides several resources for staff and long-term care (LTC) patients to help address and prevent concerns of elder abuse:
  - National Center on Elder Abuse
  - Eldercare Locator
  - National Institutes on Health/National Institute on Aging
  - National Long-Term Care Ombudsman Resource Center

## References

1. National Institute on Aging. (2016, December 29). Elder Abuse. National Institutes of Health. Retrieved from https://www.nia.nih.gov/health/elder-abuse#types. Accessed February 25, 2018.
2. Centers for Disease Control and Prevention (CDC). (2017, June 8). Elder Abuse: Violence Prevention. Retrieved from https://www.cdc.gov/violenceprevention/elderabuse/index.html. Accessed February 25, 2018.
3. The National Long-Term Care Ombudsman Resource Center. (n.d.). News and Press. Retrieved from http://ltcombudsman.org/. Accessed February 25, 2018.

## End-of-Life Common Terms

| Term | Definition |
|---|---|
| **Palliative care** | • Focuses on relief of physical suffering for patients experiencing illness or chronic disease.[1] Patient does not have to have terminal illness.[1]<br>• Uses life-prolonging medications.[1] |
| **Hospice** | • Available for terminally ill patients most commonly with life expectancy of less than 6 months.[1]<br>• Focuses on patient's comfort and quality of life.[1]<br>• Does not use life-prolonging medications.[1]<br>• Care can be given in hospital, nursing home, hospice center, or at home.[1] |
| **Medical power of attorney** | • Type of advance directive in which you name a person to make decisions for you when are you unable to do so.[2,3,4]<br>• Legal document.[2] |
| **Living will** | • A written legal document that spells out medical treatment you would or would not want to be used to keep you alive (e.g., ventilator, tube feed), as well as decisions around pain management and organ donation.[2,3,4] |
| **Do-not-resuscitate (DNR) order** | • Medical order.[2,3]<br>• Declines cardiopulmonary resuscitation (CPR) or electrical shock for resuscitation in event of cardiac arrest.[2,3,4] |

## References

1. Centers for Medicare & Medicaid Services (CMS). (n.d.). Palliative Care vs. Hospice Care. Retrieved from https://www.cms.gov/Medicare-Medicaid-Coordination/Fraud-Prevention/Medicaid-Integrity-Education/Downloads/infograph-PalliativeCare-%5BJune-2015%5D.pdf. Accessed February 7, 2018.
2. Mayo Clinic. (2014, November 11). Living Wills and Advance Directives for Medical Decisions. Retrieved February 7, 2018, from Centers for Medicare & Medicaid Services. Palliative care vs. hospice care. (n.d.). Retrieved from https://www.mayoclinic.org/healthy-lifestyle/consumer-health/in-depth/living-wills/art-20046303. Accessed February 7, 2018.

3. Crane, M. K., Wittink, M., & Doukas, D. J. (2005, October 1). Respecting end-of-life treatment preferences. *American Family Physician,* 72(7), 1263–1268. Retrieved from https://www.aafp.org/afp/2005/1001/p1263.html. Accessed February 7, 2018.
4. Auer, P. (2008, March). Primary care end-of-life planning for older adults with chronic illness. *Journal for Nurse Practitioners,* 4(3), 185–191. doi:10.1016/j.nurpra.2007.11.015

## End-of-Life Discussions

**Angela R. Stiltner**

- Effective communication is key to all end-of-life discussions and promotes high-quality medical care including better patient outcomes and improved patient and family satisfaction with care (see **Box 13-1**).[1,3,5,11,12,15,16]
- The clinician's primary role should be to facilitate high-quality discussions that promote good decision making and patient-centered care, and establish and define goals of care.[3]
- Patients make decisions based on an understanding of the extent of disease and prognosis in the context of their individual values, goals, and preferences.[14]
- Goals of care discussions should include issues encountered in healthcare decision making, including decisions about specific treatments or therapies, intensity of care, and planning for future care needs (advance care planning).[14]
- Clinicians typically fail to initiate end-of-life discussions until late in the course of an illness. These discussions best occur early in the disease trajectory while a patient has decision-making capacity and are re-evaluated at each visit and at critical decision-making points with a patient's routine clinician. These discussions are less effective during a life-threatening crisis and when addressed by clinicians with whom the patient is unfamiliar.[2,4,5,9,10,13,14]
- Delay in these end-of-life discussions may limit a patient's experience with some end-of-life care options such as hospice care. Hospice care has been associated with better outcomes and improved satisfaction for patients, caregivers, and families.[4,13]
- Advance care planning and development of advance directives are key in the process of documenting a patient's end-of-life care goals and preferences.[9,10]
- Advance directives generally address two primary issues: who makes decisions for the patient when decision-making

capacity is lost (healthcare surrogate or durable power of attorney [POA] for health care) and specific medical interventions that should or should not be undertaken (living will or healthcare directives).[9,10]

- Advance directive documents vary state to state and may include a durable medical POA document, living will, durable do-not -resuscitate (DNR) order, Physician Orders for Scope of Treatment (POST)/Physician Orders for Life-Sustaining Treatment (POLST), and Medical Orders for Scope of Treatment (MOST)/Medical Orders for Life-Sustaining Treatment (MOLST).[9,10]
- Medical intervention discussions should include review of potential general medical interventions commonly encountered such as artificial nutrition and hydration, intubation, and cardiopulmonary resuscitation (CPR). Other more specific interventions may be relevant depending on the specific medical conditions such as intravenous (IV) antibiotics, dialysis, implantable cardiac defibrillator (ICD) or pacemaker, left ventricular assist device (LVAD), and in the case of cancer, chemotherapy and radiotherapy.[2,9]
- Meaningful medical intervention discussions occur when the patient and family have a realistic understanding of the severity of the medical condition including prognosis and consequences of initiation and discontinuation of a specific intervention.[2]
- Informed decision making requires the patient to have an understanding of the potential risks, benefits, and burdens of each medical intervention. Treatment choices may have a negative or positive impact on quantity of life and quality of life. A patient should consider these when making an informed decision.[10,12,14]
- Patients have an ethical and legal right to refuse life-sustaining treatments such as artificial nutrition or hydration. Patients also have a right to ask the clinician to withhold a treatment prior to initiation or withdraw a treatment after initiation.[10]
- A DNR order is not the equivalent of a directive to discontinue all forms of treatment. The absence of a DNR order also does not instruct the clinician to do everything.[5]

- Goals of care should not be limited in focus to end-of-life care, but should include goals for how a patient wants to live; these include the patient's hopes, wishes, values, and preferences. There should also be discussion about specific life tasks, goals, projects, and legacy work that the patient would like to complete.[3,14]
- For these end-of-life discussions, a patient should also ensure he or she has named a medical power of attorney (POA) or surrogate decision maker as part of his or her advance care planning. The POA/surrogate decision maker should attend each of these important end-of-life care discussions between the patient and clinician.[3,9,12]
- POA/surrogate decision makers become important to the care team when the patient no longer has medical decision-making capacity. If no POA or surrogate decision maker has been named, each state has laws governing who is involved in these decisions.[3,9,10]
- A POA or surrogate decision maker must make decisions considering what the patient would want if able to communicate his or her wishes and taking into consideration previously expressed values and preferences for care. If preferences were not explicitly expressed prior to the patient's loss of decision-making capacity, the surrogate decision maker bases decisions on an inferred opinion about what he or she thinks the patient would want considering his or her values and life experiences (substituted judgement) or what is in the best interest of the patient.[3,9,10]
- Successful end-of-life discussions have been linked to reductions in hospital utilization and aggressiveness of care at the end of life, increased use of hospice services, decreased family conflict, and a greater likelihood of dying in the preferred place of death.[6,7,8]
- A systematic approach to regular end-of-life discussions and communication will foster collaboration between the patient, surrogate decision maker, and clinician. As a result, these discussions improve the patient and family's ability to plan for the future, develop realistic goals in line with patient and family values, and provide emotional support.[5]

**BOX 13-1 End-of-Life Discussions Key Points**

- Effective communication is critical.
- Explore patient's hopes, wishes, values, goals, and preferences for care.
- Consider quality of life vs. quantity of life.
- End-of-life discussions should occur early in disease trajectory and become an ongoing conversation as disease progresses and prognosis changes.
- Clinicians should develop a systematic process to incorporate end-of-life discussions.
- Advance care planning should address:
  - Goals of care
    - Cardiopulmonary resuscitation (CPR) and intubation
    - Artificial nutrition and hydration
    - Specific medical interventions (e.g., IV antibiotics, dialysis, ICD, pacemaker, LVAD, chemotherapy, radiotherapy)
    - Description of a good death including place of death, specific requests, tasks, projects, and legacy work
  - Advance directives
    - POA for health care/surrogate decision maker
    - Living will addressing specific medical interventions
    - Durable do-not-resuscitate orders
    - Specific physician orders for treatment (e.g., POST/POLST, MOST/MOLST)
- Informed decision requires an understanding of the potential risks, benefits, and burdens of medical intervention in the context of disease state and prognosis.
- Patients have an ethical and legal right to refuse or withdraw life-sustaining treatments or interventions.
- Successful end-of-life discussions are linked to the following:
  - Improved patient outcomes
  - Reduced hospital utilization
  - Less aggressive end-of-life care
  - Increased use of hospice services
  - Improved patient and family satisfaction
  - Decreased family conflict
  - Increased likelihood of honoring preferred location of death
- Hospice care is associated with improved patient outcomes and satisfaction with care.

## References


1. Bertakis, K. R. (1991, February). The relationship of physician medical interview style to patient satisfaction. *Journal of Family Practice* 32(2), 175–181.
2. Bischoff, K., O'Riordan, D. L., Marks, A. K., Sudore, R., & Pantilat, S. Z. (2018, January 1). Care planning for inpatients referred for palliative care consultation. *JAMA Internal Medicine*, *178*(1), 48–54.
3. Bodtke, S. L., & Ligon, K. (2016). *Hospice and Palliative Medicine Handbook: A Clinical Guide*. CreateSpace.
4. Davison, S. N. (2010, February). End-of-life care preferences and needs: Perceptions of patients with chronic kidney disease. *Clinical Journal of the American Society of Nephrology*, 5(2), 195–204.
5. Durso, S. S. (2013). *Geriatric Review Syllabus: A Core Curriculum in Geriatric Medicine* (8th ed.). New York, NY: American Geriatrics Society.
6. Fallowfield, L. J., Jenkins, V. A., & Beveridge, H. A. (2002, July). Truth may hurt but deceit hurts more: Communication in palliative care. *Palliative Medicine*, *16*(4), 297–303.
7. Gattellari, M. V., Voight, K. J., Butow, P. N., & Tattersall, M. H. (2002, Januaray 15). When the treatment goal is not cure: Are cancer patients equipped to make informed decisions? *Journal of Clinical Oncology*, *20*(2), 503–513.
8. Hagerty, R. G., Butow, P. N., Ellis, P. A., Lobb, E. A., Pendlebury, S, & Leighl, N., . . . Tattersall, M. H. (2004, May 1). Cancer patient preferences for communication of prognosis in the metastatic setting. *Journal of Clinical Oncology*, 22(9), 1721–1730.
9. Hanks, G. C. (2010). *Oxford Textbook of Palliative Medicine* (4th ed.). New York, NY: Oxford University Press.
10. Hazzard, W. B. (2003). *Principles of Geriatric Medicine & Gerontology* (5th ed.). New York, NY: McGraw-Hill.
11. Kaplan, S. G., Greenfield, S., & Ware, Jr., J. E. (1989, March). Assessing the effects of physician-patient interactions on the outcomes of chronic disease. *Medical Care*, 27(3 Suppl), S110–S127.
12. Kinzbrunner, B. M., & Policzer, J. (2011). *End-Of-Life Care: A Practical Guide* (2nd ed.). New York, NY: McGraw Hill Medical.
13. Mack, J. W., Cronin, A., Keating, N. L., Taback, N. Huskamp, H. A., & Malin, J. L., . . . Weeks, J. C. (2012, December). Associations between end-of-life discussion characteristics and care received near death: A prospective cohort study. *Journal of Clinical Oncology*, *30*(35), 4387–4395.
14. Naik, A. D., Martin, L. A., Moye, J., & Karel, M. J. (2016, March). Health values and treatment goals of older, multimorbid adults facing life-threatening illness. *Journal of the American Geriatrics Society*, *64*(3), 625–631.
15. Roter, D. L., Hall, J. A., Kern, D. E., Barker, .L. R., Cole, K. A., & Roca, R. P. (1995, September 25). Improving physicians' interviewing skills and reducing patients' emotional distress. A randomized clinical trial. *Archives of Internal Medicine*, *155*(17), 1877–1884.
16. Wright, A. A., Zhang, B., Ray, A., Mack, J. W., Trice, E., & Balboni, T. . . . Prigerson, H. G. (2008, October 8). Associations between end-of-life discussions, patient mental health, medical care near death, and caregiver bereavement adjustment. *JAMA*, *300*(14), 1665–1673.

## Falls[1,2,3,4,5,6,7,8,9]

- Over the past decade, mortality from falls has increased by more than 42% in persons older than age 65 years, pushing falls into one of the top areas for causes of death.
- Screen older adults above age 65 years old for falls.
  - Ask patients annually if they have fallen.
  - If they have fallen, perform gait or balance tests, such as the Timed Up and Go (TUG) test.
- Potentially modifiable risk factors:
  - Chronic conditions (e.g., decompensated heart failure)
  - Medications (e.g., diuretics, benzodiazepines, opioids, anticonvulsants, laxatives, antipsychotics, antidepressants, sedative hypnotics, antihypertensives, nonsteroidal anti-inflammatory drugs [NSAIDs]); use of ≥ 4 medications
  - Any use of assistive device (e.g., trip over cane)
  - Alcohol intoxication and illicit drug abuse
  - Environmental hazards (e.g., unsafe walking surfaces, cluttered floor, poor footwear, poor lighting, loose throw rugs, area carpets)
  - Sensory and neuromuscular factors (e.g., impaired vestibular function, muscle weakness, visual field loss, poor reaction time)
  - Neuropsychological factors (e.g., depression, fear of falling)
  - Impaired balance and mobility
  - Acute illnesses
- Nonmodifiable risk factors:
  - Female sex (i.e., live longer; higher prevalence of osteoporosis leading to higher fall-related fractures)
  - Age above 80 years
  - Arthritis
  - Cognitive impairment
  - History of falls

- Fall prevention.
  - Home health evaluation after discharged from facility for home safety evaluation (e.g., instillation of grab bars in bathroom, removal of rugs, proper use of lighting).
  - Ophthalmology or optometry referral.
    - Cataract surgery reduces falls.
    - Appropriate use of eyewear lenses.
  - Occupational and physical therapy referral.
    - Home safety interventions.
    - Gait, balance, and strength training.
  - Podiatry referral.
  - Perform medication review with goal to reduce psychoactive and other medications.
  - Use of vitamin D supplementation (at least 800 IU daily) may prevent falls (i.e., improves muscle strength and balance).
  - Involvement in an exercise program.
  - Identify and treat orthostatic hypotension.
- Low bed and bed alarm reduce falls minimally.
- Avoid restraints given increased risk of falls with injury.
- Fear of falling can result in social isolation, loss of function, and reduced quality of life and more falls.

## References


1. Moncada, L. V. (2011). Management of falls in older persons: A prescription for prevention. *American Family Physician, 84*(11), 1267–1276. Retrieved February 7, 2018.
2. Moncada, L. V. (2017). Preventing falls in older persons. *American Family Physician, 96*(4), 240–247. Retrieved from https://www.aafp.org/afp/2017/0815/p240.html. Retrieved February 7, 2018.
3. American Geriatrics Society 2015 Beers Criteria Update Expert Panel, Fick, D. M., Semla, T. P., Beizer, J., Brandt, N., & Dombrowski, R., . . . Steinman, M. (2015, October 8). American Geriatrics Society 2015 updated Beers criteria for potentially inappropriate medication use in older adults. *Journal of the American Geriatrics Society, 63*(11), 2227–2246. Retrieved from http://onlinelibrary.wiley.com/doi/10.1111/jgs.13702/abstract. Accessed October 3, 2017.
4. Cadwell, S., Dearmon, V., & Vandewaa, E. A. (2017). Reducing falls in patients with dementia by reducing psychotropic medication use: Does it work? *Journal for Nurse Practitioners, 13*(4), e191–e194. doi:10.1016/j.nurpra.2016.10.018

5. Lord, S. R. (2017). Falls. In *Hazzard's Geriatric Medicine and Gerontology* (7th ed.). New York, NY: McGraw-Hill. Retrieved from. http://accessmedicine.mhmedical.com /content.aspx?bookid=1923&sectionid=144521752. Accessed February 7, 2018.
6. U.S. Preventive Services Task Force (USPSTF). (n.d.). Recommendations for Primary Care Practice: Published Recommendations. Retrieved from https://www.uspreventiveservicestaskforce.org/BrowseRec/Index/browse-recommendations. Accessed September 17, 2017.
7. American Geriatrics Society (AGS), British Geriatrics Society (BGS). (2010). Prevention of Falls in Older Persons AGS BGS Clinical Practice Guideline 2010. Retrieved from https://geriatricscareonline.org/FullText/CL014/CL014_BOOK003. Accessed September 23, 2017.
8. Enderlin, C., Rooker, J., Ball, S., Hippensteel, D., Alderman, J., & Fisher, S. J., . . . Jordan, K. (2015). Summary of factors contributing to falls in older adults and nursing implications. *Geriatric Nursing, 36*(5), 397–406. doi:10.1016/j.gerinurse.2015.08.006
9. Rosen, T., Mack, K. A., & Noonan, R. K. (2013). Slipping and tripping: Fall injuries in adults associated with rugs and carpets. *Journal of Injury and Violence Research,* 5(1), 61–65. doi:10.5249/jivr.v5i1.177

## Infection[1,2,3,4,5,6,7,8,9]

- Aging impacts the immune system in several ways, including decreased macrophage activity, decline in T-cell function, fewer amounts of complement proteins, and others.
- Factors that increase the risk of infection with aging includes malnutrition, comorbidities (e.g., stroke, diabetes, renal failure), immunosenescence, impaired mucociliary clearance, mechanical changes of the urinary tract (e.g., decreased urinary flow rate), decreased gastric acidity, and others.
- The presentation of infection in older adults present with fewer symptoms; fever, leukocytosis, and localizing signs are often absent. Symptoms seen in older adults that signify an underlying infection can present atypically (e.g., delirium, generalized weakness, incontinence, falls).
- Fever in older adults is present with an oral temperature above 100°F (37.7°C), repeated temperatures orally above 99°F (37.2°C), rectal temperature above 99.5°F (37.5°C), or a temperature ≥ 2°F (1.1°C) above baseline values. A complete blood count (CBC) can be ordered if infection suspected; a white blood cell (WBC) count above 14,000 cells/$mm^3$ indicates bacterial infection most likely.

- Older adults with fever of unknown origin (i.e., temperature above 101°F or 38.3°C for at least 3 weeks and undiagnosed after 1 week) can be diagnosed in majority of cases. The diagnosis is usually a treatable infection (e.g., tuberculosis, intra-abdominal abscess), connective-tissue disease (e.g., temporal arteritis, rheumatoid arthritis), or malignancy.
- Pneumonia and influenza are leading causes of death in older adults due to infection. Vaccines to prevent these are vital.
- Adequate nutrition should be encouraged to improve wound healing and recovery from infection.

## References


1. Agarwal, S., & Busse, P. J. (2010). Innate and adaptive immunosenescence. *Annals of Allergy, Asthma & Immunology, 104*(3), 183–190. doi:10.1016/j.anai.2009.11.009
2. Centers for Disease Control. (2016). 10 Leading Causes of Death by Age Group, United States – 2015. Retrieved from https://www.cdc.gov/injury/wisqars/pdf/leading_causes_of_death_by_age_group_2015-a.pdf. Accessed February 10, 2018.
3. Gavazzi, G., & Krause, K. H. (2002, November). Ageing and infection. *The Lancet Infectious Diseases,* 2(11), 659–666. Retrieved from http://www.thelancet.com/journals/laninf/article/PIIS1473309902004371/abstract. Accessed February 10, 2018.
4. Norman, D. C. (2000). Fever in the elderly. *Clinical Infectious Diseases, 31*(1), 148–151. Retrieved from https://doi.org/10.1086/313896. Accessed February 10, 2018.
5. Perissinotto, C. M., & Ritchie, C. (2014). Atypical presentations of illness in older adults. In *Current Diagnosis & Treatment: Geriatrics* (2nd ed.). New York, NY: McGraw-Hill. Retrieved from http://accessmedicine.mhmedical.com/content.aspx?bookid=953&sectionid=53375629. Accessed February 10, 2018.
6. Kane, R. L., Ouslander, J. G., Resnick, B., & Malone M. L. (Eds.). (2017). *Essentials of Clinical Geriatrics* (8th ed.). Decreased Vitality. New York, NY: McGraw-Hill. Retrieved from http://accessmedicine.mhmedical.com/content.aspx?bookid=2300&sectionid=178120110. Accessed February 10, 2018.
7. Delves, P. J. (2017, January). Overview of the Immune System. Merck Manuals: Professional. Retrieved from http://www.merckmanuals.com/professional/immunology-allergic-disorders/biology-of-the-immune-system/overview-of-the-immune-system. Accessed February 11, 2018.
8. High, K. P. (2017). Infection: General principles. In *Hazzard's Geriatric Medicine and Gerontology* (7th ed.). New York, NY: McGraw-Hill. Retrieved from http://accessmedicine.mhmedical.com/content.aspx?bookid=1923&sectionid=144563653. Accessed February 10, 2018.
9. Ogawa, T., Kitagawa, M., & Hirokawa, K. (2000, August 1). Age-related changes of human bone marrow: A histometric estimation of proliferative cells, apoptotic cells, T cells, B cells and macrophages. *Mechanisms of Ageing and Development, 117*(1–3), 57–68. doi:10.1016/s0047-6374(00)00137-8

## Polypharmacy

**Angela R. Stiltner**

- Polypharmacy is simply defined as the use of multiple medications, which includes prescribed medications, supplements, over-the-counter medications, and herbal therapies. The exact number of medications typical of polypharmacy varies from 5 to 10 medications in most references.[5]
- Polypharmacy most commonly references prescribed medications but it is just as important to consider supplements, over-the-counter medications, and herbal therapies, as supplement-drug interactions are also common.[7,20]
- Polypharmacy increases the risk of adverse drug events (ADEs), hospital admissions, drug-drug interactions, drug-disease interactions, inappropriate medication use, hip fractures in older adults, prescribing cascades, and poor adherence to medication regimens.[6,9,10,11,12,18,19]
- Age-related changes in pharmacokinetics and pharmacodynamics increase the likelihood of adverse health consequences associated with polypharmacy.[3]
- Age-related changes include reduced renal function with decreased drug clearance, reduced hepatic function with variability in drug metabolism, and increased body fat relative to skeletal muscle, which can increase volume of distribution of certain medications. Improper medication dosing that fails to consider these age-related changes increases the risk of ADEs, drug toxicity, hospitalization, and mortality.[9,13]
- Multimorbidity increases the risk of polypharmacy. Twenty percent of Medicare beneficiaries have five or more chronic conditions and 50% receive five or more medications.[3,17]
- Older adults often receive care from multiple providers. It is critical to review all medications including over the counter, herbal, and supplements at each visit.[9]
- Clinicians must balance overprescribing and underprescribing as multiple medications are often required to manage clinically complex older adults.[2]

- Prescribing cascades develop when an ADE is misinterpreted as a new medical condition leading to the prescribing of new medications. **Any new symptom should be considered drug related until proven otherwise**.[12]
- Adverse effects of one symptomatic therapy may be self-limited in both severity and duration; therefore any medications added to manage the adverse side effects (such as nausea at the initiation of an opioid) should be reviewed and discontinued as soon as possible.[8]
- Quality measures for medication prescribing should include avoidance of inappropriate medications, appropriate use of indicated medications, monitoring for side effects and drug levels, avoidance of drug-drug interactions, and involvement of patient, including integration of patient values and goals of care.[15,16]
- Systematic processes may reduce inappropriate medication prescribing including educational interventions, computerized medication order entry, decision support, and multidisciplinary teams led by physicians and pharmacists.[1,16]
- Careful documentation and justification of each medication targeted to specific medical condition is equally as important as the number of prescribed medications.[9]
- Often, the adverse consequences of polypharmacy are both predictable and avoidable. Following clinical practice guidelines and drug formularies can improve prescribing.[8]
- A guiding principle for appropriate medication prescribing should include framing clinical management decisions within the context of risks, burdens, benefits, and prognosis, including remaining life expectancy, time until benefit is derived, treatment targets (e.g., primary or secondary prevention or symptom control), functional status, goals of care, and quality of life.[3,16]
- For patients at the end of life, clinicians should engage patients and families in shared decision making about when to initiate, discontinue, or continue therapies taking into consideration the guiding principles of appropriate medication prescribing above (see **Box 13-2**).[14]

**BOX 13-2 Polypharmacy Key Points**

- Typically 5–10 medications.
- Increased with multimorbidity.
- Increases risk of:
  - Adverse drug events
  - Hospitalizations
  - Drug-drug and drug-disease interactions
  - Inappropriate medication use
  - Hip fractures in older adults
  - Prescribing cascades
  - Poor adherence to medication regimens
- Consider age-related changes in pharmacokinetics and pharmacodynamics.
- Regular review of all medications including over-the-counter and alternative therapies.
- Follow quality measures for medication prescribing.
- Focus on systematic processes to improve prescribing practices.
- Document and justify each medication targeted to specific medical condition.
- Avoid prescribing cascades.
- Frame clinical management decisions in context of risks, burdens, benefits, and prognosis.
- Involve patients and families in shared decision making regarding appropriate medications at the end of life.

## References


1. Alldred, D. P., Kennedy, M., Hughes, C., Chen, T. F., & Miller, P. (2016, February 12). Interventions to optimise prescribing for older people in care homes. *Cochrane Database of Systematic Review*, 2, CD009095.
2. Boyd, C. M., Darer, J., Boult, C., Fried, L. P., Boult, L., & Wu, A. W. (2005, August 10). Clinical practice guidelines and quality of care for older patients with multiple comorbid diseases: Implications for pay for performance. *JAMA*, *294*(6), 716–724.
3. Durso, S. S. (2013). *Geriatric Review Syllabus: A Core Curriculum in Geriatric Medicine* (8th ed.). New York, NY: American Geriatrics Society.
4. Ferner, R. E., & Aronson, J. K. (2006, July 15). Communicating information about drug safety. *BMJ*, 333(7559), 143–145.
5. Field, T. S., Gurwitz, J. H., Avorn, J., McCormick, D., Jain, S., & Eckler, M., . . . Bates, D. W. (2001). Risk factors for adverse drug events among nursing home patients. *Archives of Internal Medicine*, *161*(13), 1629–1634.
6. Fugh-Berman, A. (2000, January 8). Herb-drug interactions. *Lancet*, 355(9198), 134–138.

7. Hanks, G. C. (2010). *Oxford Textbook of Palliative Medicine* (4th ed.). New York, NY: Oxford University Press.
8. Hazzard, W. B. (2003). *Principles of Geriatric Medicine & Gerontology* (5th ed.). New York, NY: McGraw-Hill.
9. Lai, S. W., Liao, K. F., Liao, C. C., Liu, C. S., & Sung, F. C. (2010, September). Polypharmacy correlates with increased risk for hip fracture in the elderly: A population-based study. *Medicine (Baltimore)*, 89(5), 295–299.
10. Lu, W. H., Wen, Y. W., Chen, L. K., & Hsiao, F. Y (2015, March 3). Effect of polypharmacy, potentially inappropriate medications and anticholinergic burden on clinical outcomes: A retrospective cohort stud. *Canadian Medical Association Journal*, *187*(4), E130–E137.
11. Rochon, P. A., & Gurwitz, J. H. (1997, October 25). Optimising drug treatment for elderly people: the prescribing cascade. *BMJ*, *315*(7115), 1096–1099.
12. Rowe, J. W., Andres, R., Tobin, J. D., Norris, A. H., & Shock, N. W. (1976, March). The effect of age on creatinine clearance in men: A cross-sectional and longitudinal study. *Journal of Gerontology*, *31*(2), 155–163.
13. Shega, J. W. (2012). *UNIPAC 9: A Resource for Hospice and Palliative Care Professionals – Caring for Patients with Chronic Illnesses: Dementia, COPD, and CHF* (4th ed.). Glenview, IL: American Academy of Hospice and Palliative Medicine.
14. Spinewine, A., Schmader, K. E., Barber, N., Hughes, C., Lapane, K. L., Swine, C., & Hanlon, J. T. (2007, July 14). Appropriate prescribing in elderly people: How well can it be measured and optimised? *Lancet*, *370*(9582), 173–184.
15. Steinman, M. A., & Hanlon, J. T. (2010). Managing medications in clinically complex elders: "There's got to be a happy medium." *JAMA*, *304*, 1592–1601.
16. Tinetti, M. E., Bogardus, Jr., S. T., & Agostini, J. V. (2004, December 30). Potential pitfalls of disease specific guidelines for patients with multiple conditions. *New England Journal of Medicine*, *351*(27), 2870–2874.
17. Weng, M. C., Tsai, C. F., Sheu, K. L., Lee, Y. T., Lee, H. C., & Tzeng, S. L., . . . Chen S. C. (2013, November). The impact of number of drugs prescribed on the risk of potentially inappropriate medication among outpatient older adults with chronic diseases. *QJM*, *106*(11), 1009–1015.
18. Wimmer, B. C., Cross, A. J., Jokanovic, N., Wiese, M. D., George, J., & Johnell, K., . . . Bell, J. S. (2017, April). Clinical outcomes associated with medication regimen complexity in older people: A systematic review. *Journal of the American Geriatrics Society*, 65(4), 747–753.
19. Wold, R. S., Lopez, S. T, Yau, C. L., Butler, L. M., Pareo-Tubbeh, S. L., & Walters, D. L., . . . Baumgartner, R. N. (2005, January). Increasing trends in elderly persons' use of nonvitamin, nonmineral dietary supplements and concurrent use of medications. *Journal of the American Dietetic Association*, *105*(1), 54–63.

# Index

Note: Page numbers followed by 'f' and't' refers to figures and tables respectively

## I

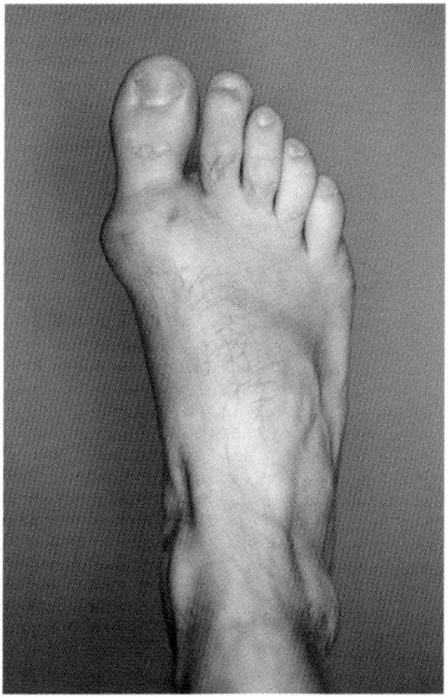

**Figure CP-1** Gout (***Figure 7-1***, page 194)



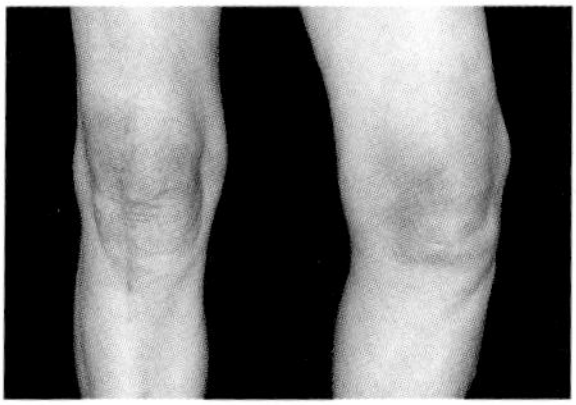

**Figure CP-2** Osteoarthritis (***Figure 7-2***, page 199)



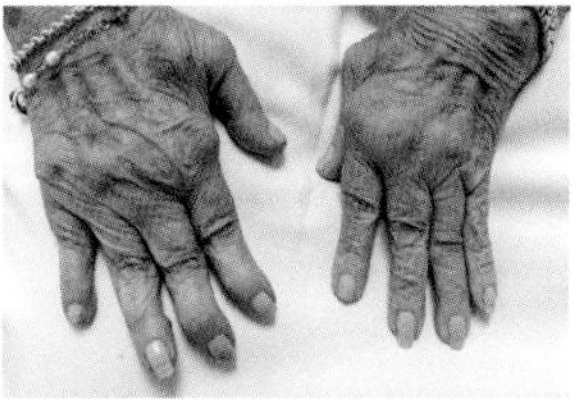

**Figure CP-3** Rheumatoid Arthritis (***Figure 7-3***, page 210)

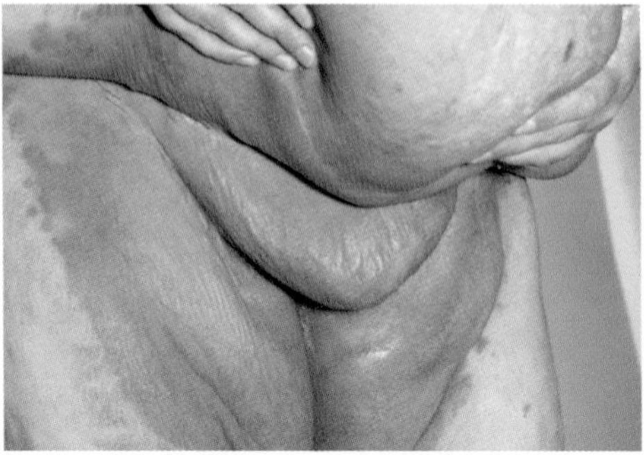

**Figure CP-4** Candidiasis (***Figure 8-1***, page 223)



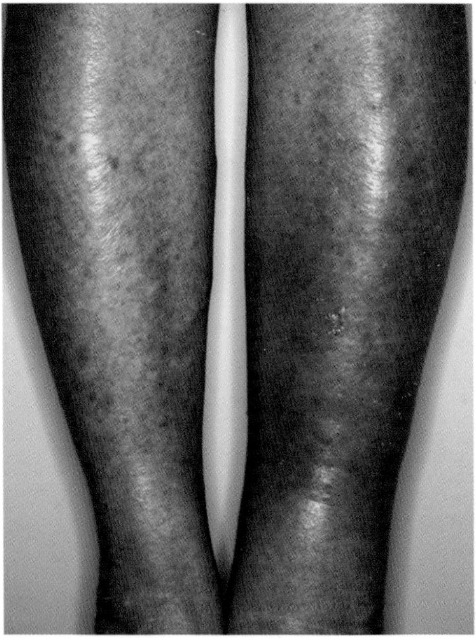

**Figure CP-5** Cellulitis (***Figure 8-2***, page 228)

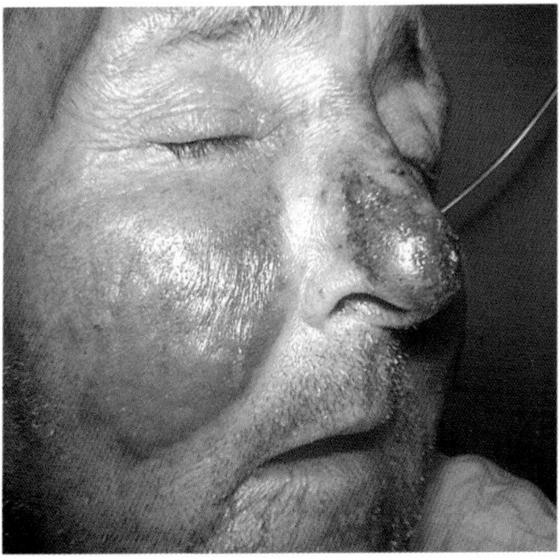

**Figure CP-6** Erysipelas (***Figure 8-3***, page 229)

Courtesy of Dr. Thomas F. Sellers, Emory University/CDC.

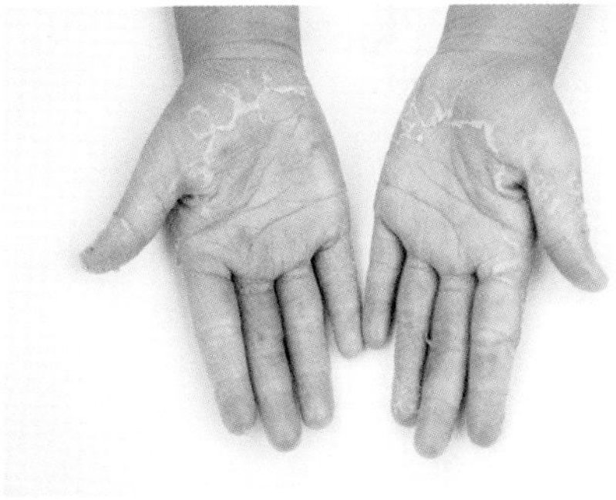

**Figure CP-7** Contact Dermatitis (***Figure 8-4***, page 233)

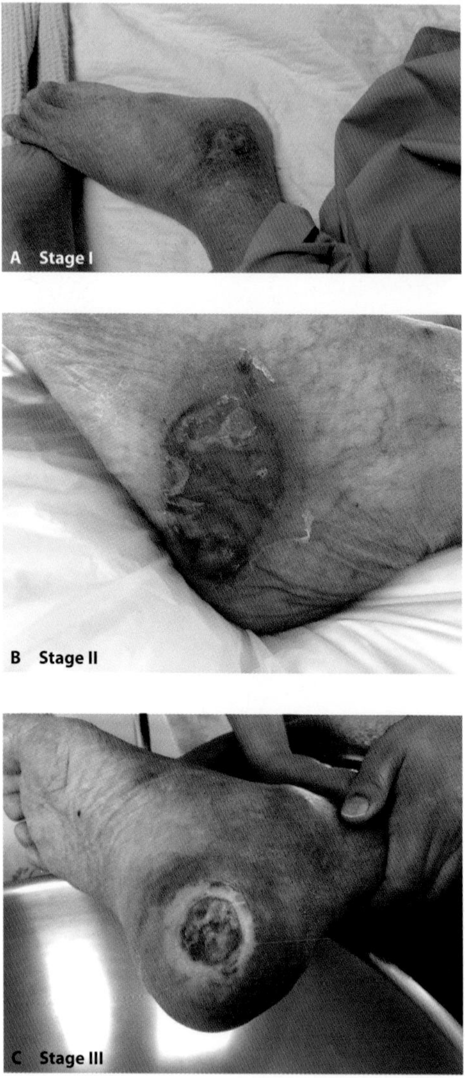


**Figure CP-8(A-C)** The Four Stages of Ulceration (***Figure 8-5A-5E***, page 240)

(a) Casa nayafana/Shutterstock; (b) and (c) © Duangnapa Kanchanasakun/Shutterstock.

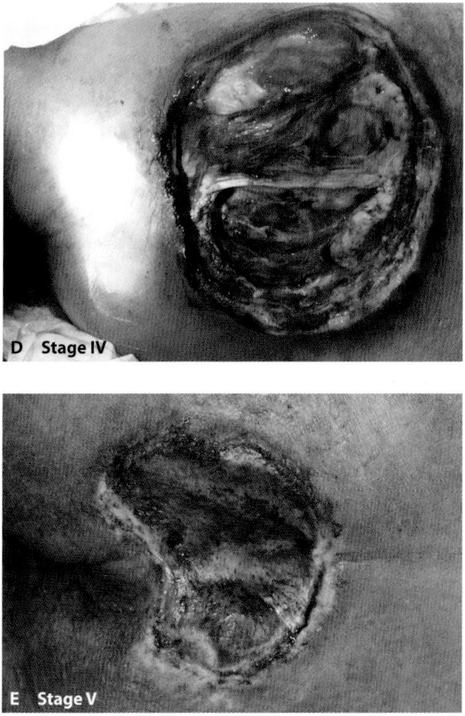


**Figure CP-8(D-E)** The Four Stages of Ulceration (***Figure 8-5A-5E***, page 240)

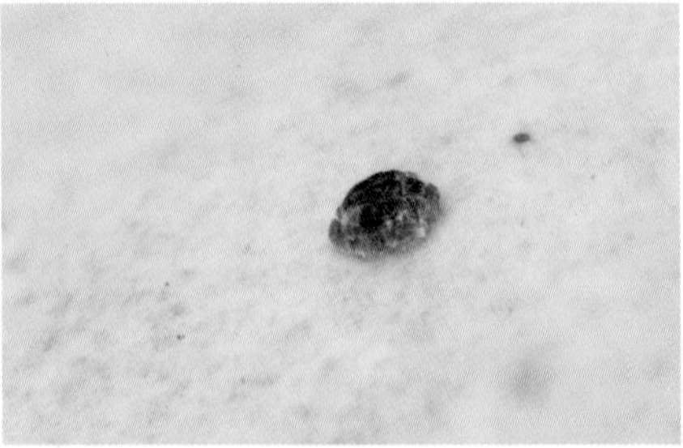

**Figure CP-9** Seborrheic Keratosis (***Figure 8-6***, page 246)



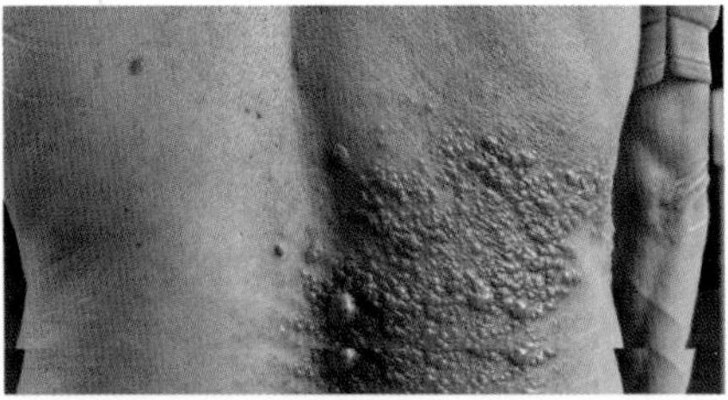

**Figure CP-10** Herpes Zoster (***Figure 8-7***, page 249)



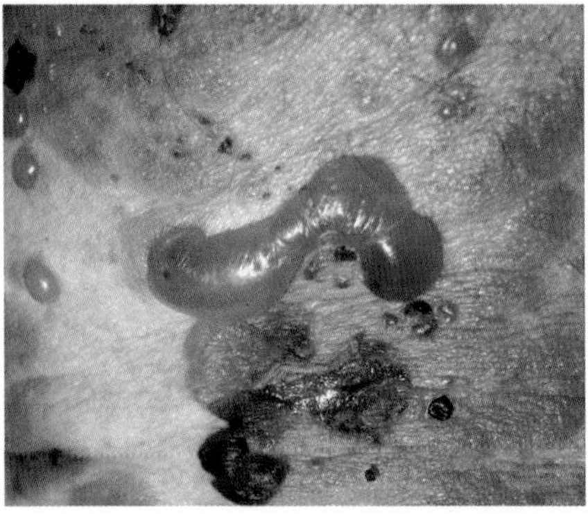

**Figure CP-11** Bullous Pemphigoid (***Figure 8-8***, page 254)

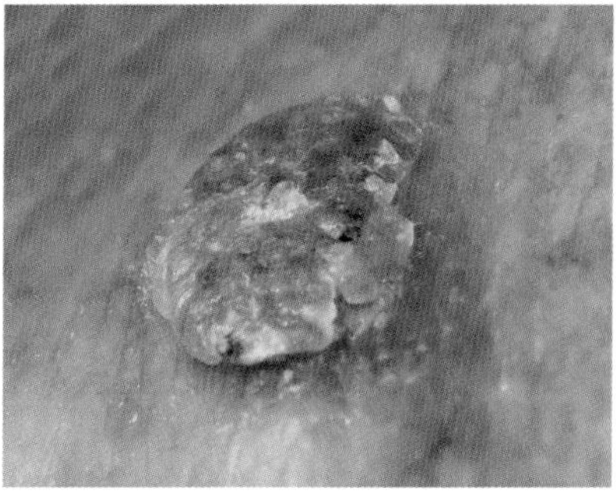

**Figure CP-12** Actinic Keratosis (***Figure 8-9***, page 260)


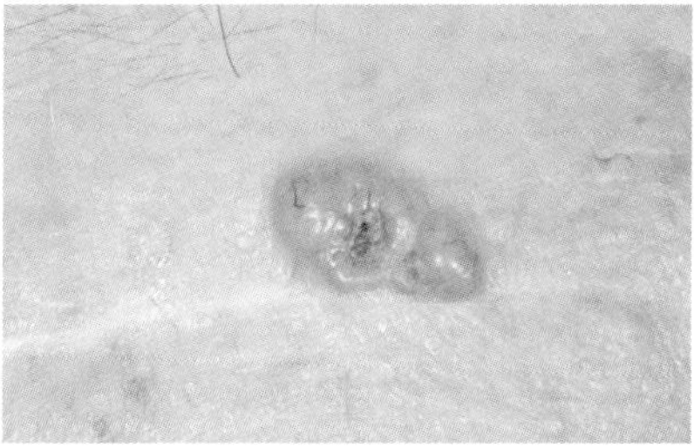

**Figure CP-13** Basal Cell Carcinoma (***Figure 8-10***, page 263)


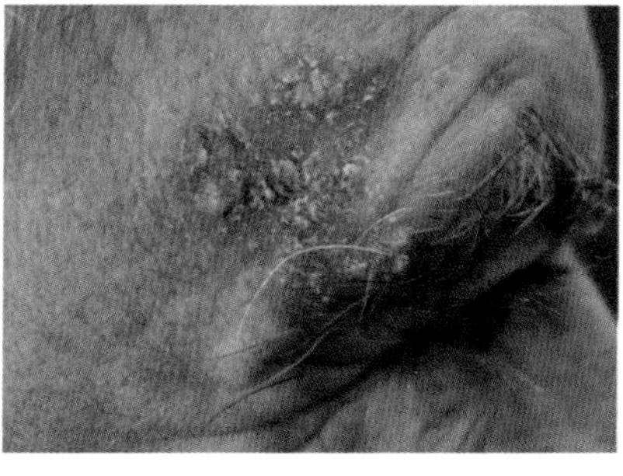

**Figure CP-14** Squamous Cell Carcinoma (***Figure 8-11***, page 266)

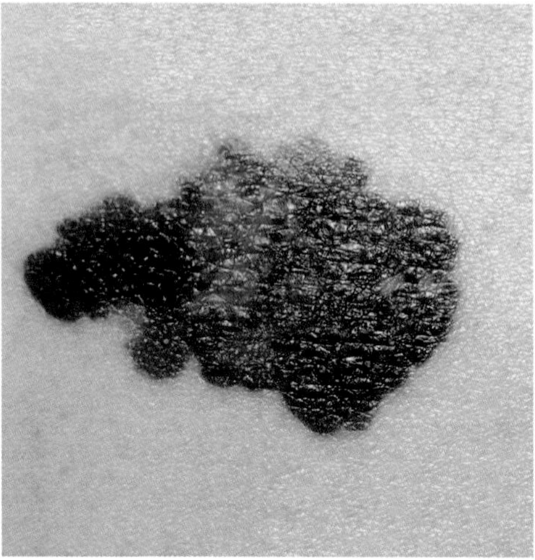

**Figure CP-15** Malignant Melanoma (***Figure 8-12***, page 268)



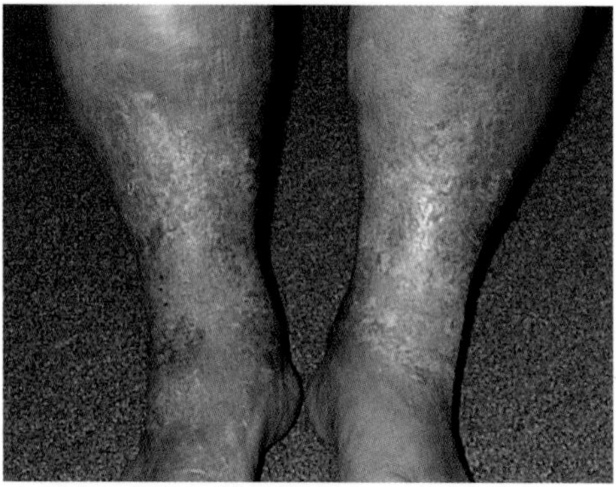

**Figure CP-16** Stasis Dermatitis (***Figure 8-13***, page 271)